THE
MYOFASCIAL
SYSTEM

THE MYOFASCIAL SYSTEM

in Form and Movement

Lauri Nemetz

Foreword by David Lesondak

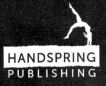

HANDSPRING PUBLISHING

First published in Great Britain in 2023 by Handspring Publishing, an imprint of Jessica Kingsley Publishers
An imprint of Hodder & Stoughton Ltd
An Hachette UK Company

Front cover image source: David Gilliver, www.davidgilliver.com.

Disclaimer: To the maximum extent permitted by law, neither the Publisher nor the Authors assume any responsibility for any loss or injury and/or damage to persons or property arising out of or relating to any use of the material contained in this book. It is the responsibility of the treating practitioner, relying on independent expertise and knowledge of the patient, to determine the best treatment and method of application for the patient.

A CIP catalogue record for this title is available from the British Library and the Library of Congress

ISBN 978 1 91208 579 8
eISBN 978 1 91208 580 4

Printed and bound in Great Britain by Ashford Colour Press Limited

Jessica Kingsley Publishers' policy is to use papers that are natural, renewable and recyclable products and made from wood grown in sustainable forests. The logging and manufacturing processes are expected to conform to the environmental regulations of the country of origin.

Handspring Publishing
Carmelite House
50 Victoria Embankment
London EC4Y 0DZ

www.handspringpublishing.com

CONTENTS

Foreword by David Lesondak — vi
Acknowledgments — vii
About the author — ix
Contributors — x
Preface — xvii
Orientation keys — xx

PART 1 Myofascial material: The scaffolding and space of the moving body

CHAPTER 1 The form of fascia — 3

CHAPTER 2 The shape of movement/human evolution in motion — 46

CHAPTER 3 The body in motion and emotion — 66

CHAPTER 4 Different ways of seeing—game rules, game plans, and body analysis — 78

CHAPTER 5 The essential corners in a round world — 97

CHAPTER 6 Spirals — 114

CHAPTER 7 Concepts of core — 119

CHAPTER 8 Arms, oblique connections, and active movement — 133

PART 2 Fascia and the dynamic body: Spatial use and coordination

CHAPTER 9 Yoga — 147

CHAPTER 10 Pilates — 158

CHAPTER 11 Training, weight work, and sports specifics — 164

CHAPTER 12 Aging process—myofascial efficiency throughout life stages — 179

CHAPTER 13 Environmental matters—internal and external space and how we perceive and use it — 191

Epilogue — 211
Appendix Building a tensegrity model — 212
Index — 213

FOREWORD by David Lesondak

There is a well-known quote (attributed to at least three different people) that "writing about music is like dancing about architecture." It's relevant here because that more or less accurately sums up my feelings about most books about movement and form.

Perhaps my bias is inherent in the medium. Form, as defined by height × width × depth, occurs in three dimensions. And it could be argued that movement occurs in at least four dimensions, as it's the movement of that form across space, but also over time. Now, despite what happens in your mind, reading words on a page is a resolutely two-dimensional experience. But it does take time to read a book.

The Lauri that I know wears many hats—dance therapist, photographer, yoga teacher, hiker, writer, adjunct professor, kayaker, nature enthusiast, and dissector par excellence, to name a few. For her these are not separate activities at all. Each of them exists in relationship with and is informed and enhanced by the other. She also loves collaboration, recognizing that insight, innovation, and integration often best occur in a collegial, communal environment.

As in her life all of these qualities are abundant in her book. Including her love of pure movement. While seemingly organized like a more traditional textbook, *The Myofascial System in Form and Movement* also offers you, the reader, many different branches and byways so that you can literally choose how to "move" through the book.

First there's Lauri's text itself, revealing her encyclopedic knowledge base. Then there are the series of thematic, color-coded boxes which offer you the opportunity to sit and reflect, get up and move or stretch in a specific way or sequence, get the viewpoints from dozens of experts, or look at the inner and outer world differently. I could easily imagine someone wanting to take a day and work through all the movement labs. Or reading through the chapter and then going back to the boxes. There are myriad ways to approach this book—think of it as a "choose your own adventure" fascia book!

Lauri has put a tremendous amount of thought, care, and big tent sensibility into crafting a book that invites movement in many dimensions, so I hope you will take your time and go on an adventure with this book. I assure you it will be time well spent.

David Lesondak
University of Pittsburgh Medical Center
Pittsburgh PA, USA
July 2022

ACKNOWLEDGMENTS

There is always a lot more behind a book than the final words on the page. There are so many threads and stories that have created the body of work before you. If all goes well, these words will inspire more thoughts and changes towards growth. This book is gloriously imperfect, and yet somehow has come into its own form.

To my family, love through all the waves that life creates. There have been some huge ones. The challenges of the past several years included losses small and large, personal and professional. There were emergency surgeries, wounds to heal, both physical and metaphoric. We have gone through all of them as best we can.

My friends and colleagues—I am beyond thrilled that each and every one of my "guests" in this book said "yes" enthusiastically to being part of this, and "yes" again even as the book shifted. I thank each and every one of you! A huge thanks to the photographers, models, and our donors that appear in these pages and the many unnamed people that are nevertheless so dear and important to me. I am deeply grateful.

To Sarena, who followed me through this journey from the first suggestion to get me to write a book, to watching me at conferences from Harvard Medical and more recent presentations online during the pandemic. You did tell me authors have unexpected things happen during the writing process! I don't think I could possibly have guessed what was to come.

To Tracey Mellor, who shared my adventures through the FNPP (Fascia Net Plastination Project) and also helped me through *many* tea talks about this book project. Your support means so much. To Jihan, besides being an excellent dissector and partner in crime, we had the best laughs during those days in Germany and bike riding will always bring smiles. To more collaborations to come. To the rest of the FNPP team I offer many profound thanks, especially to Gary and Rachelle and the entire group of amazing friends and colleagues.

To Vladimir, through our dissection time in Guben to working on an article (still coming!), thanks for sharing this adventure. To Robert Schleip, for your generosity of spirit, always. To Gil, thanks for early dissection exploration, and for giving me respect as a friend and colleague.

To James Earls, thanks for agreeing to present with me several years ago at Oxford. What a joy that was. More recently you helped me grieve and see larger sandboxes.

Chris and Ann Frederick get a special shout out for inviting me to play in their world and stay at their home during a crazy hot week (114°) in Arizona. To Leslie and Lydia too for giving me a space to grow and for finding a way to teach together after decades of knowing each other.

To David Lesondak, thank you for sharing a sense of humor and wonder simultaneously. Our friendship really developed during this crazy pandemic and I am grateful. From sharing photo conversations to adventures in several cities, thank you for sharing as a colleague and friend.

To great thinkers, from the late Barry Lopez to Bill T. Jones, who sparked questions and creativity, I give profound thanks. To Dr. James Williams, who opened his lab at Rush Medical and took a gamble on a non-traditional anatomist, a grateful and profound thanks for letting me explore.

ACKNOWLEDGMENTS *continued*

While time and circumstances have created separations, I still hold deep threads to Robert (Van de Peer) and Tom, passionate sailors both. I realize I have had a small appearance in both of their major works, an art piece of mine in Robert's book on master printmaking, and my fascial hearts and kidney (ghost organ) in Tom's well-known third edition tome. Both served as early guides and from both I learned how to read the metaphoric charts, and then navigate my own waters. To Todd I give an acknowledgement for artistic skill and giving the space to explore.

The body is incredible at changing shape. I have been lucky to dissect and see the fascial scaffolding of hearts and the pericardium that encloses them. It was in a lab that I first heard about broken heart syndrome, or cardiomyopathy, sometimes known as Takotsubo cardiomyopathy. This condition is a shape-change response to intense stress. Takotsubo is a Japanese fishing trap that the enlarged left ventricle of the heart resembles in this syndrome. Under the care of a doctor, the good news is that the heart can often heal and change shape again. So this final acknowledgement is to those whose hearts have been broken and who work hard at changing their shape for themselves and others. We are in a time of many challenges, but we are also capable of more good than we often know. Changing any part of the system affects it all. Thanks to all of the movers and thread connectors out there and you, the reader, as an important part of this web.

ABOUT THE AUTHOR

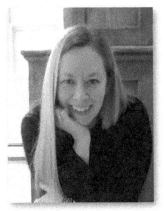

Laurice (Lauri) D. Nemetz, MA, BC-DMT, LCAT, ERYT500, C-IAYT

Lauri considers herself a guide for other explorers and sustains a healthy curiosity for seeing and learning things in new ways. She is an Adjunct Professor at Pace University (Pleasantville, NY), a 2020 recipient of the President's Award for Outstanding Contribution; a visiting Associate Professor in the Department of Physical Medicine at Rush University Medical Center (Chicago, IL); and an anatomical dissector and lead teacher with several projects including the Fascial Net Plastination Project (FNPP) and KNMLabs with Leslie Kaminoff (*Yoga Anatomy*). She was a senior faculty member and dissection assistant for Anatomy Trains® from 2010 to 2020, certified by Thomas Myers. She is a New York licensed creative arts therapist (LCAT), an active member of the American Association for Anatomy, a board-certified member of the Academy of Dance/Movement Therapists, a certified yoga teacher at the 500-hour level, a Stott Pilates instructor, and certified yoga therapist (C-IAYT). Lauri has exhibited her artwork internationally with themes of anatomy and movement and also kayak guides occasionally, in addition to being a dedicated trail walker and runner. She loves creating spaces for growth and learning.

More information at www.wellnessbridge.com.

Constantly regard the universe as one living being, having one substance and one soul; and observe how all things have reference to one perception, the perception of this one living being; and how all things act with one movement; and how all things are the cooperating causes of all things which exist; observe too the continuous spinning of the thread and the contexture of the web.

Marcus Aurelius, *Meditations*, Book IV

CONTRIBUTORS

Jihan Adem

Jihan is a myofascial manual therapist specializing in a technique called *Bowen Therapy*. She has been teaching Bowen in and around the UK and Europe since the early 2000s, both introducing courses to new students and delivering specialized postgraduate training.

In her private practice in the southwest of England, Jihan utilizes the versatility of Bowen to work with a variety people presenting with many and varying symptoms although her passion lies in working with sleep-related breathing disorders. As one of the few female fascial dissectors currently in the UK, Jihan brings a somatic understanding of tissue densities when leading dissection labs. As principle of Bowen College UK, this grounded knowledge brings for a fascinating educational stance.

Madeline Black

Madeline's life pursuit is the discovery of how the human body moves. Over 30 years in the field of movement, her curiosity explored all aspects of movement in dance, Pilates, yoga, Gyrotonic®, fitness training, and from studies of human biomotion, human cadaver dissection labs, osteopathic and manual therapies. Madeline is the author of *Centered: Organizing the body through movement theory, kinesiology, and Pilates techniques*; the second edition was published by Handspring Publishing in Winter 2021. Madeline developed the Madeline Black Method™, a method teaching movement teachers to use assessment skills, movement sequences and manual techniques to help people achieve their fullest movement potential. Madeline Black offers her program, Madeline Black Method™, online and live workshops, for all movement teachers at www.madelineblack.com. Madeline has filmed many workshops and movement classes for Pilates Anytime and Fusion Pilates EDU Online. She has a private practice in Sonoma, California, USA.

Nile Bratcher

Nile Bratcher is a health and performance specialist, dancer, and surgical technologist. Nile continues to serve his clients through self-awareness, variability, and compassion. He can be found at www.nilebratcher.com.

Dr. Vladimir Chereminskiy

Dr. Chereminskiy is an Assistant Professor at the Department of Pathology and Anatomy, Eastern Virginia Medical School. Dr. Chereminskiy is also the Director of Anatomy and Plastination at the von Hagens Plastinarium in Guben, Germany. He has been pivotal in the Fascial Net Plastination Project (FNPP).

Rachelle Clauson

Rachelle Clauson is a Nationally Certified Massage Therapist with a private practice in San Diego, California, for the past 18 years. Since January 2018, she has been working as a volunteer dissector and photographer with the Fascial Net Plastination Project (FNPP). She co-produced *Fascia in a NEW LIGHT: the Exhibition* with Gary Carter in Berlin at the 5th International Fascia Research Congress and has helped organize webinars, written articles, and created videos and media content to continue to help share the project. Rachelle is passionate about the creation of more visual representations of fascia to better convey its organization and function to movers, touch therapists, and body-oriented practitioners worldwide.

Holly Clemens

Holly Clemens, PhD, LMT, is a Professor of Sport and Exercise Studies, Health, and Physical Education at Cuyahoga Community College in Cleveland, Ohio, where she specializes in teaching exercise physiology, kinesiology, motor learning, and exercise prescription and program design. She also provides neuro-myofascial based movement training and strength and conditioning programming for the athletic teams at the college. Holly was the recipient of the Ralph M. Besse award for Teaching Excellence at her college in 2016. She has been involved in the health and fitness industry for 30+ years writing health and fitness articles and presenting a variety of fitness, health, wellness, and movement-based programs and workshops at the local, state, and national levels. In addition to teaching, Holly is an Anatomy Trains® Certified Teacher, ACSM-Exercise Physiologist, NSCA-Certified Strength and Conditioning Specialist, Fascial Stretch Therapist-Level III, Yoga-Tune Up Certified Teacher, ERYT500, and served as a dissection lab assistant for Thomas Myers Anatomy Trains® from 2016 to 2020.

Mary M. Copple

Mary M. Copple is a Certified Laban Movement Analyst and assists teaching the EUROLAB Certification Programs in Laban-Bartenieff Movement Studies in Berlin. In the 1970s, she gained a Diploma of Dance in Education from Dartington College of Arts and has been conducting movement workshops that explore Laban's conception of "dynamic space" with architecture and design students since 2016. Mary also gained a Magister in French Philology (Linguistics major) and Information Science from the Freie Universität Berlin in 2002 and works as a translator in the fields of gesture research and language philosophy.

Michol Dalcourt

Michol Dalcourt is an internationally recognized industry leader in health and human performance. He is the founder and CEO of Institute of Motion (www.instituteofmotion.com), inventor of VIPR and VIPR PRO (www.vipr.com) and co-founder of PTA Global (www.ptaglobal.com). As an international lecturer and educator, Michol has authored numerous articles on human design and function. Michol has done extensive work in the areas of health and human performance, and consults with many of the fitness industry's biggest companies, including Equinox, Microsoft, and Nike, amongst others. Michol has contributed to programs for general health as well as athletes of all levels.

Dennis Dunphy

Dennis's first endeavor as a fitness professional began in 1999 at 24-Hour Fitness and soon after he started his own training business. Many of his clients are people aged 40+ who experience physical issues and pain, and his greatest reward comes from helping others improve physically and mentally. His journey has led to an ever-increasing insight into the human body and how all the body's systems work in unison. This knowledge led him to co-create Stick Mobility in 2015 to help others achieve better movement and health. www.stickmobility.com

James Earls

James Earls is a manual therapist with a background in functional, comparative, and evolutionary anatomy. His passion is to make anatomy understandable and contextual. James has written a number of books, including *Born to Walk* and *Understanding the Human Foot*. He lives and practices in London, UK, and teaches for www.BorntoMove.com.

Fascia Net Plastination Project (FNPP)

The Fascial Net Plastination Project (FNPP) is a collaboration of the Fascia Research Society, the Plastinarium, and Body Worlds. The FNPP's achievements have come into being because of a shared vision to highlight fascia in a full body plastinate and willingness to take risks. Under the directorship of Robert Schleip, Vladimir Chereminskiy, Rurik von Hagens, and Angelina Whalley, the remarkable individuals of the advisory board and volunteer team come from Austria, Australia, Brazil, Canada, England, Finland, Germany, Israel, Singapore, Switzerland, and the USA. Because of their willingness to share their expertise, resources, and time they have brought the vision into reality. www.fasciaresearchsociety.org/plastination

Mike Fitch

Mike Fitch is an innovative fitness educator and movement coach with 21 years' experience in the fitness industry. As the founder of Global Bodyweight Training, he has developed multiple skill-based bodyweight programs, including the popular Animal Flow practice. He has taught thousands of fitness professionals in more than 20 countries, has appeared on the cover of numerous fitness magazines, and is frequently featured in print and digital media. In 2019 he launched the Animal Flow On Demand platform, expanding the program into the direct-to-consumer market. He makes his home in Boulder, Colorado, where he spends time snowboarding, hiking, and practicing Animal Flow.

Chris Frederick

Chris Frederick co-directs the Stretch to Win Institute in Arizona, where he teaches certification courses in Frederick Stretch Therapy™ (FST™). Previous to becoming a physical therapist in 1989, Chris's professional dance career was cut short due to injury. He subsequently became a dance medicine specialist working with the New York City Ballet and other dance companies.

Chris currently specializes in the integration of manual and movement therapy with FST. He is author of the books *Stretch to Win* and *Fascial Stretch Therapy*, as well as numerous articles and book chapters covering variously inter-related topics on manual therapy, fascia, and movement evaluation and treatment. Chris practices living a Taoist lifestyle and has taught group class Taiji and Qigong which he currently integrates in his clinical, teaching, and writing work.

Johannes Freiberg Neto

Johannes Freiberg Neto has been a Professor of Physical Education since 1983 at the University of São Paulo (USP). He was an athlete and coach of the Brazilian karate team with titles of national champion, Panamerican and 3rd place in the 1998 World Cup (Paris). He has been Structural Integrator of the Rolfing Method and Master Trainer in Fascial Fitness since 2017, a member of the Fascia Plastination Project since 2018, and a Master's student in Aging Sciences at Universidade São Judas Tadeu (USJT).

Carrie Gaynor

Carrie Gaynor, RN, uses bodywork and movement to help people move well and be well. Through her business, *Modern Nature Bodyworks*, she works with clients of a wide range of ages and abilities, offering sessions in Anatomy Trains® Structural Integration, Fascial Stretch Therapy™, and Gray Institute Functional Movement. Carrie also teaches *Yoga for the Health of It*, incorporating Functional Movement and TriYoga Flow. Carrie is a senior teacher and popular presenter of Anatomy Trains® courses. She has published articles on Structural Integration through the International Association of Structural Integrators. Her website is www.modernnaturebodyworks.com.

Julie Hammond

Julie Hammond is the director and lead teacher of Anatomy Trains® Australia; she has been in the bodywork industry for over 20 years and still runs a busy practice in Western Australia. She is a self-confessed anatomy nerd with a passion for the pelvic floor and jaw anatomy and dysfunction. Through her clinical practice observations, Julie became interested in the link between the diaphragms in the body and how focusing on a more global approach achieved more significant results with her clients. Julie contributed a chapter to David Lesondak's new book *Fascia, Function and Medical Applications*. Julie is currently studying human and medical science with a strong focus on research. julie@anatomytrainsaustralia.com

Gil Hedley

Gil Hedley, PhD, has been teaching his integral approach to anatomy via dissection labs, public lectures and online since 1995. He is the producer of The Integral Anatomy Series and the author of several books. Presently Gil is based in Colorado Springs, Colorado, at the Institute for Anatomical Research, where he presides over its board of directors and conducts in-depth anatomical studies.

Michael Jacobs

Michael Jacobs is golf instructor and biomechanical researcher based in Manorville, New York. In addition to his work coaching players at every level from elite professional major champions to everyday amateurs, Michael conceived and designed with Dr. Steven Nesbit the Jacobs 3D sports movement analysis system, which measures and evaluates the forces and torques in athletes' bodies and the implements they use. A member of *Golf Digest*'s 50 Best Teachers and *Golf Magazine's* Top 100 Instructors as well as a recipient of multiple PGA of America section teaching and coaching honors, Michael is based at Rock Hill Golf and Country Club on Long Island.

Travis Johnson

Travis has been a professional coach in Tokyo, Japan, since 2007. He owns and operates a performance facility with his wife in central Tokyo, serving individuals from all walks of life. Travis has acquired over a dozen industry accreditations and teaches professionals as a DVRT Master Instructor, Original Strength Instructor, and Gray Institute Course Instructor. A graduate of the 2010 Gray Institute Functional Transformation program, his applied knowledge base covers the spectrum from rehabilitation to injury prevention to performance. Travis has developed Strength and Conditioning programming for professional rugby and soccer teams and has taught extensively throughout Japan.

Leslie Kaminoff

Leslie Kaminoff is a yoga educator inspired by the tradition of T. K. V. Desikachar. For over four decades he has led workshops and developed specialized education in the fields of yoga, breath anatomy, and bodywork. Leslie is the co-author, with Amy Matthews, of the best-selling book *Yoga Anatomy*. Leslie is the founder of The Breathing Project, a New York City-based educational non-profit dedicated to advancing educational standards for yoga teachers and other movement professionals. He has also partnered with Lauri Nemetz and Lydia Mann to create KNM Labs (www.knmlabs.com), offering unique, dissection-based anatomy trainings.

Sue Lembeck-Edens

Sue Lembeck-Edens began practicing Dance/Movement Therapy with older individuals over 30 years ago. A passion to serve older populations powered Sue to create inclusive programming in therapeutic exercise and complementary health education. Sue currently directs the fitness programming at Juniper Village, a life care retirement community in State College, Pennsylvania, where her classes in yoga, t'ai chi, qi gong, strength training, Pilates, and dance are adapted to fit the needs of residents at all levels of ability. A co-creator of RE*fresh* Mind, Body, Spirit – Juniper's wellbeing program for residents and associates – Sue brings her background in meditation and expressive movement to enhance both the individual and community spirit. She maintains a private bodywork practice, serves as a Dance/Movement Therapy mentor, and teaches continuing education in anatomy, professional development, and ethics to students of massage therapy and holistic health practices.

David Lesondak

David Lesondak is an Allied Health Member in the Department of Family and Community Medicine at the

University of Pittsburgh Medical Center (UPMC). He is the author the international bestseller *Fascia, What It Is and Why It Matters*. David is also the editor of *Fascia, Function, and Medical Applications*, as well as the host of the podcast *BodyTalk*. He maintains a private practice at UPMC's Center for Integrative Medicine where he helps people with chronic pain, injuries, pre- and post-surgery issues and more using an array of fascial and myofascial techniques, often coupled with specific movements.

Tracey Mellor

Tracey Mellor is a Movement teacher, primarily Pilates, Fascial Fitness and yoga. A studio owner for almost 20 years in the south of England, she divides her time between following her fascination for fascia, applying fascial research in the movement teaching environment, teaching exercise professionals the principles of The Fascial Fitness exercise modality and teaching clients with chronic physical and neurological conditions in her studio. Building self-awareness and somatic self-confidence are the cornerstones of her teaching style.

A founding member of the Fascial Research Society and part of the Fascial Net Plastination project, Tracey is constantly curious about the human body, always open and ready to listen to new concepts, particularly if it can benefit a client's wellbeing or can bring an understanding of fascial anatomy to a wider audience. Tracey edited *Pilates for Children and Adolescents* (Handspring Publishing 2014).

Gail O'Reilly

Gail O'Reilly teaches several styles of yoga and also coaches running that integrates and applies the science, physiology, and psychology of yoga. Since 2004 she has taken extensive training in yoga, including Hatha, Kundalini, Nidra, and Restorative, and has taught thousands of hours of classes. Her passion for sports inspired her to create a running program that focuses on coaching that is formulated with the principles of yoga and includes mental, physical, and energetic aspects. Her training methodology has helped recreational and competitive runners. Gail previously created the Cycling with a Yoga Mind program and training DVD in 2009. www.Zenergy.Live

Fiona Palmer

Fiona has been a movement therapist for the last 25 years and a bodyworker for more than 20 years. Fi's background is in clinical Pilates, pelvic floor dysfunction, and low back pain. She found that improved breathing helped those with back pain and pelvic floor problems and became interested in the links between the diaphragms. Outcomes for clients significantly improved by taking a global approach to a local problem. Fi runs a clinic in Suffolk and an online Pilates and hypopressive breathing and postural exercise business. She is one of the Anatomy Trains® teachers, allowing her to share her passion for anatomy and the body.

Dr. Rebecca Pratt

Dr. Rebecca Pratt, PhD is currently a Professor of Anatomy at Oakland University William Beaumont School of Medicine in Rochester, Michigan, USA. Her present adventure has her teaching dissection-based clinical gross anatomy and medical histology across medical years M1, M2, and M4. She completed her PhD in Cancer Cell Biology from Purdue University in Indiana, USA. She currently resides on the Board of Directors for the Fascia Research Society. She has been recognized multiple times by the American Association for Anatomists for excellence in teaching, scholarly activity, and service to the discipline. Dr. Pratt writes for the National Board of Osteopathic Medical Examiners and was twice honored as Item Writer of the Year. Dr. Pratt shares her excitement for fascia every chance she gets.

Rebekah Rotstein

Rebekah Rotstein is the creator of the medically-endorsed Buff Bones® system, with hundreds of trained instructors around the world. She presents at conferences, hospitals, and studios worldwide on topics of integrated movement, Pilates, and bone health. She has participated in eight cadaver dissections and completed programs and coursework in fascia research, somatic studies, and visceral manipulation. Rebekah was one of the first visiting instructors at Pilates Anytime, is a long-standing ambassador for American Bone Health and worked as a partner of the US Department of Health and Human Services.

Dr. Robert Schleip

Dr. Robert Schleip is currently at the Technical University of Munich (TUM) Department of Health Sciences as well as having directed the Fascia Research Group at Ulm University, Germany. After several decades practicing and teaching Rolfing Structural Integration and the Feldenkrais Method, he transformed into a curiosity-driven laboratory scientist, exploring the surprisingly alive cellular dynamics of the fascial net. His work on "active fascial contractility" was honored with the Vladimir Janda Award for Musculoskeletal Medicine. Robert served as driving force behind the first Fascia Research Congress (Harvard Medical School Conference Center, Boston, MA, 2007) as well as the subsequent events of that congress lineage. He is Vice President of the Fascia Research Society and Research Director of the European Rolfing Association. More about him at: www.somatics.de and www.fasciaresearch.de.

Dr. Emily Splichal

Dr. Emily Splichal, Functional Podiatrist and Human Movement Specialist, is the Founder of EBFA Global, Creator of the Barefoot Training Specialist® Certification, author of Barefoot Strong and CEO/Founder of Naboso Technology. With over 20 years in the fitness industry, Dr. Splichal has dedicated her medical career towards studying postural alignment and human movement as it relates to barefoot science, foot to core integration and sensory integration.

Jason Spitalnik

Jason Spitalnik has been practicing Thomas Myers's Structural Integration since 2007 and teaching Anatomy Trains® Structural Integration since 2010. He was also a teacher for students continuing on for an Associate's degree in health and life sciences. Jason is trained in many different therapies, such as structural integration, osteopathic cranial techniques, visceral manipulation, and neuromobilization. Jason has also been doing research on collagen and collagenase for several years. Jason runs a practice with massage therapists and an acupuncturist.

Marla Sukoff

Marla L. Sukoff, MD (BC-PM&R), RYT-500 is a former modern dancer, an MD (board certified physical medicine and rehabilitation specialist), lifelong student of integrative and functional medicine, a yoga teacher (RYT-500), and pelvic floor educator. She has developed a program of Pelvic Floor Health for Women – Pelvic Floor Balancing, where she has been integrating a variety of approaches for pelvic floor awareness and training (anatomic, myofascial, embodiment, yoga therapy, pilates, PT). She explores the myofascial connections of the pelvic floor throughout the body for both optimizing movement function and therapeutics. Her workshop classes are taught "in and around the chair," and she applies these principles to her yoga flow classes as well. Marla teaches both locally, through the North Castle Library (New York), as well as online through presentwisdom.com.

Dr. Neil Theise

Neil Theise is a physician-scientist and Professor of Pathology at NYU Grossman School of Medicine. Within and around and through that, he is a liver pathologist, a stem cell researcher, a gay activist, a complexity theory geek, a JuBu (senior student at the Village Zendo in NYC), a shamanic initiate, a philosopher of science (so he's been told, though he usually denies it), an anatomist (see "interstitium"), an entrepreneur in pharma and med device technologies, and probably some other things. For some of that, unclear which parts, he received an honorary doctorate from the University of Bordeaux in 2010.

Laura Victoria Ward

Laura Victoria Ward is a Laban/Bartenieff Movement Analyst, Registered Somatic Movement Educator and maximalist. She is the artistic director of Octavia Cup Dance Theatre, a multi-generational contemporary ballet company, and she plays violin, guitar, and sings with the punk rock band Dick Pinchers. She has worked in dance, theatre, fitness, somatics, and the creative arts for over 30 years. Laura's fascination with fascia began in 1996 when she studied Connective Tissue Therapy with Theresa Lamb and continues to the present day following the work of Gil Hedley.

Thanks to the talented photographers, artists and models who also made this book so special in addition to those listed above: Kelly Kamm (photographer extraordinaire and beautiful yoga teacher and person), Sondra Lorring (model who also lent her profound words), Barry Knittle (thanks for strapping my kayak paddle with lights!), Benjamin Feinstein (my older son, artist, and photographer), Doug Feinstein (brother-in-law for the glial photo), the lovely Lydia Mann for images from our dissection (knmlabs.com) and also to Nada Khodlova (with her beautiful quote), Karen Rider, Lori Officer and her sisters, Stacie Bird, Ingeborg Miller, Paula Bisbey, Patty Goodwin, and Jared Kaplan.

A final thanks...

The largest contributors here are the body donors from various programs that continue to teach us and gave permission during their lifetimes to have their images used for education. Please respect their wishes to view them with consideration that their forms continue to shape how we perceive our own movement in life.

PREFACE

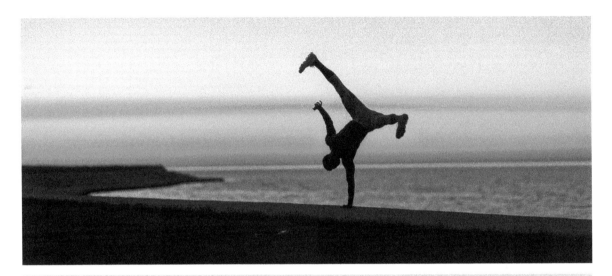

FIGURE PREFACE.1 The myofascial system in movement. "At times throughout history, artists have possessed more knowledge of the human body than physicians and their studies have given them a profound view into the structures of the body. The skills they developed in dissection transferred onto their stunning artwork depicting the human body. The art I create has always been through dance. Dancing centers me and reconnects me to who I am as an individual and the innate connection I share with creation, music, movement, and healing. At the same time, my passion has also been the study of anatomy and physiology. My personal dissections, just like the artists of old, have helped me advance as a dancer, health coach, and surgical technologist."—Nile Bratcher

Image courtesy of Nile Bratcher.

Welcome to the conversation

I love good conversation and questioning how we see the world. As I have explored deeper into areas of movement, art, and anatomy, I have become interested in the structure of fascia and how its form embodies the larger way nature expresses itself in both shape and connection. Life is, after all, about movement and we carve our lives through our actions, whether in a planned athletic practice, or the way we repeatedly hug a loved one, or routinely negotiate the way to the local food market or corner cafe. Life shapes us and we shape it as well. Fascia, a biological organizing matrix, may be having its moment because it is a reflection of the larger discussions in the world today. Isolating anything, whether it

be anatomical structures, elements of architecture, or social groups, changes its meaning and context. Environment is both the medium and milieu. In these pages, I have turned my eye to address in broad strokes some of the micro and macro levels of fascia, from what we know currently from the latest scientific research to the more esoteric reaches of metaphor in connection.

Along the way, I've invited several friends to come join our discussion and spark conversations. Some of the best dinner guests in science and movement are present as well as you! I ask you to engage with others in this topic with intelligence and openness to what we know, and what we are still learning. Science, after all, is never about absolutes. It is all about the willingness to test an idea and change course as new information reveals itself and to additionally communicate that information. We all have experienced places where communication is challenged, whether it is between friends, work relationships, or transmitting force across scar tissue in fascia. Fostering good conversation creates resiliency (or even the newer concept of "anti-fragility"). Most of us welcome the chance to have more possibilities in body and life. While a stress-free life sounds appealing to many, we actually need some healthy stress, both in our psychology and in our tissues, to create more resiliency to the unknowns that lie ahead.

I usually describe my own work as that of a guide (whether in education, yoga teaching, movement therapy, dissection lab, or kayak guiding on the water). What do I mean by that? I have hiked some metaphoric trails, including extensive training in movement therapy, theory, practice, and observational systems. Through my trainings and knowledge, I can often point a student or client to a shortcut or an efficient way to "travel." You as the reader and a mover in life need to do your own work, but having guides can help transverse rough terrain quickly to help get you get there. Still later, you can choose to get out your own metaphoric shoes and forge a new trail.

Starting in college with esoteric academic studies as an art historian, I then went on to graduate work in dance/movement therapy, continuing to anatomy and academia with some financial challenges that also had me learning how to speak across class differences, as well as a woman both in a female- and then male-gender-identified-dominated disciplines (and only just now are conversations widening to include transgender and others marginalized historically). Learning in all of these subject areas has given me bridges between seemingly separate fields, which often keep themselves quite far apart from each other. I enjoy seeing how shapes, patterns, and form all express themselves on micro and macro levels in movement from art to psychology to anatomy. When I came across myofascia, it made sense to me to look

at the relationship between the parts in connection, rather than as isolated parts. This is a lot like good conversation. We take dives and weave between threads of thought and ideas. Above all, we want to keep conversation moving forwards, while nodding to past history. However, if we dwell in past patterns, there isn't room for growth or change.

The body in reality only knows holism. In short, it can be a game changer for anyone in sports, movement, therapeutics, and more. It is also a place to have a conversation, whether we ultimately agree or disagree on the specifics of systems themselves. I also invite the concept of dualism. It is entirely possible, for example, to recognize the holism of the body while simultaneously observing places where the body is named differently. Both can have a place of truth.

This book has transformed greatly since it began as a focused reflection on one system of myofascial theory applied to movement. At that time, I thought I knew the ending of the story and just needed to unwind it with the same care I approach an anatomy dissection where I know what I plan to reveal, or the path of my daily trail run, or in teaching a class or workshop. All of those, of course, have a myriad of possible challenges that make the path quite different every single time. In training for resiliency on either a biological or psychological level, we are told to expect the unexpected pathways. The pandemic has had even larger plans for this particular book and made me rework this story through multiple lenses. With all great respect to places I have been, and people that have served up platters of wonderful ideas, I decided to take on the role of "hosting" my own virtual dinner gathering.

In the times of COVID, we've learned how to communicate in different mediums and platforms, although many of the issues of needing connection remain the same. Looking for context from past history, I have become interested in *The Decameron*, by the Italian writer Boccaccio (1313–1375), written during the time of the Black Death. The book looks at a group of young women and men, gathering in the countryside to wait out the plague by telling stories to each other. History professor Martin Marafioti has discussed this book commenting, "Boccaccio's prescription for an epidemic was a good dose of 'narrative prophylaxis.' That meant protecting yourself with stories. Boccaccio suggested you could save yourself by fleeing towns, surrounding yourself with pleasant company and telling amusing stories to keep spirits up. Through a mixture of social isolation and pleasant activities, it was possible to survive the worst days of an epidemic" (Spicer, 2020).

So, as with any good book, fiction or non-fiction, this is about gathering our friends and storytelling ideas of myofascia applied to movement. Stories help us both make sense of the world and connect in profound ways. Maybe the stories will serve as narrative prophylaxis for you. I'm not presuming any medical advice, of course, but ideas are powerful players in life and can help us shape our strategies for health and healing, whether we are self-reflecting or taking this into our world of clients and people we encounter.

Boles and Newman (1992), in writing on universal patterns, reflected on the danger of forgetting the larger whole. To note,

This world is of a single piece; yet, we invent nets to trap it for our inspection. Then we mistake our nets for the reality of the piece. In these nets we catch the fishes of the intellect but the sea of wholeness forever eludes our grasp. So, we forget our original intent and then mistake the nets for the sea. (p. x)

Here is perhaps my strongest word of caution: even our holistic myofascial connections, literally in netlike form, are not the entire picture. The world is full of giant sandboxes to play in and even in our enthusiasm for fascia, form, and movement, we still need to step back to take in the ocean.

I hope these pages spark a conversation for you. It must be noted that everyone is welcomed to the table. Bodies come in many colors, sizes, gender identifications, and ages and this is the time to celebrate our connected body!

References

Boles, M. and Newman, R. (1990) *The Golden Relationship: Art, Math & Nature.* Bradford, MA: Pythagorean Press.

Spicer, A. (2020) 'The Decameron – the 14th-century Italian book that shows us how to survive coronavirus.' *The New Statesman,* March 9, 2020. www.newstatesman.com/2020/03/coronavirus-survive-italy-wellbeing-stories-decameron

Further reading

Lu, M., Uchil, P. D., Li, W., Kwong, P. D. *et al.* (2020) 'Real-time conformational dynamics of SARS-CoV-2 spikes on virus particles.' *Cell Host & Microbe 28*, 6, 880–891.e8. https://doi.org/10.1016/j.chom.2020.11.001

Lynch, K. (2005) *The Image of the City.* Publication of the Joint Center for Urban Studies. Cambridge, MA: MIT Press.

Taleb, N. N. (2012) *Antifragile: Things That Gain from Disorder.* New York: Random House.

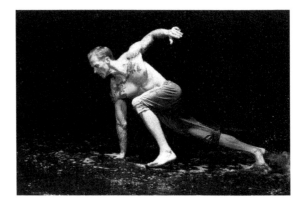

FIGURE PREFACE.2 The fascial system is fibrous but also fluid in nature. Training fascia creates increased possibilities for movement and expression by encouraging multiple choices available to the system.

Image courtesy of Mike Fitch, Animal Flow.

ORIENTATION KEYS

This book is designed to be user friendly whether you wish to thumb through or settle in deeper. As we start our journey, we will borrow from the visual and architectural concept of "way-finding" which is a way to organize the external environment. In the spirit of way-finding, we will use color and symbols to orient to the following ideas and concepts utilized throughout this book:

Breakout box

Written by guests at our metaphoric table, some of the brightest thinkers and movers in the myofascial world, these boxes provide insight into a wide range of work. Enjoy the opportunity to hear "sound bites" directly from some of my favorite friends and colleagues and experience their unique perspectives on direct areas of fascia and movement.

Thought box

Take these opportunities to pause and reflect on a focused idea. These thought boxes are idea seeds for further discussion and a place to pause and reflect on a focused idea. Many are from me, and some come from our guests to spark your own thoughts for reflection. In some we will explore new ways of conceptualizing language around fascia and movement or how applications can be applied. If you are looking to be sparked by an idea, look for the light bulb. These are moments of "food for thought" and sometimes short "sound bites"—a taste into a concept.

Movement lab

Try out movement ideas through our "lab" which is a place to experiment with you as the movement scientist. These are suggestions for movement play. Take care of yourself with any adaptations you need and feel free to experiment as you think of additional applications. As with any scientific investigation, feel free to repeat in any manner that you wish, and note the results.

Design principle

Design principles highlight areas that explore design reflected in architecture, either internal or external. Most principles of design used in human design take elements from the natural world.

Why Fascia, Why Now?
David Lesondak, author

The question was asked of me: "Why fascia, why now?" As a relatively early adopter, my first reaction was more, "What took you so long?"

The sea change in fascia awareness came home to me while watching the 2018 Netflix reboot of "Lost in Space." In the first episode, after being trapped half-underwater for hours, one of the Robinson family members develops life-threatening compartment syndrome in her lower leg. Her younger sister then saves her life by using some high-tech medical implement to release the pressure by cutting through her fascia.

I was really annoyed. First off, that's not how compartment syndrome works. The second and deadliest error? They pronounced it "fay'sha." I almost stopped watching right then and there. Still, I realized I may have seen the first mention of fascia in popular entertainment. That has to be a good thing, right? For the record, I eventually stopped watching. For a story about a family of scientists, the Robinson family exhibited a profound lack of critical thinking. And the writers got a lot of basic science totally wrong. And while I stopped taking it personally, I changed the channel and never went back.

The history of science is full of popular bad ideas and knowledge that, looking back, was little better than belief. Greco-Roman culture forbade dissection on humans, but it was okay on animals. They reasoned that human bodies and animal bodies were ostensibly the same, which no doubt misinformed a lot of early medicine. Likewise, geocentrism comes from that era and the great thinker Aristotle. Geocentrism held sway for over 1,000 years until 1543 when Copernicus first published his hypothesis that the earth orbits the sun. Galileo was jailed in 1630 for popularizing this heresy. From there, Johannes Kepler developed the Laws of Planetary Motion and, building on those ideas, Isaac Newton did the math in 1687 and "suddenly," heliocentrism (and gravity) was obvious.

Closer to our times, the enteric nervous system, our gut brain, was first discovered in 1907. It was subsequently ignored/forgotten three times before that reality gained traction. Now it's here to stay. The first writing I've been able to find about fascia being more than biological packing peanuts comes from the early 1800s. Such is the process and progress of science. Ideas and theories rise and fall. Some tenaciously endure, and eventually thrive.

There are poetic parallels that we're becoming aware of just how thoroughly our own body is interconnected while becoming aware of how we are interconnected environmentally on this planet we call home, while becoming further interconnected to each other via the internet; but I hesitate to ascribe this connectivity to some cosmic or spiritual significance. Perhaps the answer is more mundane. Maybe it is just fascia's time.

David Foster Wallace told the story of two fish going about their day. As one swims past the other, he says, "How's the water?" and the other fish responds, "What is water?"

For many centuries the biological sciences have obsessively studied everything in the water while ignoring the water—the viscous, living water that is our fascia. Slowly over time enough scientists have finally studied the water itself and reported so many fascinating things about it that water can no longer be ignored.

So maybe now is the perfect time for a bath. Come on in, the water is fine.

1

Myofascial material
The scaffolding and space of the moving body

In this first section, we explore the design of the moveable body in relationship to the perspective of myofascia: the joining together of muscle (myo) and fascia (definitions to be explored!).

The form of fascia   3

The shape of movement/human evolution in motion   46

The body in motion and emotion   66

Different ways of seeing—game rules, game plans, and body analysis   78

The essential corners in a round world   97

Spirals   114

Concepts of core   119

Arms, oblique connections, and active movement   133

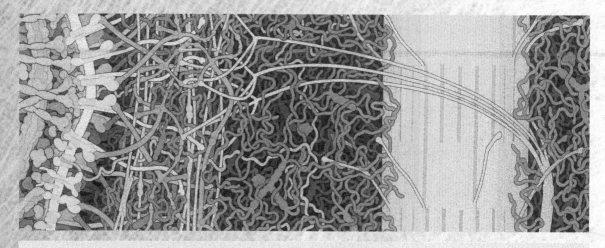

FIGURE PART 1.1 "A network of fibrous proteins and polysaccharides form a structural matrix between cells in our bodies. In this cross section, a cell surface is at left. A dense basal lamina braces the outside of the cell, composed of long collagen fibers, cross-shaped laminin proteins, and snaky proteoglycan molecules. Other forms of collagen help to strengthen the extracellular matrix, including huge collagen structural fibrils (at right in yellow) and anchoring fibrils (arching molecules in yellow). This painting was created as part of the celebration of the 50th anniversary of the Protein Data Bank, and is adapted from Figure 6.3 of *The Machinery of Life*."

Credit: Illustration by David S. Goodsell, RCSB Protein Data Bank. doi: 10.2210/rcsb_pdb/goodsell-gallery-033

We cannot live for ourselves alone. Our lives are connected by a thousand invisible threads, and along these sympathetic fibers, our actions run as causes and return to us as results.

Herman Melville

When the pandemic hit, the world simultaneously became both much smaller and wider for all of us. For me, spending more time at home, I often took my walks or runs at the crack of dawn, exploring the 508 acres of a nearby park and its varied surfaces, which ranged from gravel to pavement to the sandy shoreline of the Hudson River. This peninsula was inhabited by Native Americans possibly as far back as 7,000 years ago but much more recently was a huge landfill that accumulated 10.4 million cubic yards of garbage. It was a wasteland, severely damaged and scarred. However, in the early 1990s some leaders with foresight had an idea to repurpose this landfill and close it off, and amongst many other things, reseed the top of the garbage hill with over five *tons* of seed. Now it is thriving and teeming with wildlife. These days, I am out there in every type of weather, climbing the garbage hill. Seems poetic, somehow.

Just like the structures of the body, we are impacted by everything around us, and just like nature, we are amazingly resilient if we allow and make space for growth to happen. Fascia and movement share a common purpose of connection. It is fascia's framework that makes sense of its relational shape in the body. Movement has meaning, whether functional or expressive, through how it connects. It is a shifting support for life, providing the ability for movement in certain areas and creating restraint in others. A healthy fascial system is shaped in response to our daily actions but needs to be challenged in order to be responsive and resilient for the unexpected. Systems, both micro and macro, are interconnected networks, and organized frameworks. If we can understand our fascial system better, we can conceptualize how it works in larger spheres of thought such as myofascial connections (myo = muscle and fascia together) and concepts of fascia as part of our emotional response and sensitivity to the larger world around us, which is itself highly connected. Take away that milieu, however, and fascia loses its context and meaning for the moveable body. So, this amazing environment is something that has been so omnipresent, and yet in many ways neglected. So why has "fascia" been in and out of our awareness for so long?

In simple terms, it matters if it is part of our daily conversation. When we name or "see" something, our awareness of that expands, whether it is a word or concept. The writer Robert Macfarlane noticed the importance of naming when he noticed

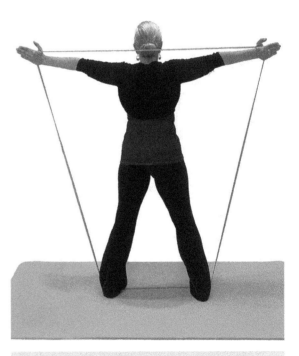

FIGURE 1.1 The body comes in many shapes and forms. Additional use of tensioned props can enhance the proprioceptive response of the fascia system. How we perceive our own body's form is evolving in relationship to the new concepts in fascia and its relationship to our movement on micro and macro levels.

that the 2007 Oxford Junior Dictionary was dropping familiar words about nature, including the common weed, the dandelion. He created a book celebrating those "lost words" (Macfarlane 2018) so that in speaking and thinking about these things, children would keep and celebrate these parts of nature. In other words, what we name or can visualize does matter to our understanding and appreciating it. We understand what we can perceive. Expand that perception, and new ways of problem solving and thinking are possible.

Many of our anatomical atlases are based on dissections, and the history of what we see and can perceive has changed dramatically depending on what we are able to dissect at definite points in history (Nemetz 2020). Stories abound that, in labs, students are traditionally told to discard anything that looks like fascia. Far from being inert, fascia is the connector and coordinator of movement. In fact, often the fascial surfaces between muscles are where movement in the living body occurs. If we toss that away, we are missing part of our understanding of why we might feel stiff in the morning or how that rocky trail impacts our tissue.

The etymology of "anatomy", after all, comes from the Greek meaning to "take apart" and separation is the main object of dissection. Perception of our understanding of the human body and its function in movement have changed every time we "see" differently through a reflection in our anatomical drawings, largely based the changes in dissection techniques over time. In part, techniques in the anatomy lab have changed what we can observe in fascial tissues. Due to the rapid need to quickly progress in a dissection, the outer layers of the body and adipose usually were burned off in a manner known as écorché (Singer 1957) in order to reveal the muscle layer underneath. The muscle and bone names have become almost fetishized and instilled with the magical powers of being most important in a mechanical levered system. Some biomechanics do come into play, but the body is endlessly more complex.

More recently, techniques from decellularization to plastination have allowed a perceptual shift, where we can focus on those areas that were previously taken out of the picture. However, modern techniques in medical training have traditionally relied heavily on formaldehyde-preserved tissues, which offer a means for one or more classes to work over a body for several weeks. At the same time, physical dissection lab hours are decreasing, and many doctors enter their practices with only one cadaver dissection under their belts, and a preserved tissue one at that. Computer models and interactive cadaver boards also have impressive visuals, but sacrifice some of the reality and texture of the body.

The origin of the word "fascia" is often attributed to the Latin *fascis* (to bundle), but likely had its root in the more ancient Greek ταινία (taenia) which has some overlapping meanings, according to anatomist Sue Adstrum (personal communication, 2022). The Greek word describes bandages and ribbons, and taenia is used to describe a type of genus of parasitic tapeworms. This is an apt image as banded myofascial connections are created of linked segments creating a ribbon-like whole like the tapeworm bearing its name. In the later Latin, the symbolism of a bound group of sticks together came to represent authority and strength as bundled groups of sticks together creates strength where a single twig is easily broken.

Medical descriptions of fascia made their way into literature, including the relatively recent description in 1814 (Mackesy) which described bands of connective tissue as fascia that influence the support for movement of the body, in this case damaged by a leg fracture. A casual search on sciencedirect.com for published articles on fascia listed 1,539 titles in 2001 and, as of 2022, 111,809 results (and growing).

Fascia is part of the vibrant, living body, and a net and network for communication surrounding all of our living cells and provides a framework and the environment for the rest of the body. It is a part of neurology, proprioception, and wound healing. It is also a spring force for efficient movement. Motion and movement are tied into spatial changes in position (proprioception), on both an ideological and a physical level. If I want to express my views on a social concept, I might join a movement that often expresses itself physically (think of a march for justice). As an athlete, if I want to run up a hill with more efficiency, I can learn to use the elastic properties of fascia. However, these concepts only make sense in the broader overlapping systems as part of the larger whole. Fascia additionally is used today as an architectural term to describe a banded area under a roof that is sometimes used to secure building and is often decorative in its nature.

Why is fascia conceptualized as fabric, nets, and tissues?

Fascia is conceptualized as a biological fabric or a large net, capturing and containing, but also allowing a degree of openness in the body system. If we continue the metaphor, it explains a lot in terms of wound healing and scar tissue as well. A poorly re-stitched tear in the fabric of the body will likely create areas of immobility and pull further threads toward the center of the injury. A skilled seamstress or knitter will not see a hole in a sweater and simply stitch it closed but will try to re-weave the torn fabric to create more integrity.

Of course, we are not here to be system selective, as the entire body has its part to play in how and why we move, but we have particular love for this previously neglected area of anatomy. Fascia has often been called our "Cinderella tissue" (Schleip 2003) for, like Cinderella, it was not sufficiently valued for what it is and what it can do. Fascia, like fabric, has a type of weave. Though often considered inert and disposable in many medical training programs, fascia's functions include wound repair, force transmission, and sensory functions. In terms of movement, fascia is both a connector of

the body system and reflective of coordination or distress in the movement system.

So let's go back to our metaphor of the fascia as biological fabric that keeps our cells from sliding apart. Just like fabric, the individual fibers of fascia are not strong, but organize them together (in a woven sense) and you get strength. As with fabric, we have a certain level of stretch or give and an end-feel and place where that give is finished. The bundling of fiber gives the strength to this mobile scaffolding. Fascia is also responsive to training in both short and long term, and is also involved in many injuries or ease in the body system. Without the organization of fascia, muscle does not have continuity. Beyond that, fascia is a regulatory system like our other systems. It has structure and shape, but it is also formed and re-fashioned by how we engage it. A channel for force transmission, fascia plays a role in our sensing of the body, and a connector that makes sense of our movement form.

As stated by Jaap van der Wal (2009):

Connective tissue-saving dissections create a different type of artifact. Fascia dissected into individual 'parts' can only be properly understood if the relationship between the connective tissue septa and layers and adjacent muscles is already known. It may come as no surprise that these relationships can only be seen and determined during the dissection procedure itself. In other words, one must know the architecture of the fascial system. Architecture is different from anatomy. Anatomy informs us where. Architecture tells us how. (p.6)

It is partly for this reason that van der Wal is against the terminology of "anatomical preparations", as there is the desire not to delete the relationship between connective tissue and the adjacent muscle. Our process in movement is about continuously shaping into form and a constant gesture of creation.

With a great appreciation to our holism, we can also speak to the ingredients that create our fascia buffet. If we ask the chef why ingredients matter in cooking, we can begin to understand that food can be merely functional, or transformative in skilled hands that can maximize moisture retention, quality, and so on.

The basics

At its most basic, fascia is essentially a simple mix of cells, gels, fiber, and water. Stir them loosely with more water and you may be creating more of a dinner soup; add more fiber and you have a heartier dish, so to speak.

Cells: fibroblasts and creating fascial architecture

Fibroblasts are the most common cell in fascia and connective tissue. They make a trail of collagen that becomes the scaffolding of the system, and some people have a lot more than others. If you have a lot of fibroblasts in your body system, your body will be inflexible but stable. On the other side of the coin, if you're looser, you'll be less stable due to lower numbers of fibroblasts. Fascia actually has less elasticity than we might think, because we need some stiffness to transmit force.

You also need glide. In healthy fascia, about 30% of the fibroblasts are specialized cells known as fasciacytes and may have to do with stimulation and load. As noted in Carla Stecco's *Clinical Anatomy* article (2018):

Hyaluronan occurs between deep fascia and muscle, facilitating gliding between these two structures, and also within the loose connective tissue of the fascia, guaranteeing the smooth sliding of adjacent fibrous fascial layers. It also promotes the functions of the deep fascia. In this study a new class of cells in fasciae is identified, which we have termed fasciacytes, devoted to producing the hyaluronan-rich extracellular matrix. (Stecco 2018)

Fiber

Fascia can be seen as the web that holds the body together and is the substance of its shape. The fibers have different compositions in different parts of the body. The iliotibial band, for example, has a different composition that is less mobile. In dissection lab, we look at the structure as being like packing tape, with strong stability. Other areas, like the fascia in the breast, are much looser of a weave, allowing for freedom of movement around a muscle.

Water, bound and free, and the gels that love them

Our watery, ocean-like bodies have both free and bound water, and these differences are important. Bound water is held in the body by macromolecules or organelles whereas free water is not. We are fluid both in terms of our water nature, but also in how that water content changes over our lifetime, with our young bouncy baby selves consisting of about 90% water whereas those over 80 years may be only about 50% water (Watson *et al.* 1980). Bound water is what keeps our tissues resilient. Glycoaminoglycans (GAGs) are long linear polysaccharides and are hydrophilic, attracting and binding water. In essence, they serve as both a shock absorber for the body as well as a lubricant, which helps glide in the body. This arrangement is similar in a wood cell where bound water is chemically attached to the cellulose, whereas in free water the liquid is found in the empty spaces. Dried wood is the loss of moisture first in the free water, and then in the bound water. This creates distinct shrinkage of the system. Very importantly, the amount of bound water decreases in age, and with that comes an increase of tissue stiffness. If we can retain the bound water, there may be a delay of age-related diseases (Kerch 2020). On the other hand, free water gets extruded during movement and manual work like a sponge being wrung out, allowing for a relaxation of collagen fibers and more pliable tissues. Additionally, water unbinds during an injury creating the swelling of knee, or ankle, for example.

We can think of fascia in terms of movement and health. Healthy fascia shows a lot of mobility between layers with a high proportion of proprioceptive receptors. Where there is a build-up of dehydration, fascia adhesions will increase. When there is too much hyaluronan (the polysaccharide found in the extracellular matrix) the tissue gets sticky and loses some of its ability to bind water. As a non-Newtonian fluid, hyaluronan is thixotropic; it changes its viscosity in response to loading conditions. Take ketchup as an example. If the ketchup isn't used in a while, it becomes solid and immobile. However, if you shake the bottle, the viscosity is changed, and with that change comes more mobility. The increased hyaluronan may happen as a response to stress and trauma, including high levels of exercise. Agitation, in the form of movement or in the form of manual pressure, influences the viscosity of the hyaluronan.

Fascia and categories

The fascia community has labelled fascia just about every fibrous connective tissue in the body except the submucosal layers (think linings in the body) and the dermis (the "true skin" with all its vessels and structures), which, for other of our traditional scientist friends are the entry points into this tissue.

Fascia is often categorized into three major types: superficial, deep, and visceral (having to do with the organs). However, Langevin and Huijing (2009) created a list of twelve terms to describe the different types of fasciae. These are: dense connective tissue, areolar connective, superficial fascia, deep fascia, intermuscular septa, interosseous membrane, periost, neurovascular tract, epimysium, intra- and extramuscular aponeurosis, perimysium, and endomysium

Kumka and Bonar (2012) have chosen to classify via their functional categories: 1) linking (tissues with high amounts of collagen type 1 which are active in active stabilization and passive continuities); 2) fascicular (multidirectional fascia bundling vessels); 3) compression (densely woven, multidirectional connective tissues that provide compression and enhance proprioception); and 4) separating fascia (compartmentalizes organs, etc., and provides support and shock absorption).

These are all based on fascia-related terminology as categorized in the *Terminologia Anatomica*, the standard book for human anatomical terminology, with its most recent edition published in 2019. In their thought process, fascia in its various types helps to improve musculoskeletal efficiency in the entire body system (Federative Committee on Anatomical Terminology 1998). Work is continuing to update this terminology as our discussions between anatomical groups continue to refine ideas in classifications as well the public's rapidly growing interest in fascia.

The rise of myofascial links, chains, slings, and other named things...

Shape expresses itself in health. Curiously, this is what we see in the changes of structure and shape resulting from cancer and other disorders. Is it possible that illness is the forgetting of shape and form? Shape seekers of all sorts historically have come to the myofascial system in looking for answers to health questions. In biology, the structure and form of creatures is studied under the concept of morphology. Links, chains, slings, nets, lines, and other ways of describing myofascial connections have come about as largely observational responses in a desire to explain relational connections and also to have a predictive tool for helping others.

Andrew Still, DO (1828–1917), founded the modern field of osteopathy in an effort to make medical reforms and to construct an idea of treatment that focused on holism and regaining a balance in physical form and health. Still (2017, p.403) in his work often cites fascia. Findley and Shalwala (2013) commented on Still's description of fascia as "vital for organism's growth and support, and it is where disease is sown." Still's ideas have helped in understanding fascia's connection to pain and perception in the body and continue to influence modern myofascial anatomy.

Raymond Dart was a student of the Alexander Technique, which focuses on alignment and

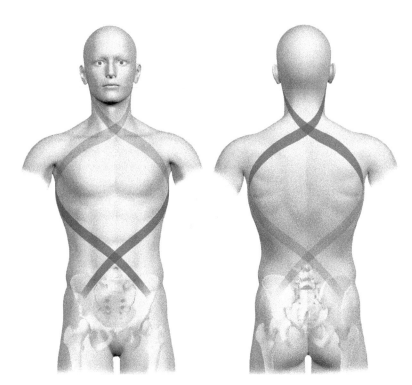

FIGURE 1.2 Dart's original concept of the double spiral was a shape that predated and also was an inspiration for Thomas Myers's Anatomy Trains® Spiral Line. Illustration after Dart 1996.

movement ease. Dart (1893–1988) was both an anatomist and an anthropologist and a member of the 1924 dig that uncovered the famous fossil of *Australopithecus africanus*, part of the close genealogical tree of hominid to human. He recognized the cross patterns of what he conceptualized as a double spiral arrangement. The diagonal directionality of these connections helped to pull the body into movement as well as lifting upwards in posture (Dart 1996). This double spiral arrangement (Figure 1.2) influenced Thomas Myers's Spiral Line, the first in his outlined system of Anatomy Trains® connections, which he conceptualized as myofascial meridians, ribbon-like in their representation.

The world of fascia would be incomplete without a nod to Ida Rolf who was revolutionary in thinking about the holism of the body rather than individual parts, and balancing the human body in a sense of whole relationship. She called her particular system Structural Integration. She also looked at reduction of rotational forces and organizing the structure of the body along its vertical axis in relationship to gravity. She encouraged length as a way to gain more freedom and possibility in movement and Rolf's work can be seen as an influencer of sorts to many fields and practitioners including Feldenkrais, Active Release Technique, Myofascial Release, Judith Aston, Hellerwork, Thomas Myers's Anatomy Trains®, and more. Throughout her teachings she expressed the idea that fascia is an organ of form and that working with this system can change postural patterns. Interestingly, scientifically we are still debating exactly what is being affected and how that holds change, whether fascial, neurologically, or some combination of it all.

The concept of muscle connections as well as myofascial connections, or that of linking myo (muscle) with fascia continues to widen in popularity. However, without an agreed upon precise definition, as each myofascial visionary understandably has their own set of rules, and often, treatment applications as well. Interestingly, as their popularity as a concept has grown, many students assume the myofascial lines are the reality, and often mistakenly cross names of different systems, or utilize a specific system's name as generic. Myofascial lines, meridians, slings, etc. are a construct, and if that construct proves useful in movement, treatment, or in other areas they do indeed have value. Of course, even an unproven concept has value if that system can help provide potential healing strategies, but reality and religious zeal for systems can sometimes overwhelm thoughtful reflection on evidence-based connections.

Any of the named myofascial connections are a pathway that is often understood as a line or area of force transmission. Myofascial connections work a balance of stability and healthy mobility and response. In engaging long myofascial chains, there is the concept of coordination between these areas in exercise, work, and pleasure, or in other words, in all aspects of the moving body in life. Movement is a combination of controlling a body in relationship to its environment, as well as creating stiffness or freedom as suitable to the situation. Fascia acts as both link and space for movement.

It is also important to conceptualize these as being conduits for areas of force transmission rather than actual physical lines that suddenly appear when we dissect a body. This has been shown in the work of myofascial pioneers including Leopold Busquet and Paul Chauffour, Andry Vleeming, Herman Kabat, MD, and Godelieve Struyff-Denys, Kurt Tittel, Ingrid Wancura-Kampik, Thomas Myers, and the Steccos amongst others.

Up and down (vertical) connections are described in systems such as Vleeming's slings, Meziere's work, or Myers (Anatomy Trains®). Visceral work through neurovascular connections includes thinkers like Shacklock. Side-to-side connections (areolar force transmission) are the domain of Huijing, and ligamentous connections (or dynaments) have developed from the work of Van der Wal. Many of these types of directional connections were noted by Myers (2020) himself. Over the years, there has

been much interest in possible crossovers in myofascial meridians to eastern medicine. Dr. Helene Langevin has furthered a lot of the thought processes in understanding fascia and stretch mechanisms in movement and acupuncture. Her studies with mice essentially being placed in a yoga-like up-dog position showed a slowing of cancer in breast tissue cells. Her work has also theorized that the Asian meridians, particularly in acupuncture, are likely following fascial planes. Additionally, the twist of an acupuncture needle turns collagen fibers along with hydrophilic proteoglycans wrapping around the needle like spaghetti noodles around the tines of a fork. This twist appears to stimulate and stretch the fascia. In a paper review in 2011, Bai *et al.* looked at the anatomical basis for the idea of traditional Chinese medicine (TCM). As noted, "the histological structures where an acupuncture needle acts are fascia connective tissue containing nerve endings, capillary vessels, fibroblasts, undifferentiated mesenchymal cells, lymphocytes, and so forth. Acupuncture points are traditionally believed to be sites that produce strong reactions when stimulated" (Bai *et al.* 2011).

In many definitions, fascia is considered a moveable, shaping, fluid structure. One of the recent definitions that caught my eye comes from Blottner *et al.* (2019), who note:

The fascia receives more and more attention as a functional component of the body in fundamental and applied human life sciences on Earth. As a shaping element of the human movement apparatus the fascia comprises a multicellular three-dimensional layer of connective tissue components (collagens, fibrocytes/-blasts, extracellular matrix), more specialized fibroblast-derived cells (fascia-, telocytes), contracting myofibroblasts, mechano- and propriosensors, and nociceptors. Fascia is a multicellular/multicomponent biological material for human body structural and functional integration as well as serving as a sensation organ in terms of movement and performance adjustment, body awareness and control.

So why study any of these systems? Maps are useful tools in planning a trip, understanding the geography, and ultimately where to go to next. We just need to remember to get the latest updates, or sometimes throw them out completely and go exploring for ourselves.

Seeing the form of fascia

There is no perfect way to see fascia as a whole form or system in itself. It is a substance of connection, and those connections run deep through skin, in muscle, and into cells on many levels. So why bother looking at the form of fascia as a highlighted area of interest? It is important anytime we shift perspective and perception. Art is known for doing so, and why not the same for anatomy? We can appreciate that the Arts and Crafts style of architecture expresses one aesthetic, or that the Impressionist movement of painting was about perceiving the world in a new way. Neither is an absolute expression of either architecture for humans or painting the world in absolute colors. Just as different art helps us to see the world differently, different anatomical ideas help give us insight into what makes our bodies function.

Are we reducing fascia to the same parts and pieces of anatomy as the reductionist muscle and bone naming that has happened for many centuries? The answer isn't so easy. Attend any fascially focused anatomy dissection, and while separation inevitably occurs, the whole is what is honored first and foremost. We are also shifting how all of us see and perceive the body and highlighting common threads, rather than the separate pieces that are the mainstay of modern anatomy. As noted in my own past research, "Dissection can reveal or obscure aspects in our understanding of the human body. Destroying one part of the connected form in order to reveal a particular perception of the body system is, by nature, part of dissection technique" (Nemetz 2020).

Jean-Baptiste Marc Bourgery, who lived in the nineteenth century, created a comprehensive anatomy textbook with the artist Nicolas Henri Jacob (Figure 1.3) that remains a well-known atlas, published originally in eight comprehensive volumes. These are among the first clear images using a figure–ground shift in perception of our visual focus. This term of figure–ground perception is from the visual arts, where the "figure" is what our eye focuses on while the "ground" is the backdrop to that. If we have a figure–ground reversal, we are suddenly seeing what was previously background. In these images, and the images that follow from the Fascial Net Plastination Project (FNPP), the fascia and myofascial connections are now the highlighted forms, and with that awareness we start to be able to see things afresh.

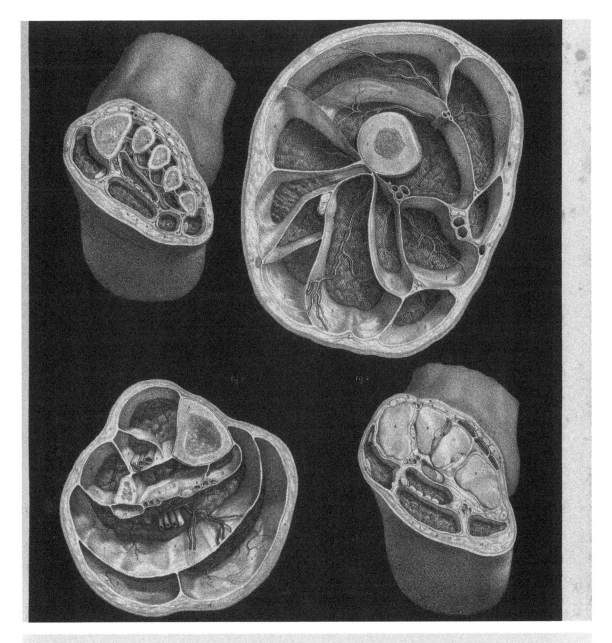

FIGURE 1.3 Fascia septa in the body give shape to the muscle compartments and provide pockets of shape within the overall connective system. One definition of fascia is that of a "a sheath, a sheet, or any other dissectible aggregations of connective tissue that forms beneath the skin to attach, enclose, and separate muscles and other internal organs" (Stecco and Schleip 2016).

Credit: Traité complet de l'anatomie de l'homme comprenant la médecine opératoire: avec planches lithographiées ... / par N.H. Jacob. Wellcome Collection. Public Domain Mark.

Chapter one

Fascial Net Plastination Project—Seeing is believing

Rachelle L. Clauson

If you have studied the myofascial system, you have some awareness of the huge role fascia plays in how our bodies move, get injured, and recover. As the living scaffolding that connects, separates, and organizes all our parts, we literally could not exist without our fascia. To understand fascia's function, including its energy storage capacity, adaptability to load patterns, and relationship to muscle coordination, we first need a road map of where it lives, what it looks like, and how it relates to the whole body. How else can we even begin to perceive fascia in our own bodies, or in our clients' bodies? But road maps of fascia, a.k.a. images and models, have not been easy to come by until recently.

A major leap forward in making fascia more visually accessible came when two giants in the fields of fascia research and three-dimensional anatomy joined forces. In 2018, the Fascia Research Society and the Plastinarium, the creators of the internationally acclaimed BODY WORLDS, collaborated to form the Fascial Net Plastination Project (FNPP) with the goal of creating the world's first 3D human fascia plastinates. Plastination is a preservation technique that infuses human cadaveric tissue with plastic polymer which halts decay, permanently fixes the tissue, and enables anyone to study true human anatomy in three dimensions. Four years later, the FNPP completed ten fascia plastinates and one female, whole-body plastinate highlighting the fascial system and how it interconnects throughout the entire body. The following images (Figures 1.breakout.1–9) are the results of this groundbreaking collaboration.

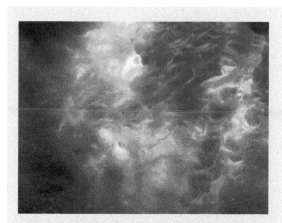

FIGURE 1.BREAKOUT.1 Superficial fascia of the abdomen plastinate.

With friendly permission of www.fasciaresearchsociety.org/plastination. www.vonhagens-plastination.com.

When viewed as a whole-body system, fascia begins just beneath the skin with the superficial fascia, or *fascia superficialis*. The varying thickness of superficial fascia all over our body gives us our silhouette and shape, which can change over time. Even though this tissue is manipulated at first depth before ever reaching muscle, superficial fascia is often overlooked in movement and hands-on therapy anatomy education. Commonly recognized as simply the "fat layer", deeper study reveals a complex organization with significant clinical relevance. Dividing walls called skin ligaments or *retinacula cutis* organize the adipose into thousands of little pockets and create a fascial bridge from the skin to the deeper tissues of the body. In this image of backlit plastinated superficial fascia from the abdomen you can clearly see the bubble wrap-like texture. Cellulite becomes less of a mystery with a better understanding of the organization of this tissue. Sometimes creating a rippling on the surface of the skin, our superficial fascia's "scaffolding" is always there and is essential to our form and function.

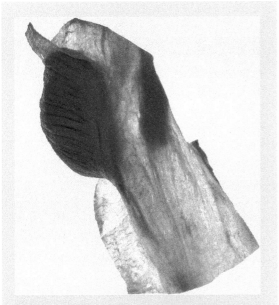

FIGURE 1.BREAKOUT.2 Deep fascia of the thigh plastinate.

With friendly permission of www.fasciaresearchsociety.org/plastination. www.vonhagens-plastination.com.

Deep fascia, or *fascia profundis*, is closely associated with the muscles and can be divided into two categories: aponeurotic and epimysial. In the limbs, epimysial fascia surrounds individual muscles while aponeurotic fascia surrounds groups of muscles. Both tend to be thinner than their superficial counterpart (averaging less than a millimeter in thickness). Aponeurotic deep fascia can look a lot like strapping tape because of its highly organized collagen fibers, it can transmit force over a distance, and it can change in thickness and organization based on how it is loaded over time. In this image you see plastinated aponeurotic deep fascia of the thigh called the fascia lata. The cylindrical structure completely envelops the thigh and has septa which dive to the bone creating three distinct muscular compartments. This fascial specimen has been divided at the medial thigh and laid flat. The fascia lata is continuous and embedded within the gluteus maximus muscle and the tensor fascia lata muscle, so we included them in the specimen to show their intimate relationship. You can also see in this image that the IT band, or iliotibial tract, is not a band at all, but rather a reinforcement and thickening of the lateral aspect of the fascia lata which occurs over time with repeated loading from walking and running.

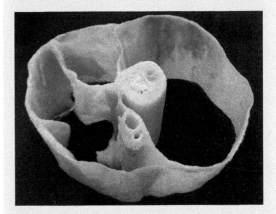

FIGURE 1.BREAKOUT.3 Deep fascia cross section of the thigh plastinate.

With friendly permission of www.fasciaresearchsociety.org/plastination. www.vonhagens-plastination.com.

Aponeurotic deep fascia fully envelops our limbs like a stocking or a sleeve, but unlike clothing it also dives inwardly to the bone longitudinally, creating walls of fascia called septa that separate the muscles into groups. In this image of a plastinated cross section of the thigh, all the muscles have been removed leaving behind only the surrounding aponeurotic deep fascia, the septa, and the femur bone. It is easy to see this "wagon wheel" arrangement of fascia creating three primary compartments—anterior, medial, and posterior—which would normally contain the quadriceps, the adductors, and the hamstrings. Understanding the relationship of the muscles with these deep fascial structures helps us better appreciate the stability our fascia provides from the inside out.

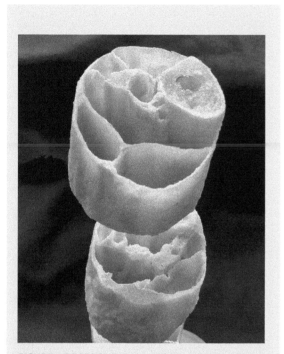

FIGURE 1.BREAKOUT.4 Deep fascia cross section of the lower leg plastinate.

With friendly permission of www.fasciaresearchsociety.org/plastination. www.vonhagens-plastination.com.

Highlighting the fascial system, instead of the more familiar muscular system, we create a completely different view of the body where the muscles are only visible as negative space. The three plastinated cross sections of the lower leg in this image have been stacked together and spaced apart on an acrylic rod to give an inside view of the fascia cruris, the deep fascia which envelopes the lower leg and divides it into compartments. The three large, empty spaces toward the bottom and left in the plastinate on top previously contained the two heads of the gastrocnemius and the soleus muscles. With the tibia, fibula, and neurovascular bundle still in place, the relationships of bone, vessel, nerve, and muscle are mapped out in 3D.

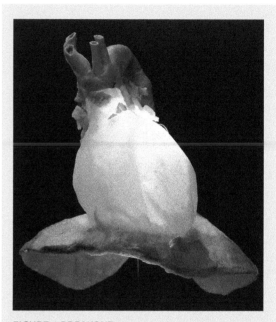

FIGURE 1.BREAKOUT.5 Visceral fascia of the heart plastinate.

With friendly permission of www.fasciaresearchsociety.org/plastination. www.vonhagens-plastination.com.

The only visceral fascia the FNPP created in this first plastinated fascia collection is of the fibro-serous pericardium and the respiratory diaphragm. Up lit, the empty pericardium defines the space where the heart once lived, and the diaphragm muscle forms the "skirt" at its base. The two structures are completely connected at the diaphragm's central tendon. This fascial connection is rarely seen anatomy books which would typically isolate the heart and the diaphragm in their illustrations. Seeing the intimate relationship of the pericardium and diaphragm here, suspended and delicately lit from beneath, can be a profound experience. Views of anatomy like this one can subtly influence our perceptions of self as we integrate our understanding with our movement and breath.

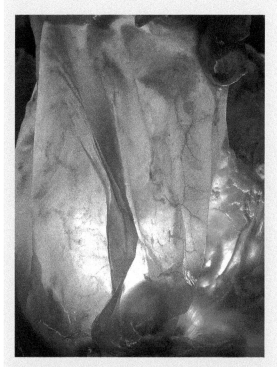

FIGURE 1.BREAKOUT.6 Pericardium dissection.

With friendly permission of www.fasciaresearchsociety.org/plastination. www.vonhagens-plastination.com.

Early on, the FNPP dissection team began experimenting with light to better see the architecture of the fascial tissues. We were intrigued by the new view the light provided and, ultimately, were inspired to name the FNPP exhibit *Fascia in a NEW LIGHT* because of it. This image of the fibroserous pericardium was taken right after the heart had been removed from a formalin-preserved cadaver. This strong, but supple, bag-like structure surrounds the heart, providing support and uninhibited movement for the heart as it beats. The golden sunset colors of the tissues are naturally occurring when white light is shone through them.

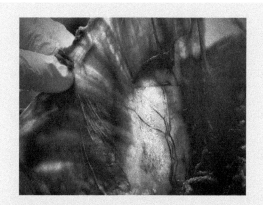

FIGURE 1.BREAKOUT.7 Respiratory diaphragm dissection.

With friendly permission of www.fasciaresearchsociety.org/plastination.

The respiratory diaphragm is the primary muscle used in breathing. Lying just below the heart and lungs, this dome-shaped muscle spans the entire circumference of the torso, separating the thoracic cavity from the abdominal cavity. In this image we see just one half of the muscle from a formalin-preserved cadaver. It is easy to identify the contractile muscle tissue fibers shooting outwards in all directions like petals of a daisy. The middle area is the central tendon where no muscle fibers exist. By back lighting the tendon, you can see veins and arteries as they pass through to the muscle. Because of the unique shape of the respiratory diaphragm's musculature, it can be sometimes difficult to conceptualize. Images like this help us better understand its structure and function.

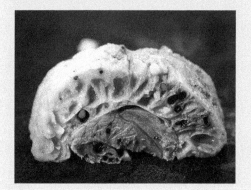

FIGURE 1.BREAKOUT.8 Lower leg cross section dissection.

With friendly permission of www.fasciaresearchsociety.org/plastination.

Like an MRI, viewing the body in cross section gives us the opportunity to see all the tissues, superficial to deep, at the same time. This specimen was dissected from a formalin-preserved cadaver to show the superficial fascia, deep fascia, and muscle in the posterior half of the lower leg. Only the skin has been removed from the surface exposing the thick arc of tissue on the top of the muscle, the superficial fascia. Comprised of both fibrous and adipose elements, superficial fascia connects the skin to the deeper structures of the body. In this specimen, the fibrous septa called skin ligaments, or *retinacula cutis*, have been highlighted by removing some of the adipose tissue, leaving the empty, honeycomb-shaped pockets behind. The bright red you see is polymer plastic which was injected into the arterial system and then hardened to give a better view of the vasculature throughout. Just above the muscle tissue you can see a thin, strong white membrane called the fascia cruris. This is the aponeurotic deep fascia that surrounds the muscles of the entire lower leg. Seeing the tissues in cross section like this can help us better understand the depths of what we touch when working with clients or moving and massaging our own limbs.

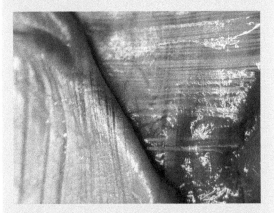

FIGURE 1.BREAKOUT.9 Latissimus dorsi dissection.

With friendly permission of www.fasciaresearchsociety.org/plastination. www.bodyworlds.com/FR:EIA.

Fascia comes in many shapes and sizes. In some areas it is loose, slippery and slide-y, in others it is dense, fibrous, and tough. Though differing in type, arrangement, and organization, no matter where it lives, one of the primary fibers in all fasciae is collagen. This image from a formalin-preserved cadaver allows us to see the tightly packed, parallel collagen fibers in deep aponeurotic fascia up close. On the left, we see a section of the left latissimus dorsi muscle and fascia which has been separated from the spine on the right and folded back to highlight the glistening, pearly-white collagen fibers. This fascia is quite logically classified as dense, regular connective tissue and transmits the contraction of the muscle to the spine as a flat tendon. The right half of the image shows the mostly transparent serrati fascia which creates a gliding surface between the latissimus dorsi and the erector spinae muscles beneath. Some white collagen fibers are visible in the serrati fascia which are extensions of the serratus posterior inferior. Looking through the serrati fascia, you can identify the erector spinae muscles and fascia by their longitudinal fiber direction, parallel to the spine. Images like these can quickly fill in gaps in our understanding when learning how deeply the muscle and fascial systems are interconnected with one another and how the myofascial planes of tissue are free to glide in different directions.

Further reading

BODY WORLDS. www.bodyworlds.com/FR:EIA.

Fascial Net Plastination Project.
    www.fasciaresearchsociety.org/plastination.

Otocast. app.otocast.com (search FNPP).

Plastinarium. www.vonhagens-plastination.com.

Holistic body systems (Figures 1.4a,b and 1.5a,b) are formed from tube-like networks and create the shape of the body (Myers 2020). These include the nervous system (the neural net which is involved in timing), the circulatory system (with bodily function) and the fascial system (involved with spatial organization, and therefore with proprio and interoception). Being able to see them reveals the shape of the body system and the extent of their reach into every corner of the body points to the importance of each of these systems. Shape is a great communicator, and all of these systems show the form of the individual human in all of their complexity.

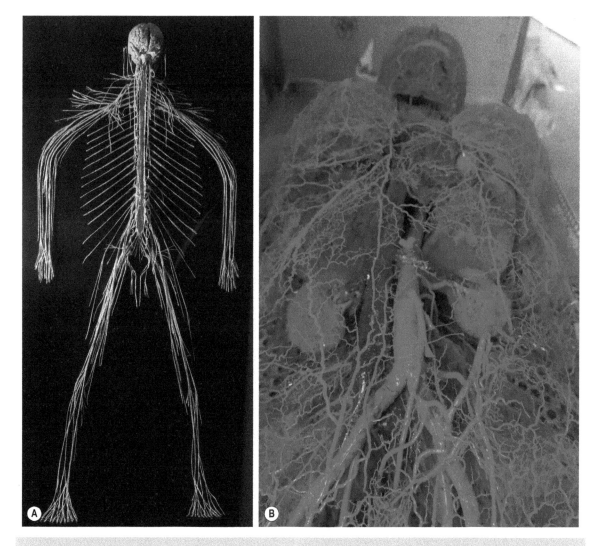

FIGURE 1.4 (a) The central nervous system and the peripheral somatic nervous system have been extracted from the cranial cavity, spinal canal, and surrounding soft tissues of the human body. The nervous system specimen is schematically representing the nervous distribution throughout the body. This plastinate allows tracing the emergence of the cranial nerves from the brain, the roots from the spinal cord, formation of the trunks and plexuses with subsequent originations of the peripheral nerves. b) The full human body arterial corrosion cast represents the negative replica of the arteries and arterioles (Figure 1.4b). Liquid thermosetting polymer methyl methacrylate (BioDur®) was injected through the incision into carotid the artery of the cadaver with subsequent polymerization within blood vessels. The tissues surrounding solid polymer were broken down by means of KOH and HCL solutions, thus exposing the finest configuration of the vascular system of the entire human body. In the photograph we can distinguish the largest artery of the body—the aorta, which branches out and gives arteries, which are also dividing and subdividing, forming a three-dimensional imaginary configuration of the body organs and parts. Systems photos and text by Dr. Vladimir Chereminskiy PhD, Director of Anatomy & Plastination, von Hagens Plastination; with kind permission.

A form of fascia: FR:EIA (Fascia Revealed: Educating Interconnected Anatomy)

Dr. Vladimir Chereminskiy

FR:EIA is the first whole-body plastinated specimen ever which solely emphasizes on the portrayal of various fasciae. It was designed to bring the understanding of fascia in a simple way to the general public and professionals. The design of the body incorporates all of the possible types of fasciae, from its superficial layers to the deep ones.

On the right side of the body, you can see the integumentary system: the protective covering of the organism, serving as an important window into the body. The next layer, the superficial fascia, which is important for aesthetic and kinematic reasons, also functions to house lipids. There is a strong relationship between skin and the subcutis, which exists throughout the entire body by means of vertical fibrous connections (retinacula cutis). Fascial constructs in weight-bearing areas are always better developed. Examples of this can be seen in the lower portion of the gluteal region, in the heel of the feet, or palm of the hand.

The deep fascia has been displayed on the medial and left side of the body, showing both the aponeurotic and epimysial types. The myofascial compartments, the neurovascular sheaths, have been demonstrated on the upper and lower extremities.

The internal fascia of the thoracic cavity and the visceral fascia of the mediastinum are shown through the window in the anterior-lateral part of the left side of the thoracic wall.

Head and neck dissection displays a clinical relevance of fascial compartments and sheath during head injuries, inflammatory processes, and reconstructive surgery.

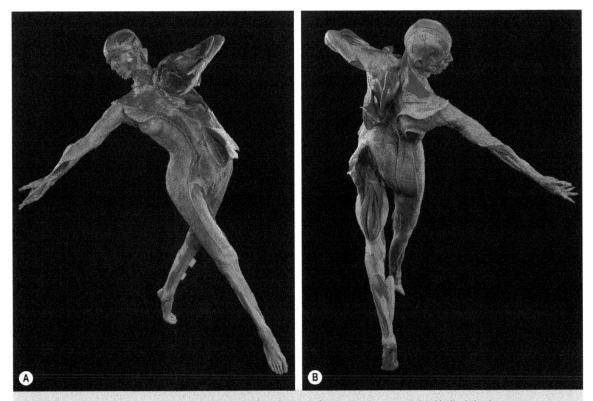

FIGURE 1.5 Front a) and back b) view of FR:EIA, the first full body fascia plastinate, and third holistic body system.

Credit: Photo courtesy of BODY WORLDS: www.bodyworlds.com/freia.

Communicating anatomy is something that has historically been done through art in many forms from engravings to wax models. Preserving the whole human body for education has been experimented with from applied vanishes to 18th century anatomist Honoré Fragonard's écorchés which, like modern plastinates, were placed in life-like poses so that the viewer could "see" inside the workings of the body.

As a member of the FNPP, I worked on the international dissection team on a number of pieces as well as being part of the teaching team for the final workshop of the project in January 2022. One of the absolute highlights though was spending the summer of 2019 as part of the extraordinary volunteer team that produced the first fascial plastinate known as FR:EIA (Figure 1.5a). Under the direction of Dr. Robert Schleip and design by Dr. Vladimir Chereminskiy and Gary Carter, this has become the first full body plastinate highlighting the fascia. I spent much of my time initially on the superficial fascia, which differs in density, in general appearing thinner toward the distal areas of the body. Superficial fascia helps provide support for the skin above it and surrounds many of the superficial nerves, like the cluneal nerves that when entrapped can cause lower back pain. Highlighting the Superficial Back Line (one of the Anatomy Trains® lines) provides a peek into windows showing the connections from the plantar fascia, Achilles tendon, calf muscles to hamstrings on upwards to the erector spinae muscles and the epicranial fascia. Diving down deeper are windows highlighting the visceral fascia inclusive of suspensory ligaments that hold the organs in their space, among them the pericardial sac. Meningeal fascia includes the fascia in the brain, such as the glial (gluey) cells. Deep investing fascia is both aponeurotic and epimysial. Often organized in pattern, this includes areas like the iliotibial band (IT band) that structurally looks like packing tape and has a stabilizing function. Deep fascia adheres to the fibrous capsule in joints and can help perceive both movement and joint positioning and is important in the body's perception of movement and spatial relationship.

In January of 2022 I got to visit FR:EIA at the Berlin BODY WORLDS Museum with Gary before helping as part of the teaching team for the final segment of projects in the FNPP. Spending time alone with FR:EIA, and then with a workshop group, allowed me to watch how others reacted to seeing this new plastinate which is an amalgamate of the donor herself along with the vision of not only the team but the fascia experts whose ideas are incorporated in this form. First the visual shift from muscle to the whiter and blue tinged fascia caught people's eye. Then, I watched as several interacted with the displays nearby, applying fascial concepts to movement. More details of the specific areas of this dissection and the team's entire work are part of the pre-conference presentation (Nemetz, Carter and Clauson) at the Fascia Research Congress (2022) and will be in further articles and lectures as time continues. It is hard to fully predict who will be impacted by seeing FR:EIA or images of her. She, and the entire team of volunteers that worked on her have become part of fascial history. The form of FR:EIA is important because her human and feminine shape is familiar, but new in highlighting the connected and curving lines of myofascial continuities.

Compartments, circles, spheres

Shape is maximized in circles, spheres, and more, whether we are discussing the fascial enclosures seen in a cross section of the thigh (Figure 1.6) or the design of a traditional anatomical theater (Figure 1.7) containing concentric ellipses. Even our planet Earth is often divided into spherical categories: the lithosphere containing the core to Earth's crust, the hydrosphere containing the water of the planet, the biosphere, containing the living ecology of the planet, and the atmosphere, containing the air.

Any system relationship in shape teaches us about the relativity between parts. In the case of the traditional dissection theater, the design allows the maximum ability to view the dissection in the

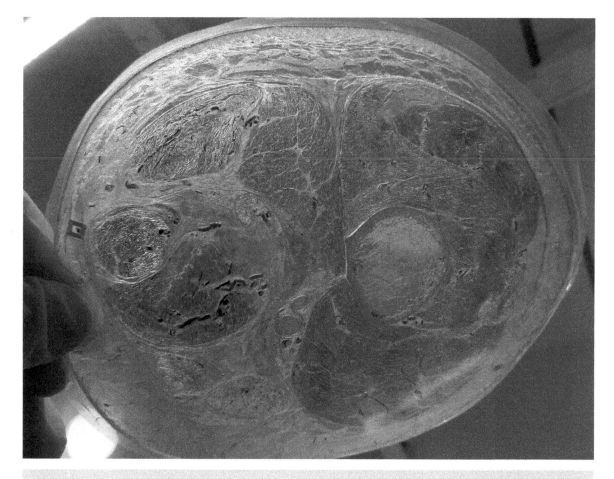

FIGURE 1.6 Plastinated cross-section of the thigh. The 1.5 mm thick slice plastinated and stained, using a technique which mainly discriminates lipids of the loose connective tissue (semi-transparent) and elastic and collagenous fibers of the fascia, aponeuroses, and tendons, which are stained in red. It also demonstrates the compact bone tissue, trabecula of the bone cavity, and the semi-transparent bone marrow of the femur. The epimysial fascia envelops the quadriceps femoris muscle group and their tendinous components are stained in light red. Each group of muscles of the posterior and medial compartments has its unique fascial sheath. Thus, the slice demonstrates the unaltered anatomy of the musculofascial compartments of the thigh. The polymer-injected arteries and arterioles demonstrate tissue vascularization.

Photo and text with kind permission; Dr. Vladimir Chereminskiy, PhD, Director of Anatomy & Plastination, von Hagens Plastination; Assistant Professor, Department of Pathology and Anatomy Eastern Virginia Medical School.

most efficient use of space for spectators. The cross-section plastinated slice allows a viewpoint of fascial compartment relationship in a likewise efficient use of space.

In traditional medical language, fascia is a broad area of tissue such as plantar aponeurosis (commonly known as plantar fascia), Scarpa's fascia (with a nod to the need to step back from medical eponyms which usually highlight male medical professionals only), fascia lata, and so on. Fascia can be classified under connective tissue, but not all connective tissues are fascia. This is an important distinction as it is easy to equate the two, but connective tissue includes broader categories.

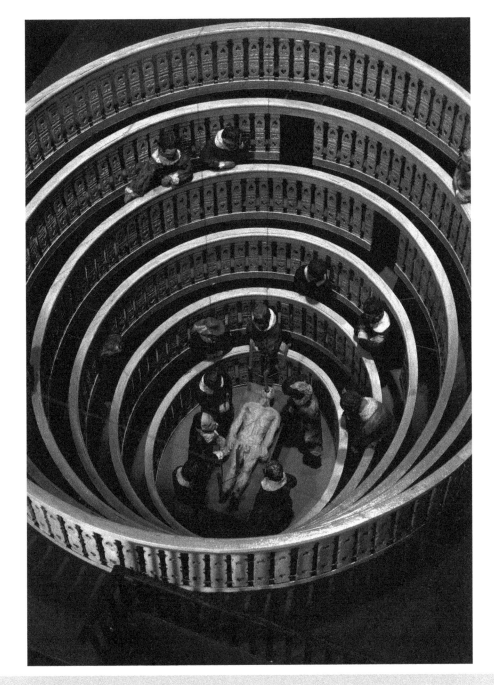

FIGURE 1.7 Scale model of anatomy theater built at Padua in 1594, showing a dissection taking place. The architecture of the anatomy theater is designed to maximize spatial relationship, allowing viewers to observe the anatomical dissection from a ringed and steep vertical succession of levels.

Credit: Wellcome Collection, Science Museum, London. Attribution 4.0 International (CC BY 4.0).

Set aside the complexity of fascia within the human body for a moment and present the larger community with the familiar. An orange (Figure 1.8): a beautiful example of how fascia dictates structure and function. Show an orange to your patient or class and initiate discussion by asking them how they would peel the fruit. Knife? Fingernail? Some may understand that "softening" the orange by applying pressure to the outer rind of the fruit and rolling it on a hard-flat surface first makes the rind *much* easier to peel. This teaching moment explains that by pressing on the orange and rolling it in multiple directions you are disrupting tiny fibers that connect the rind to the deeper fascia compartmentalizing the pulp of the orange. When the rind is removed, remnants of the orange's superficial fascia can be observed (and picked off) leaving the pulp arranged in circular sections. In order for sections to be separated, the loose investing fascia must be detached between wedges. These fascial planes and the potential spaces formed between the two loose layers of connective tissue allow each orange slice to be individually shared.

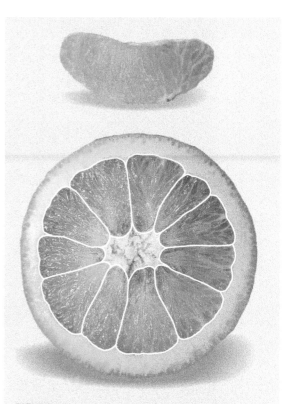

FIGURE 1.8 The organization of the orange helps us simplify the complexity of fascia for the greater community. By engaging your patients in the conversation of how best to peel an orange you are getting them to buy in to dynamic stretch, flexibility and whole-body care because after all, an orange is much easier to remove once the attachments between the skin and the fruit capsule have been broken.

First, we can classify the four major categories of tissue: nerve, muscle, epithelial, and connective. Out of all the cells in the body, connective tissue is the most varied. Specialized connective tissue includes blood, cartilage, adipose, reticular, and bone. The connective tissue (CT) proper includes loose and dense tissues, which both consist of fibroblast cells, collagen fibers in dense, irregular, or loose connections. This connective tissue "derives its name from its function in connecting or binding cells and tissues. It is ubiquitous in the body and can be considered the 'glue' that holds the body parts together" (Stecco and Hammer 2015, p.1). Connective tissue is, as its name suggests, a connector and structural supporter of other tissues in the body.

The natural world again gives us a shape-map for the similar tissues in our bodies. Cacti have a "skeleton" really more similar to our "fascia." It is created by the vascular cambium whose interior xylem that "comprises thick cell walls reinforced by lignin, a highly branched and compressively stiff (but brittle) polysaccharide (De Vivo *et al.* 2020, p.214). The living cactus's flexible system-wide internal structure becomes rigid upon its death (Figure 1.9). This structure is so intriguing

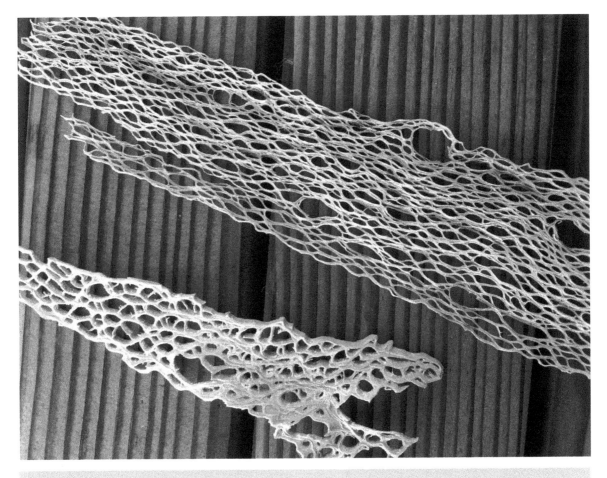

FIGURE 1.9 Cactus extracellular matrix. Fascia, in addition to human and animal anatomy, is also utilized as a term in subjects including architecture and botany (Online Etymology Dictionary 2022). Even the word fascination is related to "fascia." Photo by the author.

to scientists that it is being explored for its combination of lightness and torsional strength.

So where does our fascia come from?

The cells that create fascia are largely fibrocytes (myofibroblasts and fibroblasts) and adipocytes. Our early life starts from a fertilized ovum that divides and splits into stem cells. These cells then differentiate into the three layers of ectoderm (creating the epidermis and nerve cells), mesoderm (muscle cells specializing in contraction) and endoderm (epithelial cells that create the inner lining of the lungs or digestive tracks

and make and secrete enzymes and hormones). Connective tissue cells do two major things in the body, one of which is providing protection from outside invaders and the other building the shape to come for the rest of the cells and so the function of movement can happen. Even at about the beginning of the third week of embryological development, the web of reticulin fibers (an immature collagen) starts to appear and is what shapes our form.

Spatial relationships as the body is being formed determine quite a lot. In the brain, for example, the neocortex is a six-layered structure where connective tissue cells are the organizing highways for the cells that are laid down. It might be possible to conceive of the idea that structural change can impact a person in different ways whether we conceive of this as neurological or spatial in the way it is expressed.

Ghost organs and finding the architecture of the fascial body

"Ghost" organs are so named for their appearance, devoid of color and more importantly, stripped of the blood and muscle tissue associated with organs and their functions. The shape, or design, of the organ has been understood as the most important feature in theoretically creating viable organs or tissue for the human body that could be reseeded with healthy tissue on the framework of the actual organ (Ott *et al.* 2008). This part left behind is the extracellular matrix or ECM, the fibrous components of the fascia that also contain the nutrient-rich ground substance and additional lymph. It is what is made from the cells that are excreted into the space in the tissues. The ECM "works as a molecular store, catching and releasing biologically active molecules to regulate tissue and organ function, growth and regeneration" (Zügel *et al.* 2018). We can think of the ECM as layers of woven fabric in colloidal slippery glue. Think of papier-mâché strips of woven fabric swimming in that mixture of glue, flour, and water that you may have played with as a kid.

When I first heard about fascial organs, I followed the lab work of Doris Taylor, who has been working with hearts reseeded with stem cells. My goal was to create similar fascial organs with the purpose of having a teaching model that could be recreated during a day or two in the lab. I started my exploration in 2015 and 2016 with hearts, followed up with five additional hearts, and then a kidney (Figure 1.10).

Since I was not working on a surgical level, I could use less expensive lab solutions and I came up with a 20-step procedure, which I liken to old darkroom photography, where the chemical processes start and stop at different stages. I used sodium laurel sulfate, a common ingredient in shampoo, as a literal detergent. At other points, salt was added to weaken the cell walls, and water to stop the process from going too far.

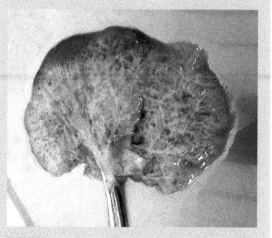

FIGURE 1.10 Ghost kidney. The ECM is the essential membrane of the body; it holds and weaves together our structure and shape. The kidney ECM interestingly creates its classic shape when placed in a watery environment. Without that environment, the ECM loses form. Photo by author with thanks to Anatomy Trains® and Laboratories for Anatomical Enlightenment.

Helene Langevin *et al.* (2013) looked at the ECM in terms of fibroblast regulation. In other words, when tissue is stretched, the fibroblasts actively remodel the matrix and may help to protect against swelling. This may have a connection to lymphatic functioning in particular, which could have implications for cancer research. Collagen fiber, along with elastin, are considered important parts of the ECM (Mercer and Crapo 1990) and in studies of both rats and humans is considered important "as the principal load-bearing elements of the lung parenchyma." In terms of spatial use, elastin forms rings around each alveolus. Tomoda, Kimura and Osaki (2013) published that collagen fiber as part of the ECM is critical in maintaining the shape of the lung and furthermore "suggests that collagen fiber orientation in the human lungs is markedly related to the mechanical properties." In other words, the respiratory movement is linked to the orientation of the collagen fibers.

What are some other purposes of the ghost organs? As noted by Lesondak (2018), they shift our understanding such as in the case of osteopath Gunnar Spohr's work which looked

> ...at the heart as a myofascial unit, in this case one without a clear origin or insertion, we move away from a purely mechanical model of heart function to a more kinetic, biotensegrity-based model. This further suggests that what we think of as a heartbeat might really be the inherent fascial property of elastic recoil." (p.109)

Additionally, I found that my fascial kidney was an interesting educational model—it kept its classic shape and form when submerged in water, but immediately lost its spatial identity when it was taken away from that environment. In the future, I plan to refine the procedure so that it is easier for others to replicate. Additionally, we can wonder at what other organs would lend themselves to the process, such as the fascial bladder.

Shapes in other natural forms of organic living tissue have a similar make up. Consider a leaf (Figure 1.11) whose cellulose structure also gives flexible form to a plant.

Taking architecture and form from the humble leaf... If you have ever taken a stroll in the fall, you have probably seen several leaves stripped of their main covering, leaving the scaffolding of their structures on display. Gershlak *et al.* (2017) noted that decellularized plants could serve as a type of conduit for human endothelial cells that could utilize the shape of the vascular system of the plant. In short, the authors (and credit to their sense of humor here) wanted to develop a "green" means of tissue engineering to help create a vascular network that was literally bioengineered and available for grafting to humans. The vascular network, structured like tree branches, is remarkably similar across nature whether in the plant or animal kingdoms.

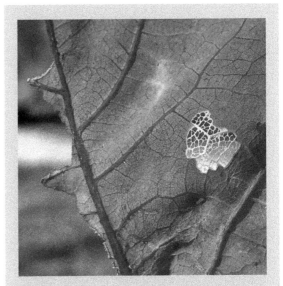

FIGURE 1.11 A lovely example of leaf fascia, a.k.a cellulose. Photo courtesy of Jared Kaplan.

 Building a web of fascial connection from a ball of yarn

I often look for ways to creatively connect people in a physical sense in the beginning of a workshop. Tossing a yarn ball is an exercise that can be useful in various settings, from modern dance workshops to corporate team building programs. Around 10 years ago, I started carrying a ball of yarn in my bag as an extra prop to emphasize connections in a warm-up, especially since it helps build understanding of how fascia impacts the whole system (Figure 1.12).

Hold one end of a large ball of yarn and pass the ball to different participants in your group (toss it to a new friend and introduce a name) until everyone has at least one part of the string to hold. Then lower the whole structure so that it is flat on the floor. This is similar to seeing the fibers of the collagen flattened, without the interstitial space, like how preserved tissue often flattens our perspective. Now have some participants standing and some seated so you can see the different levels, but also the three-dimensionality of the fibers. As a teacher, I might pull on a string, and see the repercussions in the connected "myofascial" lines. Likewise, if I tighten an area or pull a bunch of strings together, the resulting tension is similar to scar tissue.

We are training the fascial system all the time. Any time we shift how we train or move the body, we are affecting the fascial system. We start to think about how we can train the fascia with more intelligence.

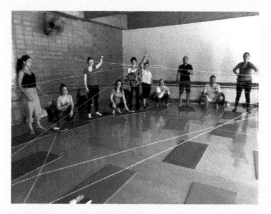

FIGURE 1.12 The threads of collagen fiber and the spatial relationship of myofascial connections can be represented in string. Flatten the connections down to the ground and it is similar to seeing embalmed tissue, which loses the interstitial space.

Collagenase, what it is, what it does and how to affect it
Jason Spitalnik

We do not have "fibroclasts" to break down older or unused or damaged collagen fibers.

The body has specific cells that produce the enzyme collagenase, responsible for breaking down collagen fibers. There are three types of collagenases under the larger category of protease enzymes called matrix metalloproteinases (MMPs), all of which break down specific types of collagen or assist during different stages in the collagen breakdown process.

Collagenase is an MMP enzyme that is secreted from the same fibroblasts that produce collagen fibers. In other words, fibroblasts produce both collagen and collagenase.

Collagenase is an enzyme capable of solubilizing insoluble fibrous collagen by peptide bond cleavage under physiological conditions of pH and temperature. And just like other cells produce specific types of collagens, fibroblasts are not the only cells that produce MMPs. There are also macrophages (those toxin-eating Pac-Men), keratinocytes (skin cells), chondrocytes (cartilage cells), and even smooth muscle cells. Breaking down the extracellular matrix proactively is a distributed phenomenon, and these enzymes are very specific to which types of collagens they break down.

Collagenase does not work alone, at least in wound repair. Cytokines (which induce production of collagenase, from fibroblasts and osteoclasts) and growth factors play an important role in repairing and remodeling. Like collagenase, these are also secreted from the many types of cells listed above, including fibroblasts.

Wagner's *Collagenase* (1972) shows the difficulty in finding collagenase in mammals: "In 1961 ... mammalian collagenases were still sought in vain; we now explain our failure to detect these enzymes, by educated hindsight, on the basis that the enzymes appear to be produced de novo, on demand, possibly triggered by hormones." Under normal healthy conditions, is it possible collagenase production and secretion are triggered by chemical signals, specifically hormones, or mechanical ones, or both?

Collagenase works in an aqueous environment. In other words, in the presence of water. "The center of the collagen molecule is hydrophobic which [could be why] fascia takes a long time to remodel, as collagenase and water have a hard time getting to the center" (Brett 2003, p.23).

Is it possible the "Gordian knot" of scar tissue creates a large hydrophobic area as well as a different degree of hydroxylation? Is this why it takes so much time to break down scar tissue? Although it is scar tissue, it is "new" collagen and therefore "healthy", just not as functional. Perhaps manual therapy helps expose the hydrophobic center, which will no longer be hydrophobic if it is exposed, by unfolding and fraying of the newly formed but rather dysfunctional collagen. Would this allow collagenase and other MMPs access and accelerate the breakdown process?

References

Brett, D. W. (2003) *Topical Enzymatic Debridement*. New York, NY: The McMahon Publishing Group, Chapter 3, p.23.

Uitto, J., Chu, M., Gallo, R. and Eisen, A. (2008) *Fitzpatrick's Dermatology in General Medicine* Vol. 1. New York, NY: McGraw-Hill Medical Publishing, Chapter 61, p.528.

Wagner, B. (1972) *Collagenase*. New York, NY: Gordon and Breach, Chapter 1, pp.1 and 3.

Location, location, location: In defense of layers and naming location... and when not to

The skin is no more separated from the brain than the surface of a lake from its depths; the two are different locations in a continuous medium... To touch the surface is to stir the depths.

Deane Juhan, *Job's Body*

I have had conversations with many of my colleagues on whether or not the concept of layers in fascia is useful or even accurate in a continuous form. However, the idea of the whole of the form can also exist simultaneously with the idea of layers. Instead of one or the other, we can conceptualize

the body in terms of both. Certainly, it is important to recognize that myofascial connections don't immediately reveal themselves when we go into dissection lab. However, there are places where the scalpel divides more easily. The geography of the body is like the layers of rock and earth that form strata, the multiple layers of rock or even series of layers in the Earth's "body." It's the same in the sky, where the clouds are part of a larger environment, and yet form distinct shapes and structures.

To extend this concept to the fascial web or the fabric of the body, we know that the reality of the anatomical body is the unity; the separation is artificial. However, there are areas that lend themselves more easily to differentiation than others. Often the places that my scalpel (or even a finger) easily separates in a body are where the fascial layers are working in movement.

Fascia is the contextual milieu for the entire body and is one unified connection from about day 14 of embryological development until the moment of death. In basic terms, we can conceptualize the epimysium as the fascia around the individual muscles and is a good force transmitter from one to the other. Perimysium wraps the individual subsegments into more bundles of fascia called fascicles. The endomysium is the fascia closest to the cell and wrapping individual fibers. While the terminology of layering is still somewhat controversial in the fascial community, these layers have some important characteristics and form differences visually in the same way that a cross section of soil may be a continuous blend, but still have distinct strata when looked at in cross section. Spending time with the body in dissection can make cases for both the conception of layers and complete integration throughout the body system.

Lancerotto *et al.* (2011) described the strata that are sometimes seen in the adipose layer, which I've personally observed several times in dissection lab. The layer of adipose immediately under the skin is sometimes a single layer but is often two layers separated by membranous tissue. In their research, Lancerotto and team discovered that they could identify three layers in the subdermal tissue of the abdomen: the superficial adipose tissue (SAT), a membranous layer, and the deep adipose tissue (DAT). In the SAT layer there is a high degree of both elasticity and structural stability. In obese individuals, the SAT has substrata layers. From my observations in lab, I've wondered if these developed after large weight gains and serve to connect a large area of adipose as an extra layer of reinforcement. Perhaps also the body thought that this was a final "layer" only to have another weight gain at another time. It is almost like looking at rings on a tree trunk, where one can observe thicker or thinner rings depending on years of feast or famine.

We can make a distinction of the interstitium that is within fascia, versus that which is between the layers of fascia. A dense and stiff layer may be able to support a layer and can support weight while layers that are in-between that are looser or areolar cannot. This can all be fascia, and yes, connected, and not have different properties, especially in the living, moving body.

Loose connective tissue—the body's site for immune responses

Dr. Rebecca Pratt, PhD

The fluid-like state of the interstitium supports biochemical signaling throughout the body thus allowing an information network of all tissues. These signals communicate to our cells how to respond to internal stimuli (e.g. hormones) and external factors (e.g. muscle contraction). Interstitial fluid flow within the fascia therefore has a key role in inflammation, edema, and tissue remodeling. Because of its high abundance of ground substance (an amorphous, clear, Jell-O-like substance of water loving proteins), loose connective tissue is home to a large number of our wandering immune cells (white blood cells). Therefore, various types of loosely organized fascia can swell considerably in regions of our body where foreign substances are continually being encountered and offered to immune cells. Interstitial fluid flow helps transient cells within our blood vessels arrive in fascia. The fluid-like state of the interstitium supports our immune cells as they crawl through the jungle of collagen fibers to seek out battles waged by foreign bodies.

Neutrophils are the most numerous white blood cells and are quite motile; often migrating into fascia to act quickly. They respond immediately to biochemical cues released from our damaged tissue. Neutrophils are specialized to engulf bacteria and other infectious agents at the site of inflammation. To make a long cytokine story short, a fever is a consequence of massive amounts of neutrophils accumulating in your fascia and bombarding pathogens.

Eosinophils are white blood cells more commonly located in regions of our connective tissue exposed to chronic inflammation (such as the mucosa of large bowel) or allergies (such as lung tissue in patients with asthma). Inflammation as well as wound healing also involves monocytes. Monocytes migrate from our blood into loose connective tissue and differentiate in the ground substance into macrophages. Now in the fascia they can gobble up presented antigens and foreign bodies. When macrophages encounter large foreign bodies, they can join forces and fuse together as a foreign body giant cell and engulf pathogens!

Another wandering cell type is the mast cell. Mast cells are especially numerous in the fascia just underneath the surface of our skin as well as in the mucous membranes of our nose and mouth close to tiny blood vessels. These cells permit, at times, disruptive effects like edema due to allergic reactions. It is the mast cells' secretory products that mediate inflammation and are responsible for the variety of symptoms and signs characteristic of allergic reactions. In summary, the fluid running through our fascia effectively removes excess interstitial fluid (edema), dissolved nutrients and proteins, cellular debris from inflammation, and white blood cells. Without loosely organized, high aqueous fascial types, our immune responses would not be nearly as effective.

Healthy crimp, glide, and shear

When we think of fascial movement, we can think in terms of the shape and quality of movement in the tissues of our bodies. Let's look at why crimp, glide, and shear are important in healthy fascial functioning.

Crimping creates small folds or ridges in a substance. Natural fibers have rotation and twist to them, so that threads are actually longer than the fabrics

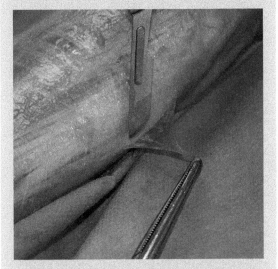

FIGURE 1.13 Author's dissection, showing how the fine layers of the fascia can be teased apart. Movement between layers is helped by hyaluronin that lubricates the space particularly between muscles and deep fascia. Photo by Lydia Mann (KNMLabs).

they are part of. Crimping synthetic fibers helps to give them a bit of the wave found with natural fibers. Fascial crimping works in much the same way, allowing for varied fiber lengths and a more efficient use of space, which gives more potential for varied movement.

Glide is needed to promote movement (Figure 1.13), and the lack of fascial glide may be a contributor to immobility, pain and congenital joint contractures known as arthrogryposis, literally a "curve of the joints." With less glide, blood flow may be restricted, and pain can increase with overstimulation of free nerve endings. In a global sense, to break up dry hyaluronan chains, movement as well as the techniques in manual work can help. Scars, whether by injury or surgical intervention, disorganize fascia into a knotted structure. It will often be dehydrated and matted and in need of reorganization. Think of your favorite knit sweater that gets a hole in it. If you try to stitch it to fix it, you may end up creating a thickened area that is reinforced, but unless the stitches are well integrated into the surrounding fabric, the area around the stitching becomes weak and even more prone to pulls and additional weakness.

However, nature, in all its wisdom, has made scarring a regular outcome in tissue repair. As noted by Bayat *et al.* (2003), "We hypothesise that wound healing is evolutionarily optimised for speed of healing under dirty conditions, where a multiply redundant, compensating, rapid inflammatory response with overlapping cytokine and inflammatory cascades allows the wound to heal quickly to prevent infection and future wound breakdown. A scar may therefore be the price we pay for evolutionary survival after wounding." Salamanders and early invertebrates such as starfish can regenerate limbs and forgo such scarring. Perhaps looking more toward these creatures and their fascial systems would yield further insight into skin repairs of the future.

Moving in general is both the cause and a possible distress in a body system—too much or too little or the "wrong" kind of movement can be detrimental to fascia. Helene Langevin (2011) notes, "when fascia is excessively mechanically stressed, inflamed or immobile, collagen and matrix deposition become disorganized, resulting in fibrosis and adhesions." The lack of healthy gliding in the fascia system has been seen in damaged tissues, often associated with lack of mobility. Microtears can be the cause of many fascial injuries, from plantar fasciitis to IT syndrome.

Shear

In dissection we often see a significant change in shear (lateral shift of the fascial layers) after the initial skin layer is removed, meaning that the skin is the largest contributor for maintaining muscle mechanical properties over the subsequent removal of layers such as the epimysium (Yoshitake *et al.* 2016, Wilke and Tenberg 2020).

Discovery of the interstitium

Dr. Neil Theise published an article in *Nature* about the interstitium (Benias *et al.* 2018), which was then identified as a new organ in the media. Coming from the field of cell biology, he and his research team found the interconnected fluid space of the tissue, which was previously seen as flattened collagen. They were able to do so by using unpreserved cell samples, free of the preservatives often used that flatten the structures and make it impossible to see the space.

The interstitium has made its way into popular science writing as well. In her book *Why Fish Don't Exist* (2020), Lulu Miller makes note of this in the course of her investigation of scientific and historical perception:

I read a news article about, say, a new organ discovered in the human body called the 'interstitium.' There all along but somehow missed by millennia of humans. And the world

cracks open a bit. I am reminded to do as Darwin did: to wonder about the reality waiting behind our assumptions. (pp.191–192)

I'll let Neil Theise, who wrote about his discovery of the interstitium, tell about the process of his discovery in his own words.

Real vs. artifact—the pathologist's dilemma
Dr. Neil Theise

Until the invention of microscopes, the nature of the body at the microscopic level was a matter of philosophy. Is the body an endlessly divisible fluid continuum? Or is it made of indivisible sub-units, "atoms?" There were no definitive ways to settle this debate until the microscope revealed the nature lying beyond the limits of our eyes: tissues comprised three-dimensional spaces bounded by walls or membranes, like little boxes or rooms. Such structures, if broken down further, didn't make smaller, similar spaces, they would merely be fragments of edges. So, the body was made of indivisible "atoms" and these were then called "cells" because they looked like the empty cells of prisoners in jail or of monks in a monastery, without furniture, just walls, ceiling, and floor.

Time passed and people discovered new ways of revealing components of tissues under the microscope. They could "fix them" with chemicals like formaldehyde or freeze them, making them stiff enough to cut into very thin sections to lay upon a glass slide. They could stain such sections chemically, specific colors revealing specific components that were previously invisible: so now we could see cell nuclei and contents of the cytoplasm. The "furniture" of these cells became filled in. This view, so called "Cell Doctrine," was defined by the answer to the ancient question, that bodies are made of cells and that all cells come from other cells. When we say "Western" medicine and "Western" biology, this is what we mean—Cell Doctrine.

With such techniques, the world of microanatomy was gradually revealed, the organization of cells and of the "matrix" around cells. Matrix was made of macromolecules (e.g. collagens, elastin, laminins, proteoglycans), the organizing structures of which helped cells to gather in patterns and structures that formed tissues and organs. These were essential features that allowed us to explore how our bodies work and function, the physiology whereby we live. Furthermore, we could look at how these structures changed in response to injury or disease, the microscope revealing how anatomy breaks down when infected or when cancer invades or how wounds repair themselves or how organ functions go awry.

Such views were very successful! We could confirm how micro-organisms were causes of disease, because we could *see* the organisms and how they disrupted the infected tissues. We could understand how surgical procedures could restore functioning tissue, creating macroscopic rearrangements that favor restitution of microanatomy upon which we depend. The successes of contemporary Western medicine are built on the foundation of microscopic studies.

However, we have been so successful that it is easy for physicians or scientists to forget that nothing we look at under the microscope is "real." Everything is an artifact. The moment we slice a bit of tissue away from the body to put on a slide, it already begins to change. Subtle changes commence as cells begin to die if one isn't quick enough with the fixation. The stiffness of fixed tissue lets one cut very thin sections, but the stiffness itself leads to cracks because stiff tissue crumbles or breaks a bit, too, when sliced thinly (think of how hard it is to cut a very thin slice of crusty bread compared to a thick slice). The colors with which we paint the slides are completely fake: nuclei are not blue, but clear. Cell membranes and cytoplasm are not pink, but clear. Collagen is not blue, but clear. With rare exceptions (e.g. red blood cells filled with iron-binding molecules making them *red*) the body is more like clear glass.

But in our mind's eye we picture tissues with color and light and shape. All of these are artifacts of slide making. The artifacts are essential. But they are not "real."

Recently, colleagues of mine, Petros Benias and David Carr-Locke, came into my office. They are gastroenterologists who specialize in endoscopy of the gastrointestinal (GI) tract. They look at the microscopic surface of the inside of the visceral organs with endoscopes, tubes with cameras that snake downward or upward to explore the inside of our living bodies. Their imagination of what they see with their scopes is conditioned by how they were trained to imagine microanatomy from textbooks filled with pictures from microscopes. And it usually looks pretty much like what they would expect. But then one day they got a new kind of endoscope, one that could see *into* walls of the tissues they were studying, not just the internal surface lining. They would inject a fluorescent dye into a patient's vein, it would circulate through all the fluid of the body, and through its glow, the 'scope could see internal detail.

To their surprise, in the wall of the bile duct, a very thin structure, they saw spaces, not the dense wall of collagen that they had been taught to look for, and because they were revealed by the fluorescent dye, they were fluid filled spaces. Confused by this, they asked me, the pathologist down the hall, to explain the finding—only I couldn't! We puzzled over this for months until we devised a way to sample the tissue they were seeing while keeping the fluorescent dye from leaking out and then getting the tissue on to a microscope slide *fast*. And what we saw was a surprise: the dense wall of collagen—with the artifactual cracks we were used to seeing—was not a dense wall at all—it was a fluid filled space supported by bundles of collagen forming a vast lattice. What we had thought was a "wall" was an artifactual collapse of the collagen lattice after the fluid drained out when the tissue was sliced; the cracks we thought were artifact were in fact the remnants of the real fluid filled spaces after being dehydrated. Real vs. artifact, artifact vs. real!

Eventually, in the months that followed, we "discovered" that was the case with virtually all fibrous connective tissue of the body, a completely "novel" finding according to our standard, Western, allopathic training and this was published in our own literature to great fanfare. Within hours, however, we discovered that there were other cultures of healing and wellness practice, more broadly within our own culture and in other cultures as well: osteopaths, fascia scientists, healers in Rolfing and cranial-sacral traditions, Chinese, Tibetan and Ayurvedic practitioners, on and on. The clinical intuitions and scientific insights from these communities were what we were catching up with—and then adding to with some refinements from our own practices (that "fascia" now encompasses fibroconnective tissue *within* all the visceral organs and the entire dermis). We called this vast tissue network "interstitium" because we found it by way of injecting a fluid dye into the interstitial spaces of the body—the word fascia emphasizes the fibroconnective tissue structures and networks that create and support the spaces. Neither word captures the whole of it. But through rethinking how we see what's "real" we are all starting to see more than ever before.

There are many lessons from this experience in terms of how we "see" and what we think we understand. It is easy when receiving teachings to reify those concepts as real, though they are always conditional on the possibility of future insights that may be come to light because of no technologies and new ways of thinking. We have barely begun to unpack the full nature of living bodies (of all species); we should remember that and remain humble about our theoretical certainties.

And then there's the most common question journalists asked me when our work went viral: what else is there about the body we haven't discovered? To which of course I answered: If I knew that I'd have discovered them? My suggestion for anyone claiming to be a scientist or a healer contemplating anything at all about a biological system—from cells to bodies to ecosystems—is to reflect on a favorite quote from the Nobel Prize winning geneticist Barbara McClintock:

> There's no such thing as a central dogma into which everything will fit. It turns out that any mechanism you can think of, you will find—even if it's the most bizarre kind of thinking. Anything... So if the material tells you, "It may be this," allow that. Don't turn it aside and call it an exception, an aberration, a contaminant... That's what's happened all the way along the line with so many good clues. (Korzybski 2010, p.179)

Every spear of grass—the frames, limbs, organs, of men and women,

And all that concerns them,

All these to me are unspeakably perfect miracles

Walt Whitman, Leaves of Grass

The shapes around us

Tensegrity

The word "tensegrity" is a portmanteau of tension and integrity. Although popularized by Buckminster Fuller, it was his student Kenneth Snelson who created the tensegrity structures well known today among fascia enthusiasts looking for a different model of the body (Figure 1.14).

What is a tensegrity structure? Basically designed with hard elements floating on elastic or string elements, the tensegrity structure mimics the bones of the body floating in the push and pull of myofascial tension. Any structure in the universe is put together through tension and compression with the idea that everything is related to everything else. As elements are moved apart, the entire

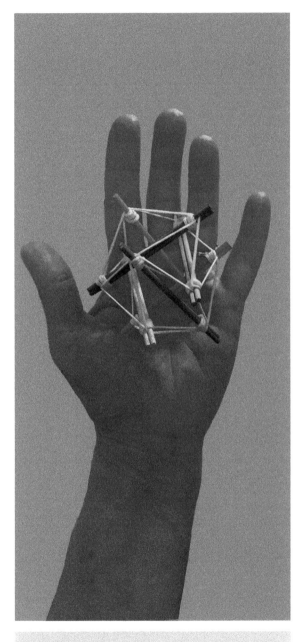

FIGURE 1.14 A homemade tensegrity model using small wooden dowels and elastic band. This is a simplified model of a body that not only distributes strain but also is simultaneously remodeling due to the information from mechanoreceptors, which provide feedback to the body about vibration, pressure, and touch.

structure expands. The same idea may be applied to the human body. As we release the structure, the body creates space, becoming more expansive. It also responds to a localized stress, by making the system translate through the whole of the system. It also helps the body at large both absorb and distribute forces.

As noted in Levin (2016), tensegrity is apparent from blood cells to bones but is additionally a multiscale structure with one part affecting all others in the body system. If we look at the body as a compression structure (where load and force are directed toward the ground), our body would look more like a traditionally built house, rather than a tensegral structure. As a tensegral structure, we see that a part of the body deformed can translate into a difficulty somewhere else in the body. Tension and compression are really key concepts here, from cell embryology to our complex bodies in the world. To extend the idea further, we can imagine the structure of the body's tensegrity as apparent in larger global systems found in nature. Buckminster Fuller talked about reforming the environment, and people will reform themselves.

We are looking at the body as a tensegrity structure that can distribute strain, rather than focus it, when it is working well. This becomes an important concept. In the universe we exist by bracing or hanging in relationship to gravitational forces. For example, bending, torsion, etc. is a combination of these forces. While spiderwebs are often utilized in images of fascia, they are not a finite, closed structure and technically not tensegral in form. However, the threads are tensile cords and as such can inform us on the concept of tensile advantages. As noted by Wainwright (1988):

Tensile stiffness of the thread supports a spider as she lets herself down from a high perch. The tension a spider puts into a dragline on the ground or into a web enables the spider to detect vibrations made by the animals that stumble into these structures, because vibrations are simply minute and frequent changes in the tension of the thread. The spider interprets the patterns of vibrations and decides whether to attack, to approach amorously, or to remain hidden... Buckminster Fuller was a champion of tension and never tired of telling us that, in the design of buildings, the more loads one can support in tension, the lighter and cheaper, more soaring, and more graceful the building can be. (pp.22–23)

The idea of body as made of of "struts" or bones with the second system of "ties" or "a tensional network of the muscles and ligaments"

comes from *Origins of Form* (Williams 2013, p.41). Williams explores the theory of design and this interplay between biological and structural. Function inevitably relates to design, whether it is the human body or a piece of practical architecture like a bridge (Figure 1.15).

Predating modern tensegral bridges are organic structures, such as the root bridges known as jing kieng jri in the Himalayas, and cane bridges in other areas. In remote areas that have distinct dry

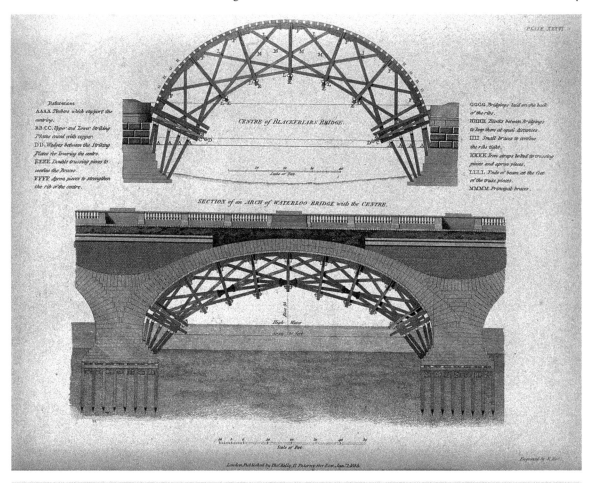

FIGURE 1.15 Bridge forms are structures that are strain distributors.

Credit: Civil engineering: wooden centring for Blackfriars Bridge (above), Waterloo Bridge (below). Engraving by R. Roffe, 1848. Wellcome Collection. Public Domain Mark.

and rainy seasons, living bridges create physical connection and access that is impossible without them. Jing kieng jri bridges are made of rubber fig tree (*ficus elastica*) saplings, known for their resiliency and springlike structure. Early in the process, the roots are coaxed to grow into and interweave with a bamboo scaffold, which supports them temporarily. The roots eventually merge together (called anastomosis) and the bridge itself becomes an ecosystem that is living and changeable. The entire system of these root bridges seems to operate in much the same way as our fascia systems grow and expand, interweaving fibers and creating a moveable structure. These bridges are particularly

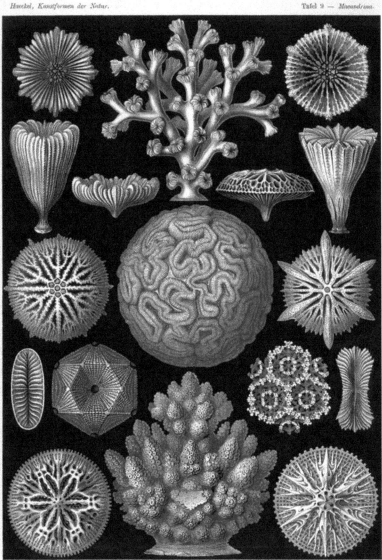

Haeckel, Kunstformen der Natur.

Tafel 9 — Maeandrina.

Hexacoralla. — Sechsstrahlige Sternkorallen.

FIGURE 1.16 *Kunst-Formen der Natur (Art Forms in Nature),* by Ernst Haeckel, 1898.

valuable as they can both handle heavy loads and survive earthquakes and other natural phenomena as long as they are well cared for.

Nature has fascinated scientists and artists alike. Form and pattern are observable in the shapes repeated in sea sponges to our internal form. The elaborate late nineteenth-century plates of Ernst Haeckel (Figure 1.16) focused on the wonder of shape in the natural world.

Biotensegrity

Orthopedic surgeon Stephen Levin came up with the term "biotensegrity" and has made the observation that the icosahedron (a 3D shape with 20 faces) can translate to a schema for modeling everything from viruses to systems in biology. He is the pioneer in applying tensegrity to the biological body and has often told the story that, while exploring the Natural History Museum in Washington, DC, he was struck by the size of the enormous dinosaur skeletons that seemed to defy regular architectural design, until he thought of their body system more like the truss-based design of bridges, rather than brick and mortar structures. Gazing at Kenneth Snelson's sculpture "Needle Tower" just outside the museum also gave him the idea that a structure could be built where the structures float without touching. As an orthopedic surgeon, he was always looking at the joints and finding that as long as the ligaments were intact, there was always space between two collagenous surfaces. Biological tissues respond in a tensegral way if we introduce stress and strain into a system. In linear structures, stress will deform the structure. However, a tensegral structure actually gets stronger and stiffer under stress and strain.

Taking this further, cell biologist Donald Ingber (2000; 2008) looked at tensegrity in terms of the building block (moveable) of the cell itself. As a student, he looked at the models from an architecture class and wondered why the concept of tensegral form was not applied to his field of study when the shape looked the same and could further explain functionality and movement of the cell in action. As noted in his work on tensegrity and mechanotransduction, Ingber writes:

This work has revealed that molecules, cells, tissues, organs, and our entire bodies use "tensegrity" architecture to mechanically stabilize their shape, and to seamlessly integrate structure and function at all size scales. Through use of this tension-dependent building system, mechanical forces applied at the macroscale produce changes in biochemistry and gene expression within individual living cells. This structure-based system provides a mechanistic basis to explain how application of physical therapies might influence cell and tissue physiology. (Ingber 2008)

So what advantages are there to looking at the body as a tensegral form? First and foremost, as a structure, the tensegrity model is a more holistic model and based on the assumption that any effect, external or internal to that structure, is going to impact the whole of the system. Second, because of the emphasis on the elastic members of the structure, the soft tissues of the body gain more profound importance than our skeletons hanging in the classroom evoke.

Fractals and form

Fractals are patterns that endlessly repeat on both large and small scales and are attributed to the mathematician Mandelbrot. The spiral pattern of sunflower seeds, for example, is a fractal (Figure 1.17), and follows the Fibonacci sequence, where each number in the pattern is the sum of the previous two (i.e. 1, 2, 3, 5, 8, 13, 21, 34, and so on). Several of our structures in anatomy, including fascia, also repeat pattern much in the same way we see these sequences in other places in nature.

If fascia is seen as being both fractal and irregular in nature, it is important to discern why anything would be designed in a complex network, which shifts the point of equilibrium. Noted in Guimberteau and Armstrong (2015), these fractal areas of biology exist in places including alveoli, vascular networks and more, noting that the body is rarely linear, but rather:

> In the fascia we see an irregular, fractal, chaotic, non-linear system... In the course of our constant search for knowledge, we have had to gradually accept that nature does not function in straight lines, and that the law of proportionality of cause and effect, which refers to the relationship of two variables whose ratio is constant, could in fact be based on non-linear rules. (pp.175–176)

As a mathematician with diverse interests, Mandelbrot was not content to see the world of math and natural science as continuous smooth lines. He looked at the natural world, which contains roughness or crinkliness, and tends to scale up or down within the body and larger systems. He self-labelled as a "fractalist" (Gomory 2010) and created the area of mathematics known as "fractal geometry", so named for its shattered or fractal form of repetition.

Remember our orange and equating the cellulose with our fascia? Just as the white of the orange lies just under the surface, and also enrobes the individual segments into smaller and smaller levels, fascia goes from enveloping large muscles to fasciculus, and so on. As noted, "animals obey power law scaling both *within* individuals, in terms of the geometry and dynamics of their internal network structures, as well as *across* species, they, and therefore all of us, are living manifestations of self-similar fractals" (West 2017).

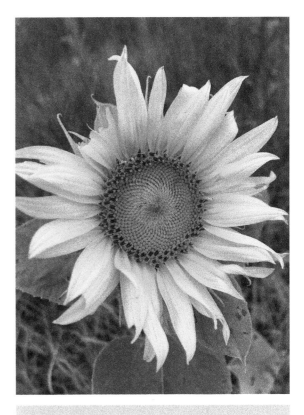

FIGURE 1.17 The sunflower's center is a fractal, with each seed twisted. Additionally, the seeds create two spiraling patterns in opposite directions, called parastichies. All of this optimizes spatial use of the seeds. Good design expressed in beautiful form is a common thread in myofascial anatomy, nature, and art.

Purposeful planes
Dr. Rebecca Pratt, PhD

Generating complex yet precise movements (slipping, sliding, gliding, and contracting) between any combination of muscles, tissues, vessels, and nervous structures the body relies on fascial planes (Figure 1.breakout.10). These planes are created from healthy, hydrated fascia, which effectively produces "frictionless" structural associations. For our liver and our small bowel to move simultaneously yet independently while we jump rope, fascia must coat the organ's surfaces and every wall of the cavity they occupy. For the biceps brachii muscle to contract while the triceps brachii muscles elongates, fascia must be present at the interface of each neighboring muscle belly for this disparate movement to occur. The freedom of motion is essential to the proper functioning of all aspects of the human body. The exquisite study by Stecco *et al.* (2013) demonstrates that fascial planes glide or roll past each other on the glycoprotein hyaluronan within the extracellular matrix between adjacent structures. For example, for nerves to stretch independently across joints as muscles manipulate action or for blood vessels to remain intact as they slip deeper through contracting muscle bellies and around smaller muscle fascicles healthy fascia is essential. When hyaluronan chains between layers are short and plump with water they permit these independent yet codependent relationships to occur. Fascial planes may "disappear" when extracellular matrix is deficient due to stasis, dehydration and/or inflammation. Fascial adhesions commonly occur with wound healing, radiation therapy,

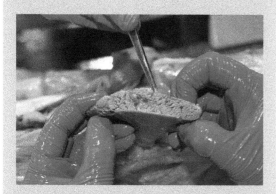

FIGURE 1.BREAKOUT.10 Photo of a right leg in prone position (posterior view, inferior to patella). Deep to the skin, superficial adipose tissue, and deep crural fascia is the discrete epimysium of the gastrocnemius muscle. Utilizing fascial planes between the gastrocnemius and the soleus muscles permits the soleus to remain fully intact during easy dissection. Hyaluronan-rich loose connective tissue permits fascial planes for neurovascular bundles. A fascial plane is also observable between skeletal muscle fascicles.

(Photo by Rebecca Pratt, PhD; OUWB 2019).

surgical procedures, and immobilization. Insults such as these generate miniscule changes to the structure of hyaluronan arranging the protein in long, sticky chains. An accumulation of adhesions and a reduction in discrete fascial planes can lead to pain, tightness, and limited mobility (Tesarz *et al.* 2011).

References

Stecco, A., Gesi, M., Stecco, C. and Stern, R. (2013) 'Fascial components of the myofascial pain syndrome.' *Current Pain and Headache Reports 17*, 8, 352. https://doi: 10.1007/s11916-013-0352-9

Tesarz, J., Hoheisel, U., Wiedenhöfer, B. and Mense, S. (2011) 'Sensory innervation of the thoracolumbar fascia in rats and humans.' *Neuroscience 194*, 302–308. https://doi: 10.1016/j.neuroscience.2011.07.066

 Functional load training and fascia

Michol Dalcourt, creator of ViPR

Vitality, **P**erformance, **R**econditioning (ViPR), and the new ViPR PRO were founded on the observation that farm kids exhibited a greater degree of Functional Strength than their gym counterparts. Functional Strength refers to the ability to be strong as an integrated body in performing task based outcomes, in symmetrical as well as asymmetrical positions. Odd position, full body strength, and stability not only help athletes, but all of us! Whether trying to reduce the risk of falls for the older population, to engaging in activities of daily living, to producing high velocity movements in sport, our bodies need omni-directional strength, stability, and motion.

Integrating the body with training exposure and mechanically stressing it with external mass (for example, ViPR PRO) introduces greater "load paths" to the body (Figure 1.breakout.11). A load path is a mechanical line of stress received by the body's tissues, which converts into the cellular activity of tissue remodeling. Using different loads, speeds and angles optimizes the conditions under which fascial remodeling can take place.

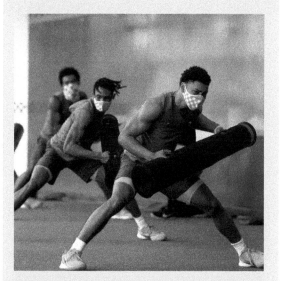

FIGURE 1.BREAKOUT.11 The load and multi-directionality in drills with ViPR PRO challenges the body in the same ways farm kids experience doing chores. This can serve as a more well-rounded means of training for fascial remodeling compared to "traditional" gym machines.

Photo courtesy of ViPR.

This was our first observation with farm kids, and gave us the idea to create the ViPR free weight tool (www.ViPR.com). Think of ViPR PRO as a bale of hay in the gym, without the mess (...it mimics the same loading inputs that our biology has interacted with for thousands of years, to induce tissue adaptations). Multidirectional loading and training offer variability in load paths to aid in omnidirectional remodeling of skin, fascia, bone and muscle (stimulating osteoblast and fibroblast activity along lines of stress...think of Davis's and Wolff's Laws). Scientifically, this is seen in the concepts of mechanotransduction. Anecdotally, this is observed when witnessing a farm kid wrestle a city kid.

Since ViPR's release, we have seen many elite athletes, fitness enthusiasts, and older adults, prehab/rehab and first responders all benefit from the inclusion of full body functional load training (Figure 1.breakout.12). It is my sincere hope that this book, the content and narrative within, serve as a clarifying resource on how to map full body load paths into training and conditioning to authenticate functional adaptations in fascia, so that our bodies can become unbreakable.

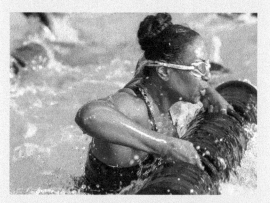

FIGURE 1.BREAKOUT.12 Full body functional load training can help people help increase adaptability for daily life and athletic endeavors. Seen here, water resistance adds another level of challenge.

Photo courtesy of ViPR.

 Triangles, folds, branches, and stars in shape, function, and form
Geometric patterns found in fascia are seen and repeated in the larger systems of nature. Robert Hooke explored shapes in nature in his book *Micrographia* (1665) and this linking of the natural world and pattern has continued to be admired by artists, architects, and scientists alike.

Triangles are utilized throughout nature and the body as a way to distribute stress and strain. If we think of triangular spaces, we can see the shape of the fibers in fascia are mimicked in the crystal structures of ice patterns, as well as in other parts of the body. The triangulation of the plantar fascia, scapula, deltoid, and similarly in Myers's named "deltoid of the hip" consisting of tensor fasciae latae, gluteus medius, and superior fibers of glut max.

Weaving

In addition to tensegrity, Kenneth Snelson was interested in weaving as a structure in the world, writing the paper "Tensegrity, Weaving and the Binary World" that appears on his website. As noted, "weaving and tensegrity share the principle of alternating helical directions, of left-to-right, of bypasses clockwise and counterclockwise" (Snelson n.d., p.16).

Folds can be thought of as building onto the shape of triangular as well as straight lines. As noted by Kemp (2016) in discussing shape in science and architecture, solids like fabric (he was thinking of cloth, but it works for the concept of fascia as well) will structurally settle into self-organization and lands:

> Into an array in which all the forces of compression and tension that necessarily exist in any construction are resolved within the "skin" of the fabric itself. Nothing is needed to hold it up other than itself—no supporting skeleton below or means of suspension to hang it from above. If we rearrange it by pulling upward one or more zones of the cloth, when released it will settle again into another stable if somewhat different configuration. Such resolution of forces is the ideal for engineers, promising both stability and economy of material. (Kemp 2016)

Branches of all sorts fascinated artist and part-time dissector Leonardo Da Vinci. As noted by Kemp (2016):

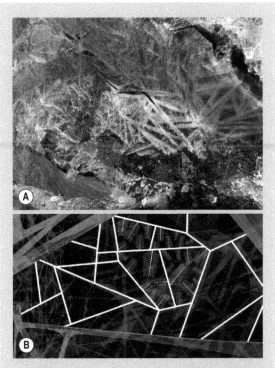

FIGURE 1.18 a) Ice crystal formations share a shape with the arrangement of glycosaminoglycans in fascia, and share a similarity with our hydrophilic fibers in fascia. b) Illustration after Guimberteau's *Architecture of Human Living Fascia* (2015), one can see the similarities between the arrangements of glycosaminoglycans (components of connective tissue) and the arrangement of ice along a shoreline.

> As always with Leonardo, a basis system discovered in one sector of nature was not isolated from the generality of that kind of system in other sectors... he draws the branching bronchi in the lungs as a marvelously coralline structure, dividing repetitively and regularly half by half in a kind of fractal array. When he dissected the "old man" in the hospital of S. Maria Nuova he identified the cause of death as the tortuosity and silting up of the old man's system of aged vessels, which no longer obeyed the

geometrical and dynamic rules that ensured efficient flow. (pp.73–74)

The shape of a glial astrocyte (Figure 1.19a) is similar to other star-like configurations, including this cactus spike (Figure 1.19b), the star shape of the suboccipitals, and even the many paths of the myofascial connections that come off the anterior superior iliac spine (ASIS). Ramon y Cajal named the original glial (meaning gluey) cells "spider" cells for their similarity to the leggy creatures. Initially dismissed as inert packing material, glial cells have gained recognized importance in caring for the neurons and their environment. Embryonically they come from the ectoderm with the microglia (important in immune functionality) being part of the mesodermal system (like fascia and muscle).

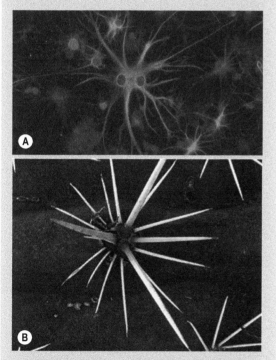

FIGURE 1.19 a) Glial astrocyte courtesy of Douglas Feinstein, PhD, Research Professor, Department of Anesthesiology, UIC. b) Spikes on a cactus, by author.

Undulations and waves

Movement qualities have a shape to them. Consider the word *undulation,* the soft rise and drop used to describe wave-like actions from the waters of the ocean to the rise and fall of hills in the countryside. If we look toward evolutionary biology, eels and snakes move by lateral undulation against a surface with resistance. In terms of human movement, undulations have been part of our movement language, especially dancing, from Middle Eastern belly dancing to dances from the African diaspora. In traditional dance forms, the undulations are often serpentine in nature. Modern dance companies such as Katherine Dunham utilized the undulations, and more movement somatic classes such as Nia also utilize undulations as part of their curriculum, most prominently featuring the movement in the sagittal plane. Hellerwork, another in the family of structural integration, is a modality that combines deep tissue bodywork with awareness and movement exercises. In the sixth session of Hellerwork, the concept of undulation is introduced, however, emphasizing the side-to-side action.

If we take the concept further, toward physics, we can conceptualize waves in terms of motion, vibrations, and actions such as sound or light waves. If you work with the traditional battle ropes, you are playing with an outside force of waves and its effect on the body itself, whether doing classic movement both in up and down waves or lateral work side to side. As humans we generally stabilize the sides of the body in order to move forwards in walking or running. However, in working ropes, the body is stationary, with the front and back stabilizing against the weight of the momentum of the waves. A study performed by Calatayud *et al.* (2015) looked at quantifying the intensity of activity. Unilateral waves in the ropes were found to work the obliques more whereas bilateral waves worked more of the erector spinae muscles. These were measured through electromyographic signals, and it would make sense to assume that the myofascial connections would be stimulated as well.

Fascia as liminal space

Liminal space is a changeover space and is where transformation takes place. Its etymology comes from the Latin "limen" which translates as a threshold, entryway, or boundary area. Used first widely in anthropological work (Turner 1967), the idea was originally linked to initiation rites into adulthood, where the adolescent is transformed into an adult. In other settings, liminal space suggests a transitional time, for example, in a hospice care setting where a person is literally on the threshold from this life into dying. Liminality, as a noun, could translate as "in-between space." So far, we have seen fascia described as a three-dimensional matrix and as the space where movement happens. Although liminal space is often used to describe subtle sensations, it links one thing to another. Our continuity of fascia exists in that threshold space—a place for movement changes.

Fascia's definition is continuing to change as we are learning more about its varied forms and the applications of this dynamic tissue. At the end of the 1800s, architect Louis H. Sullivan created the famous axiom, "form follows function" referring to designing buildings with purpose as the primary focus, instead of aesthetics. In the body we can perhaps have both as we witness the shapes and patterns fascia forms as a connector and in responding to environmental changes. We will keep the dialogue on definitions open as more professions are becoming engaged in this conversation.

References

Bai, Y., Wang, J., Wu, J., Dai, J. et al. (2011) 'Review of evidence suggesting that the fascia network could be the anatomical basis for acupoints and meridians in the human body.' Evidence-Based Complementary and Alternative Medicine 2011, 1–6. https://doi.org/10.1155/2011/260510

Bayat, A., McGrouther, D. A. and Ferguson, M. W. J. (2003) 'Skin scarring.' BMJ 326, 7380, 88–92. https://doi.org/10.1136/bmj.326.7380.88

Benias, P. C., Wells, R. G., Sackey-Aboagye, B., Klavan, H. et al. (2018) 'Structure and distribution of an unrecognized interstitium in human tissues.' Scientific Reports, 8, 1, 4947. https://doi.org/10.1038/s41598-018-23062-6

Blottner, D., Huang, Y., Trautmann, G. and Sun, L. (2019) 'Continuum linking bone and myofascial bag for global and local body movement control on Earth and in Space. A scoping review.' REACH, 100030.

Brett, D. W. (2003) Topical Enzymatic Debridement. New York, NY: The McMahon Publishing Group, p.23.

Calatayud, J., Martin, F., Colado, J. C., Benítez, J. C., Jakobsen, M. D. and Andersen, L. L. (2015) 'Muscle activity during unilateral vs. bilateral battle rope exercises.' Journal of Strength and Conditioning Research 29, 10, 2854–2859. https://doi.org/10.1519/JSC.0000000000000963

Dart, R. A. (1996) Skill and Poise: Articles of Skill, Poise, and the F. M. Alexander Technique. London: Society of the Alexander Technique (STAT).

De Vivo, L., Matsushita, A. K., Kupor, D., Luna, J. et al. (2020) 'Cholla cactus frames as lightweight and torsionally tough biological materials.' Acta Biomaterialia 112, 213–224. https://doi.org/10.1016/j.actbio.2020.04.054

Federative Committee on Anatomical Terminology (ed.) (1998) Terminologia Anatomica: International Anatomical Terminology. New York, NY: Thieme.

Findley, T. W. and Shalwala, M. (2013) 'Fascia Research Congress Evidence from the 100 year perspective of Andrew Taylor Still.' Journal of Bodywork and Movement Therapies 17, 3, 356–364. https://doi.org/10.1016/j.jbmt.2013.05.015

Gershlak, J. R., Hernandez, S., Fontana, G., Perreault, L. R. et al. (2017) 'Crossing kingdoms: Using decellularized plants as perfusable tissue engineering scaffolds.' Biomaterials 125, 13–22. https://doi.org/10.1016/j.biomaterials.2017.02.011

Gomory, R. (2010) 'Benoît Mandelbrot (1924–2010).' Nature 468, 7322, 378–378. https://doi.org/10.1038/468378a

Guimberteau, J.-C. and Armstrong, C. (2015) Architecture of Human Living Fascia: Cells and Extracellular Matrix *as Revealed by Endoscopy.* Edinburgh: Handspring Publishing Ltd.

Ingber, D. E., Heidemann, S. R., Lamoureux, P. and Buxbaum, R. E. (2000) 'Opposing views on tensegrity as a structural framework for understanding cell mechanics.' *Journal of Applied Physiology, 89,* 4, 1663–1678. https://doi.org/10.1152/jappl.2000.89.4.1663

Ingber, D. E. (2008) 'Tensegrity and mechanotransduction.' *Journal of Bodywork and Movement Therapies 12,* 3, 198–200. https://doi.org/10.1016/j.jbmt.2008.04.038

Kemp, M. (2016) *Structural Intuitions: Seeing Shapes in Art and Science.* Charlottesville, VA: University of Virginia Press.

Kerch, G. (2020) 'Role of Changes in State of Bound Water and Tissue Stiffness in Development of Age-Related Diseases.' *Polymers (Basel),* 17, 12(6), 1362. https://doi:10.3390/polym12061362

Korzybski, A. (2010) *Selections from Science and Sanity: An Introduction to non-Aristotelian Systems and General Semantics.* Forest Hills, NY: Institute of General Semantics.

Kumka, M. and Bonar, J. (2012) 'Fascia: A morphological description and classification system based on a literature review.' *Journal of the Canadian Chiropractic Association 56,* 3, 179–191.

Lancerotto, L., Stecco, C., Macchi, V., Porzionato, A., Stecco, A. and De Caro, R. (2011) 'Layers of the abdominal wall: Anatomical investigation of subcutaneous tissue and superficial fascia.' *Surgical and Radiologic Anatomy 33,* 10, 835–842. https://doi.org/10.1007/s00276-010-0772-8

Langevin, H. M. and Huijing, P. A. (2009) 'Communicating about fascia: history, pitfalls, and recommendations.' *International Journal of Therapeutic Massage and Bodywork: Research, Education, and Practice 2,* 4, 3–8. https://doi.org/10.3822/ijtmb.v2i4.63

Langevin, H. M., Nedergaard, M. and Howe, A. K. (2013) 'Cellular control of connective tissue matrix tension.' *Journal of Cellular Biochemistry 114,* 8, 1714–1719. https://doi.org/10.1002/jcb.24521

Levin, S. (2016) 'From viruses to vertebrates—A biological mechanical model using multiscale tensegrity structures.' *Conference: Multiscale Innovative Materials and Structures—MIMS16At: Cetara, Italy, Volume: Tensegrity Is Useful for Multiscale Biological Modeling.*

Macfarlane, R. (2018) *The Lost Words.* Toronto: House of Anansi Press.

Mackesy, J. (1814) 'A case of fracture, attended with symptoms of unusual violence, relieved by an extensive longitudinal incision through the fascia of the limb.' *Medical and Physical Journal 31,* 181, 214–217.

Mercer, R. R. and Crapo, J. D. (1990) 'Spatial distribution of collagen and elastin fibers in the lungs.' *Journal of Applied Physiology 69,* 2, 756–765. https://doi.org/10.1152/jappl.1990.69.2.756

Miller, L. (2020) *Why Fish Don't Exist: A Story of Loss, Love, and the Hidden Order of Life.* New York, NY: Simon & Schuster.

Myers, T. W. (2020) *Anatomy Trains: Myofascial Meridians for Manual Therapists and Movement Professionals* (4th ed.). London: Elsevier.

Nemetz, L. D. (2020) 'What you see is what you understand: how changes in dissection techniques have informed our understanding of what we perceive in anatomy.' *FASEB Journal 34,* S1, 1–1. https://doi.org/10.1096/fasebj.2020.34.s1.02793

Ott, H. C., Matthiesen, T. S., Goh, S.-K., Black, L. D. *et al.* (2008) 'Perfusion-decellularized matrix: Using nature's platform to engineer a bioartificial heart.' *Nature Medicine 14,* 2, 213–221. https://doi.org/10.1038/nm1684

Schleip, R. (2003) 'Fascial plasticity—a new neurobiological explanation: Part 1.' *Journal of Bodywork and Movement Therapies 7,* 1, 11–19. https://doi.org/10.1016/S1360-8592(02)00067-0

Singer, C. (1957) *A Short History of Anatomy and Physiology from the Greeks to Harvey.* (2nd ed.) New York, NY: Dover Publications.

Snelson, K. (n.d.). *Tensegrity, Weaving and the Binary World.* Accessed on 3/23/2022 at http://kennethsnelson.net/Tensegrity_and_Weaving.pdf.

Stecco, C. and Hammer, W. I. (2015) *Functional Atlas of the Human Fascial System.* London: Elsevier Ltd.

Stecco, C. and Schleip, R. (2016) 'A fascia and the fascial system.' *Journal of Bodywork and Movement Therapies 20,* 1, 139–140. https://doi.org/10.1016/j.jbmt.2015.11.012

Stecco, C., Fede, C., Macchi, V., Porzionato, A. *et al.* (2018) 'The fasciacytes: A new cell devoted to fascial gliding regulation.' *Clinical Anatomy 31,* 5, 667–676. https://doi.org/10.1002/ca.23072

Still, A. T. (2017) *Autobiography of Andrew T. Still: With a history of the discovery and development of the science of osteopathy, together with an account of the ... School of Osteopathy.* CreateSpace Independent Publishing Platform.

Tomoda, K., Kimura, H. and Osaki, S. (2013) 'Distribution of collagen fiber orientation in the human lung: collagen fiber orientation in human lung.' *The Anatomical Record 296*, 5, 846–850. https://doi.org/10.1002/ar.22649

Turner, V. (1967) *The Forest of Symbols: Aspects of Ndembu Ritual.* Ithaca, NY: Cornell University Press.

Van der Wal, J. C. (2009) 'The architecture of the connective tissue in the musculoskeletal system—an often overlooked functional parameter as to proprioception in the locomotor apparatus.' *International Journal of Therapeutic Massage and Bodywork: Research, Education, and Practice 2*, 4, 9–23. https://doi.org/10.3822/ijtmb.v2i4.62

Wainwright, S. A. (1988) *Axis and circumference: The Cylindrical Shape of Plants and Animals.* Cambridge, MA: Harvard University Press.

Watson, P. E., Watson, I. D. and Batt, R. D. (1980) 'Total body water volumes for adult males and females estimated from simple anthropometric measurements.' *American Journal of Clinical Nutrition 33*, 1, 27–39. https://doi.org/10.1093/ajcn/33.1.27

West, G. B. (2017) *Scale: The Universal Laws of Growth, Innovation, Sustainability, and the Pace of Life in Organisms, Cities, Economies, and Companies.* London: Penguin Press.

Wilke, J. and Tenberg, S. (2020) 'Semimembranosus muscle displacement is associated with movement of the superficial fascia: An in vivo ultrasound investigation.' *Journal of Anatomy 237*, 6, 1026–1031. https://doi.org/10.1111/joa.13283

Williams, C. (2013) *Origins of form: The Shape of Natural and Man-made Things; [why they came to be the way they are and how they change].* Lanham, MD: Taylor Trade Publishing.

Yoshitake, Y., Miyamoto, N., Taniguchi, K., Katayose, M. and Kanehisa, H. (2016) 'The skin acts to maintain muscle shear modulus.' *Ultrasound in Medicine and Biology 42*, 3, 674–682. https://doi.org/10.1016/j.ultrasmedbio.2015.11.022

Zügel, M., Maganaris, C. N., Wilke, J., Jurkat-Rott, K. *et al.* (2018) 'Fascial tissue research in sports medicine: From molecules to tissue adaptation, injury, and diagnostics: consensus statement.' *British Journal of Sports Medicine 52*, 23, 1497–1497. https://doi.org/10.1136/bjsports-2018-099308

Further reading

Alexi, J., Cleary, D., Dommisse, K., Palermo, R. *et al.* (2018) 'Past visual experiences weigh in on body size estimation.' *Scientific Reports 8*, 1, 215. https://doi.org/10.1038/s41598-017-18418-3

Berrueta, L., Muskaj, I., Olenich, S., Butler, T. *et al.* (2016) 'Stretching impacts inflammation resolution in connective tissue: Stretching impacts inflammation resolution.' *Journal of Cellular Physiology 231*, 7, 1621–1627. https://doi.org/10.1002/jcp.25263

Bertolucci, L. F. (2011) 'Pandiculation: Nature's way of maintaining the functional integrity of the myofascial system?' *Journal of Bodywork and Movement Therapies 15*, 3, 268–280. https://doi.org/10.1016/j.jbmt.2010.12.006

Dalton, E. (2011) *Dynamic Body: Exploring Form, Expanding Function.* Oklahoma City, OK: Freedom from Pain Institute.

Earls, J. (2020) *Born to Walk: Myofascial Efficiency and the Body in Movement.* (2nd ed.) Berkeley, CA: North Atlantic Books.

Huijing, P. A. (2009) 'Epimuscular myofascial force transmission: A historical review and implications for new research.' International Society of Biomechanics Muybridge Award Lecture, Taipei, 2007. *Journal of Biomechanics 42*, 1, 9–21. https://doi.org/10.1016/j.jbiomech.2008.09.027

Juhan, D. (2003) *Job's Body.* Barrytown, NY: Station Hill Press, Inc.

Kram, R. and Dawson, T. J. (1998) 'Energetics and biomechanics of locomotion by red kangaroos (*Macropus rufus*).' *Comparative Biochemistry and Physiology Part B: Biochemistry and Molecular Biology 120*, 1, 41–49. https://doi.org/10.1016/S0305-0491(98)00022-4

Lowell de Solórzano, S. C. and Levin, S. M. (2021) *Everything Moves: How Biotensegrity Informs Human Movement.* Edinburgh: Handspring Publishing.

Magnusson, S. P., Langberg, H. and Kjaer, M. (2010) 'The pathogenesis of tendinopathy: balancing the response to loading.' *Nature Reviews Rheumatology 6*, 5, 262–268. https://doi.org/10.1038/nrrheum.2010.43

Menon, R. G., Oswald, S. F., Raghavan, P., Regatte, R. R. and Stecco, A. (2020) 'T1ρ-mapping for musculoskeletal pain diagnosis: Case series of variation of water bound glycosaminoglycans quantification before and after Fascial Manipulation® in subjects with elbow pain.' *International Journal of Environmental Research and Public Health 17*, 3, 708. https://doi.org/10.3390/ijerph17030708

Nemetz, L. (2016) 'Space for well-being: understanding how humans shape architecture and why where we live shapes us anatomically.' American Anatomy Association Regional Meeting 2016, Columbia Medical School, New York, NY, USA.

Online Etymology Dictionary (2022) 'Fascia.' Accessed on 03/22/2022 at www.etymonline.com/word/fascia.

Oschman, J. L. (2016) *Energy Medicine: The Scientific Basis.* London: Elsevier.

Reeves, N. D. (2006) 'Adaptation of the tendon to mechanical usage.' *Journal of Musculoskeletal and Neuronal Interactions 6*, 2, 174–180.

Roberts, T. J. and Azizi, E. (2011) 'Flexible mechanisms: The diverse roles of biological springs in vertebrate movement.' *Journal of Experimental Biology 214*, 3, 353–361. https://doi.org/10.1242/jeb.038588

Sawicki, G. S., Lewis, C. L. and Ferris, D. P. (2009) 'It pays to have a spring in your step.' *Exercise and Sport Sciences Reviews 37*, 3, 130–138. https://doi.org/10.1097/JES.0b013e31819c2df6

Sockol, M. D., Raichlen, D. A. and Pontzer, H. (2007) 'Chimpanzee locomotor energetics and the origin of human bipedalism.' *Proceedings of the National Academy of Sciences 104*, 30, 12265–12269. https://doi.org/10.1073/pnas.0703267104

Stecco, A., Gesi, M., Stecco, C. and Stern, R. (2013) 'Fascial components of the myofascial pain syndrome.' *Current Pain and Headache Reports 17*, 8, 352. https://doi.org/10.1007/s11916-013-0352-9

Stecco, A., Stern, R., Fantoni, I., De Caro, R. and Stecco, C. (2016) 'Fascial disorders: Implications for treatment.' *PMandR 8*, 2, 161–168. https://doi.org/10.1016/j.pmrj.2015.06.006

Wilke, J., Krause, F., Vogt, L. and Banzer, W. (2016) 'What is evidence-based about myofascial chains: a systematic review.' *Archives of Physical Medicine and Rehabilitation 97*, 3, 454–461. https://doi.org/10.1016/j.apmr.2015.07.

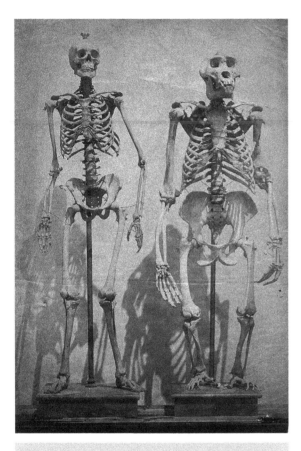

FIGURE 2.1 Skeleton of a human and a gorilla, displayed side by side. Photo by Roger Fenton ca. 1860. Humans and gorillas share 98.2% of the same DNA, but bony structure has evolved and shapes our forms differently due to the way we move.

Credit: Wellcome Collection. Public Domain Mark.

We become what we behold. We shape our tools, and thereafter our tools shape us.

Marshall McLuhan

The form of life and shape of changes

When I was younger, my family used to take weeklong vacations with the National Wildlife Federation. I learned to hike, rock rappel, canoe, and learn about nature all over North America. I observed everything from birds, animals, plants, and more, that had adapted to their environment over thousands of years. I wondered at the side-to-side movement or lateral motivation of fish as they swam, and my skinny legs that allowed me to walk through the forests. At night the "rock guy" would give all the kids a small stone of the day, a rough garnet or a piece of gneiss and tell a bit of a story of substances that predated us all.

Evolution is about movement and surviving into the next generation. Looking at the etymology, the word comes from Latin, "evolutio" or unrolling, or in the verb form, "evolvere," which means to evolve. Development is opening out into the world, and evolution in terms of our standard studies from Charles Darwin onwards speaks to changes biologically where the most adaptable (not always the strongest) survive. When working on ourselves or with clients, we are looking for capacity to change. In evolution as well, variability wins.

We share 98.2% of our DNA with the gorilla (Figure 2.1), but the difference in our anatomical architecture is quite striking, particularly in pelvic shape. Our evolutionary history often focuses on bones, in part because it is the evidence that remains behind. We are shaped by our movement interactions in the world, our environment, and genetics, which in turn affect the myofascial body and its form.

The human body owes a lot to our bipedalism, the fact that we stand on two legs. We have been discussing fascia in terms of its architecture, its spatial arrangement, and how our own movement, shapes the fascia. So, what shapes a human? The slight differences between gorillas and us demonstrates a small variation has a profound effect on the shape of our pelvis and the movement of our limbs. We are quite complex, and our evolution is an outfolding of the complex origami that we start off with as a human. In truth, many of the daily aches and pains in our current anatomical distress may be due to disconnection between our environment, shape, and myofascial anatomy all waiting to catch up to each other. An upright body has a huge number of evolutionary advantages, but also comes with challenges to the head, neck, and lower back. As humans we have had an interesting relationship with our environment, whether adapting to or trying to overcome natural environmental space. Agriculture brought a sense of safety in the domestication of animals and farming, but was also a step away from the freer engagement with the natural world. This, of course, had impact in the role of movement as a necessary means of a hunting or foraging existence, to manual labor, and more recently to factory work and then the electronics era. We need movement less and less as part of daily life. Exercise has become a responsibility for protecting health instead of a necessary part of daily life (Lieberman 2020).

As noted by J. E. Gordon (2003), "the 'design' of plants and animals … didn't just happen. In principle, both the form and materials of any structure that developed over a long period of time, in a competitive world, represent optimization regarding the loads it should carry and the economic or metabolic cost." Interest in the efficiency of bipedal gait has been noted by several authors including Bramble and Lieberman (2004), Earls (2020), Eng *et al.* (2015), and Sockol *et al.* (2007) among others. We are so myofascially efficient in our walking that our modern lifestyle, with its additional convenience in transportation and ready availability of food, leaves us prone to gaining weight. With our additional time sitting or consuming technology, we aren't moving as we were designed to evolve. The world around us appears to be outpacing our changes in anatomy.

We are also hardwired to matching rhythm to our walking or running patterns, something that is known as auditory motor synchronization. In a study by Karageorghis and Priest (2012), the authors noted, "music has a consistent and measurable effect on the psychological state and behavior or exercise participants." In other words, turning up your music tempo may indeed influence your gait and vice-versa. To note, our rhythm in walking can be reflective of our moods and vice versa. The local gym will pump up the music to increase motivation to run faster and often music is packaged to instructors with the speed of the tracks designated for optimal tempo. Walking to our own inner soundtrack can be reflective or energetic. We may also need to walk regularly in order to stimulate the body's sense of proprioceptive response.

Sea squirts, movement, and fascia

If we look to the origins of creatures that appear not to need movement, we begin to understand how our nervous system helps us to negotiate the world, from eating to moving around to finding better places to live or avoid predators. The sea squirt, a type of marine invertebrate with a supporting notocord, has no such agenda, and once the larva anchors onto its first home, its nervous system becomes quite useless; in about 3–4 days, its tail, nerve cord, and notochord are absorbed, leaving only a small mass of nerve tissue.

Humans need a more complex nervous system to coordinate our movement and to help us avoid being hurt. However, along with our complex nervous system comes some of our really ancient nervous system, tied into a body that psychologically has its challenges in leaving its worries about the past or future alone, often carrying them in postural patterns, stress, and anxiety. Back to our humble sea squirt, often described as potato-shaped. Interestingly, it is basically a fascial sack of polysaccharide cellulose over a tube with a branchial (oral) aperture and an atrial aperture. Interesting, too, that the sea squirt may actually help us with our own fascial tissues and diseases such as cancer, which appears to plague many creatures throughout the animal kingdom from mollusks to mammals. They have been found to have a role in fighting cancer through production of a substance called ecteinascidin-743, which causes tumors to shrink and continues to be studied in treating patients with myxoid liposarcomas (Grosso *et al.* 2007). Myxoid liposarcoma is a type of liposarcoma, or cancer (sarcoma) that arises in the fat cells (lipo) of soft tissue.

The sea squirt is often pointed out for its lack of mobility, but the larger lesson here may be that the sea squirt is actually very efficient at movement. After all, its larvae swim freely, and adults are able to move if needed by letting go through part of the body and then reattaching.

As noted by Beach (2010), "Fish have had half a billion years to explore lateral contraction of the body-wall for swimming. From an evolutionary perspective, all vertebrates coalesce about two primary post-cranial muscle domains: the epimere that forms the dorsal muscle groups, and the hypomere that forms the lateral and ventral muscle groups. Each spinal nerve bifurcates into a primary dorsal and ventral nerve root, with the dorsal nerve supplying the muscles of the epimere, and the ventral nerve supplying the hypomere" (p.68). Whether sea squirt, fish or human, we all have nervous systems that coordinate our choice of where we move or stay put in our environmental space.

Referencing anatomy to our shape

Much of the mythology of the ancient Greeks and Romans focused on huge mythical creatures such as centaurs, griffins, and giants. Mayor (2011) proposed that these ancient people had no historical context to understand the fossil remains of creatures such as mammoths. In order to make sense of what they encountered, they arranged the bones into creatures that seemed plausible, from the anatomy they understood. In this case, the human mind reshaped a story, and described fossils in the context of the forms they could understand.

What forms and informs us?

...form is selected from a palette of possibilities, and by selected I mean favoured by natural selection. A form that gives the organism an evolutionary advantage tends to stick.

Philip Ball (2004)

The body is shaped in much the same way that the outer natural environment shapes other things in life. Leonardo Da Vinci was fascinated with water, calling it "vetturale di natura" or vehicle of nature, believing it to be the driving force in nature. If we think in terms of fascia and its water content, we have a fabric that gains some of its context from its relationship to water, both bound and unbound in its system.

According to Myers (2020), we are shaped by several major categories: 1) genetics and DNA; 2) our interaction with the world; 3) our emotions; and 4) fluid flow (Figure 2.2) and the relationship of biomechanics in gravity. According to Wainwright (1988), shape also is linked to time and these changes happen in three time scales. "Physiological changes can happen quickly—in seconds or fractions of seconds. Developmental changes happen more slowly and can take minutes or years. Evolutionary changes are the slowest: they take generations" (p.15).

Genetics and DNA

If the code runs well, the program, in essence, goes as it should. However, just like a computer code, if there are any mutations in that system, things may run amiss. Time itself can be a factor. Like a digital file that degrades, the telomeres (ends of our DNA code) can become frayed with age. However, as humans there is a lot that can be done to fix this. The qualities of how we live our lives, from the food we put in our bodies to the environment we place ourselves in, are all part of the concept of epigenetics, the concept of what gene expression can be turned on or off.

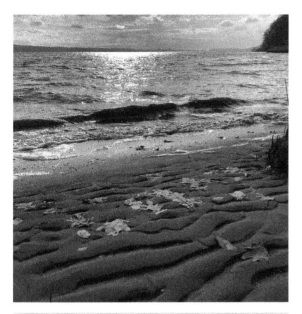

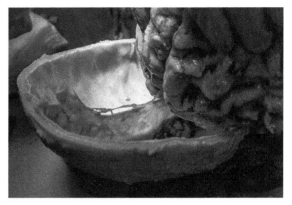

FIGURE 2.3 Falx cerebri and the dura mater. The falx cerebri (or cerebral falx) is the crescent moon shaped meningeal layer of the dura mater. The dura mater (meaning hard mother) also forms around the tubes that cover the cranial nerves and spinal column.

Photo by Lydia Mann, KNMLabs (author's dissection).

FIGURE 2.2 Fluid flow along the Hudson River, New York. Fluid flow shapes and reshapes the sand along the shoreline. Paddlers of all sorts observe the changes on the surface of a body of water to understand what may be happening underneath or in the larger system. Watching directionality of water is important in observing fluid flow and changes in current and tide. A strong eddy, for example, might indicate a rock formation underneath the surface.

Photo by author.

Embryology—the shape of folding and unfolding

All bodies are in constant change, both anatomically and psychologically. Embryology reveals the earliest stages of the nervous, circulatory, and fascial systems, which develop early on.

Spatial relationships as the body is being formed determine quite a lot. In the brain, for example, the neocortix is a six-layered structure where connective tissue cells are the organizing highways for the cells that are laid down. It might be possible to conceive of the idea that structural change can impact a person in different ways whether we conceive of this as neurological or spatial in the way it is expressed. Movement is a combination of controlling a body in relationship to environment, as well as creating stiffness or freedom as suitable to the situation, and myofascia helps with that.

The embryonic development is a dance of folding inwards and then moving outwards into the world. Form, movement, and fascia are all part of this development at the beginning of development. Why should we care about this? The dance of development is tied in profoundly with myofascial development but also with evolving and shaping our form. If we miss parts of that folding, issues can occur (such as cleft palate).

The first fold of the embryo is the **head fold,** which is a meeting of the embryotic and yolk sacs. The heart, initially sitting above the top of the bilaminar disc, folds down into its ventral position. Next, the **lateral fold** from the edges develops, the endoderm creates the tube of the gut track, and starts to also form the lungs (gastrointestinal and breathing). The mesoderm is responsible primarily for muscles, bones, and fascia. Ectoderm is the nervous system, central in the body, but coming outwards as well, forming skin and sensory perception through the skin. In this early stage, the ectoderm is surrounding the amniotic cavity and the endoderm is surrounding the primary yolk sac. In these early stages, the early split in layers divides to the parietal (somatic) layer of the lateral plate mesoderm and the visceral (splanchnic) layer of the lateral plate of the mesoderm. The last piece of origami is the **tail fold,** which begins as a backward fold, elongating the axial body and pulling the diaphragm and the associated fascial connections downwards.

The thick and collagenous membrane of the dura mater folds and creates boundaries called dural reflections. One such major area is the falx cerebri that separates the two halves of the cerebral hemispheres (Figure 2.3).

The stability of all sorts of objects, cloth dinner napkins included, lies in a principle that solid but malleable materials enjoy coming into stable configurations, particularly folds. As noted by Kemp (2016), "…all the forces of compression and tension that necessarily exist in any construction are resolved within the 'skin' of the fabric itself. Nothing is needed to hold it up other than itself—no supporting skeleton below or means of suspension to hang it from above. If we rearrange it by pulling upward one or more zones of the cloth, when released it will settle again into another stable if somewhat different configuration" (p.99).

Both technique and technology actually have quite a lot to do with the body, coming from the linguistic roots of "craft" and "treatment." Technique involves the way of doing an action. Interestingly, the French anthropologist Marcel Mauss used the term "techniques of the body" to describe both ordinary, repetitive functions of everyday movement to different forms of body training (Mauss 1973, pp.70–88). The etymology of "technology" adds a tool or machine to the equation. Fabricating a textile might be a form of early technology, as well as more modern forms of changing and manipulating the environment.

Our interaction with the world

It is not the strongest of the species that survives, not the most intelligent that survives. It is the one that is the most adaptable to change.

Charles Darwin

We tend to think of domestication as something we do to animals, but the latest scientific evidence may point to humans as self-domesticators. A University of Barcelona study (Theofanopoulou *et al.* 2017) hypothesized humans choose companions (both people and pets) with faces that are perceived as friendly. If one looks at the neural crest cells (a temporary group of cells arising from the ectoderm layer), the changes in this layer are responsible for craniofascial cartilage. Our fascia is involved in the very features that we emotionally respond to when we look at faces and it may be that we have self-selected to procreate with those that have affable faces.

Quadruped to biped

We share a lot of the same anatomy as four-legged creatures. However, our shoulder girdle differs substantially based on how we use it. For one of my clients, it was a revelation to see a human skeleton re-arranged into the quadruped position and note the same number of bones in the arms and legs, and yet the striking difference in functionality. Interestingly, the fascia has also developed differently in its relationship to its use with the ground and gravity. The plantar fascia for many can be a painful area, but the palmar fascia rarely has the same issue. Unlike other mammals, the human shoulder girdle is pushed far to the sides for brachiation, or limb to limb locomotion with our arms. Our ribcage is ovoid, with the collarbones pushing the arms out wide to the sides of the body.

However, being on a tiny base of support, we have challenges. Our ancestors with prehensile feet could not only clasp a tree branch, but also became much more interactive with the ground. Walking well can also help tone the foot in a positive way, especially the forefoot, which actually needs tone, not just stretch. This is perhaps one of the biggest challenges in rehabbing foot issues. In fact, in 2015, scientist Carolyn Eng published a study comparing the energy storage of the human IT band with a chimp's and found our energy efficiency higher, allowing for the myofascially efficient gait we retain. The segmented tent pole of our spine can support our larger head with a tiny base of support in our feet. The front of a horse for example, is weight bearing and is what is known as "gravitotal." Back legs are cursorial, and the angles are very sharp and are designed for running.

As to the pelvis, we keep analyzing the bones of the pelvis but we should be looking more at the soft tissues and their change in alignment/orientation. Particular attention has been given to the female pelvis as it is needed in birthing the next generation to survive. Bonobos and chimpanzees are less vertically aligned in their pelvis. We gain the advantage of an easier bipedal stance, but have a more difficult birth process, and also birth our children at a more vulnerable developmental stage.

"Our bipedal pattern of walking uses the movements of our hips, knees, ankles, and foot bones to propel us forward in an upright stance unlike the sprawled posture of creatures like the Tiktaalik. One big difference is the position of our hips. Our legs do not project sideways like those of a crocodile, amphibian, or fish: rather, they project underneath our bodies. These changes in posture came about by changes to the hip joint, pelvis, and upper

leg: our pelvis became bowl shaped, our hip socket became deep, our femur gained its distinctive neck, the feature that enables it to project under the body rather than to the side" (Shubin 2009, p.43).

Our foundational "floor"
Marla L. Sukoff, MD, RYT-500, Physical Medicine and Rehabilitation Specialist

I find it fascinating to view the pelvic floor (PF) through the lens of evolution. Before primates stood upright, when they were quadruped, the function of the PF was limited to elimination and sexual function. The organs were held up by the abdominal cavity and forces of stress, from four legs, were dissipated through the entire body. Once primates became bipedal, a whole new dimension arose. Now, the PF became critical for supporting the organs, as well as for stabilizing and absorbing the stress from walking and running. It became the "ball bearing" or shock absorber between the legs and the spine.

Thus, our pelvic floor has become foundational. It is the "floor" of our pelvis, and the "floor" of our core (abdominals, back, and hips). Our pelvis ("basin," in Latin) can be thought of as a "bowl" supporting our organs. Our core can be visualized as an "inner container," with respiratory diaphragm as "roof," pelvic floor muscles as "floor," and longitudinal muscles as "walls" (side walls—transversus abdominis m, posterior wall—iliopsoas m, front wall—rectus abdominis m). Given that the PF supports 70% of our body weight, its functional health is integral for achieving optimal movement and coordination.

This functional unit comes to life with our breath! When we inhale, our respiratory diaphragm descends, increasing intra-abdominal pressure. Ideally, since the joints in our bony pelvis allow movement, our bony pelvis expands with each deep "pelvic" breath. With each pelvic expansion, the "diamond" of our pelvic floor stretches due to its anatomical bony attachments. However, most of us are chest breathers, and rarely, if ever, get the breath down there! We must therefore learn to invite the breath deeper—this is key. First, relaxation of the secondary muscles of respiration, neck, and chest is crucial, followed by gradual deepening of the breath into the abdomen, then pelvis, and then down to the PF. Our PF will now begin to wake up! Through the breath, it becomes supple.

Finding our fascial connections augments this awakening. Take a moment to tune into your body—now, lift the "domes" of your arches and perhaps, you feel a concomitant "lift" in the "dome" of your PF! Next, add touching the tip of your tongue to your upper palette—does your PF lift even more?

Pelvic architecture and design principle

The shape of the pelvis is a similar shape to a helicopter propeller. If you put your finger on the top of iliac crest (your hip's top border) and another at the ischial pubic ramis, the two fingers are almost at right angles to each other. It means our pelvic design is like a twisted figure eight, like a two-winged propeller with the center at the acetabulum of the femur.

Swimming in waves

Experience the two types of movement still part of our evolutionary history. Find a large amount of space on the floor and think about your axial skeleton. The axial skeleton is named as the axis of the body including the bones of the skull, ossicles of the mid ear, hyoid bone, vertebral column, and the ribcage. Surrounding the spinal cord and ventral body cavity, as well as the brain, the axial skeleton provides protection and support. Due to the involvement of the ribcage, we can consider respiratory movements as part of this system. In movement with the axial skeleton, we have a choice in motivating side-to-side, like a fish swimming with lateral motion, or in movement in the sagittal plane, up and down, essentially porpoising, wavelike motions. The etymology of axial has roots in Latin, Greek, and Sanskrit, all related to a similar concept of the axis, or central point of a wheel. We are moving around the central part of our anatomy, the primitive central anatomy.

Our recent evolution

We have shifted greatly in going from that forest floor to the upright bipedal being we became. Our bipedalism speaks to the efficiency of standing upright in order to have energy and effort to go further. In most of the animal kingdom, the limbs are often heavy and bent. The fewer bends in our skeleton allows us to save an enormous load of calories per week (Lieberman 2018). However, our gait has a preferred walking speed at about 1.4 miles per hour (Kozma *et al.* 2018), meaning we utilize too much effort muscularly at lower and higher speeds. Utilizing fascia at the "ideal" speed, humans become quite efficient movers (Figure 2.4).

In essence, we took our similar anatomy in terms of bones, fascia, arteries, muscles, etc. and made it work, or rather we helped it work less by being more efficient. Our diaphragm functions differently and so do all of our movement motivations. We separated all of the lines that were unidirectional. Sight and movement go out forwards from the ventral part of the body and the spine and the digestive system go along the vertical part of the body. Being bipedal also gives us an anatomical advantage with the diaphragm elongated. We can pant off our heat when we endurance run, whereas other animals in quadruped position have their guts near their diaphragm, where they pant for every movement.

Often, we think we are doing a favor for the body by providing support to the foot and leg, but it is actually the process of removing the support that

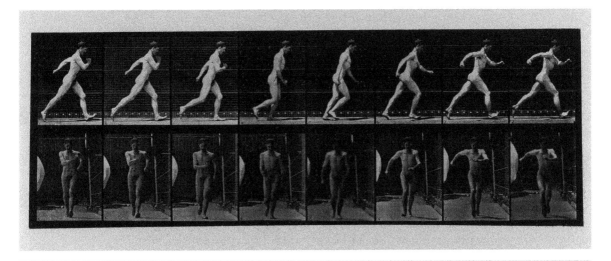

FIGURE 2.4 As bipedal creatures, our walking can be myofascially efficient, particularly if we train it to be so. Fascia (particularly in tendons like the Achilles tendon) can help provide a catapult effort that creates added force. Eadweard Muybridge created a series of roughly 20,000 photos in series in the years 1872–1885, photographing walking and other sports activities. Many other photographers such as this one, copied his style of still photos collaged together. However, as noted by Moore (2005), "isolating one moment from the natural flow actions, the instantaneous photos tended, ironically, to destroy the impression of movement."

Credit: A naked man speed-walking. Collotype after Eadweard Muybridge, 1887. Wellcome Collection. Public Domain Mark.

encourages people to strengthen their intrinsic functionality of the foot with its four layers of arch support. The first shoes are only around 10,000 years old with their primary function being to protect the foot from the environment. The foot is adaptive, and can act as a spring, or a rigid lever for push-off as well. We have been running for approximately 2 million years as bipedal beings with the longitudinal arch developing during this time. Our joint surfaces got larger, and our Achilles tendon got longer, a feature more needed in running than in walking (Bramble and Lieberman, Nature 2010).

The fascial foot and facile foot

In looking at the development of foot functionality we need to dive into its anatomy. The hinges and the rotations in the foot lead to the action of spiraling movement. Due to the offset of the heel, the heel turns medially in movement while walking. While there is a lot of concern over the height of the arch, it is really a question more of fascial responsiveness more so than flat or high arch.

Interestingly, barefoot walkers and runners are known to have thick foot calluses that offer understandably more protection for the foot while still allowing for a high level of tactile sensitivity and proprioception. Findings indicate that plantar fascia in symptomatic movers is thicker than asymptomatic. Forefoot strikers also had a significantly lower plantar fascia stiffness compared to rearfoot strikers (Chen *et al.* 2019). If we look toward design in athletic and functional footwear, the basic idea might be to design something that acts like a foot callus but doesn't limit other motions of the foot. The highly popular cushioned soles in recent shoe designs might have a feel-good factor initially, but ultimately limit the ability of the foot to respond to the environment around it. Footwear has to be changed slowly. If you switch to flat shoes and are not used to the action, the Achilles tendon will react to losing a bit of the heel found in "regular" street shoes. The more the foot is accustomed to a slight heel or being raised before running in a flat shoe, you are applying a large stretch and a lot of force transfer into the foot.

Motion control shoes have stiff pads known as heel counters, which try to reinforce the heel position and also try to prevent the foot from rolling in. When we think of running injuries, the foot impacts up to the rest of the body, particularly along the myofascial connections. There was a wave of injuries that came up in the literature from the 1970s onwards as more complicated shoes were being developed. When we think of ground reaction force it matters how we connect to the ground, or the injury will reverberate as the ground reaction force more than doubles the impact re-translated into the body.

Place a ball between your heels and slightly lift the heels and drive the heels together while pushing all the bases of the toes into the ground. This is resupination and locks the foot while working the posterior tibialis. The foot is working through plantarflexion and works the myofascial connection from the Achilles tendon to soleus, helping to pre-load the fascial tissues. The idea of fascial easiness in one part of the body obviously has effects up and down the system on the vertical level. In Sawicki *et al.* (2009), the team noted, "...mechanical work performed at other joints could be stored as elastic energy in the Achilles tendon." In other words,

everything is indeed connected to everything else. Pushing off more in muscle effort in the foot led to decreasing range of motion in the hip extension, for example. To train more of this action, training with jumps in plantarflexion helps to work elastic recoil. This can be done in upright jumps, or lying down against a jump board, as used on a Pilates reformer.

A swing of opinion

James Earls

For decades public perception of human evolution has been influenced by Zallinger's iconic image of the "March of Progress"—that line-up of hominids from knuckle-walking ape to obligatory (elegant?) biped which has been adapted, copied, and lampooned in many forms. Although most recognize this as a simplification of a complex process, the idea that we 'progressed' from knuckle-walking to bipedalism has entered the public consciousness—even though that idea was challenged long ago.

Over a decade ago, Crompton and colleagues published a landmark paper presenting considerable evidence that our knuckle-walking cousins (particularly chimps, bonobos, and gorillas) developed their locomotion strategies independently and after their split from our branch of the family tree (Crompton *et al.* 2008). If chimps and gorillas developed knuckle-walking after the separation from our *Homo* lineage, it means that arboreal suspension is more representative of our primitive locomotor strategies. The idea of our last common ancestor using overhead suspension rather than knuckle-walking is slowly making its way into the literature.

This idea of human bipedalism developing from an arboreal equivalent—walking upright along branches and holding onto those above—has received a boost from recently discovered ape fossils. Work by Böhme *et al.* (2019) reported skeletal features of a late Miocene ape (*Danuvius guggenmosi*, dated to 12 million years ago) that could use extended limbs to clamber through the canopy. Along with long straight forelimbs, other skeletal features reported in the paper include a "broad thorax, long lumbar spine and extended hips and knees."

Böhme's recent discovery supports the idea that our more distant ape cousins, the gibbons and orangutans, with their suspensory anatomy and locomotor behavior, more closely resemble our primitive state than the knuckle-walking gorillas, chimps, and bonobos. The updated understanding of human movement patterns has fed into current trends within evolutionary medicine and "primal" movement exercise regimes, leading to recommendations that we should "get back to basics" and start swinging from branches, ropes, and beams. But developing exercise and movement ideas based on evolutionary theory can be problematic and we should be cautious in our extrapolations.

Barefoot running used a comparable logic to the brachiating recommendations as it followed a similar backstory based on the evolutionary anatomy of Harvard paleoanthropologist Professor Daniel Lieberman (Bramble and Lieberman 2004). Lieberman's endurance running theory of human evolution struck many chords for those wanting a more active, simple, and natural approach to movement and exercise. However, the barefoot running movement created as many counter-arguments, shin-splints, and inflammations as it solved, and we are at risk of doing the same thing with the rise of the "brachiation theory."

The science supporting arboreal bipedalism is good; there are numerous factors that show we probably came down from the trees able to stand upright. It is easier to stand on two legs holding onto overhead branches as you walk along lower boughs. However, this is not full-on brachiation, it is suspensory locomotion. Brachiation is swinging from branch to branch, something gibbons—our most distant ape cousins—specialize in. A gibbon can reach up to 30 miles per hour gliding effortlessly between hand supports.

Humans and gibbons may have evolved a common ancestor that used suspensory behaviors of some form, but the anatomy of *Homo* has changed considerably in the 7 million years since we last shared the canopy with any of our cousins. Our arms are short relative to the rest of the body when compared to any other ape but especially when compared to the gibbons and orangutans. Likewise, our fingers are short, but our thumbs are long to assist manipulation. A gibbon's long, curved phalanges adapt perfectly to grasping and their short thumb allows a wider margin of error when reaching for a support. And while we have a relatively mobile wrist, gibbons have a ball and socket in the wrist joint to fine-tune to the angle of the next branch.

The shoulder joint shows even more divergence. The human glenoid fossa orients almost directly laterally, with the spine of the scapula nearly horizontal to the ground. This contrasts to the scapulae of all other apes, which are elongated from inferior angle to the glenoid fossa and orient more superiorly: a convenience for quadrupedal or suspensory behaviors but unnecessary for a biped. Anatomical shape, such as the shape of the scapula, is influenced by the various pressures associated with natural selection over time. Shape, environment, and locomotor abilities are entwined in the ever-present dynamic between form and function.

A comparison of scapulae from different ape species allows us to appreciate relationships between the form and function of their shoulders. A study by Young *et al.* (2015) used complex morphometric analysis tools to compare the various shapes of scapulae from a range of primate species. Although the methods are complex, the resultant output of geometric morphometrics is relatively easy to understand and can be seen in Figure 2.breakout.1. The graph created by Young *et al.* shows the principal directions of change in scapular shape between species, and also illustrates how, despite variation between individuals, each species neatly clusters together. Two directions of change are plotted on the graph. From left to right (x-axis) we see an increase in length of the scapula along the superior border and a change in the angle of the glenoid fossa from superior-lateral to almost purely lateral. On the other axis (y), we see an increase in depth in the supraspinatus fossa and an increase in size of the superior angle.

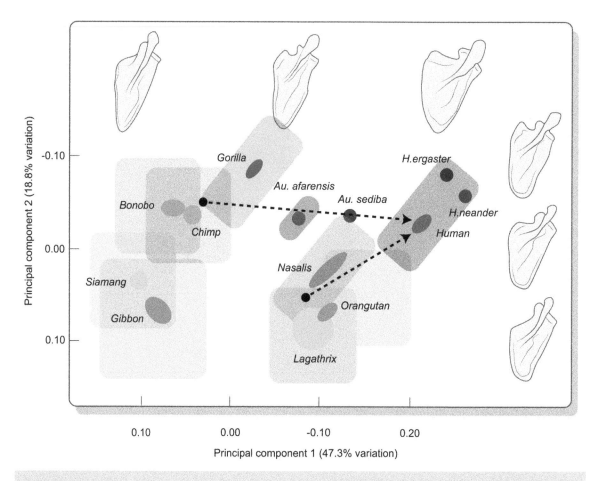

FIGURE 2.BREAKOUT.1 Individual scapulae were analyzed using geometric morphometric analyses. Results showed most of the shape variation occurred along two axes of change—angle of spine of scapula (principal component 1, explained 47.3% of variation) and borders of the supraspinatus fossa (principal component 2, 18.8% of variation). The plot shows a strong trend for species to group together according to species and, importantly, locomotor patterns. More arboreal species tend toward the bottom left of the graph and terrestrial species toward the upper right. The brachiators (gibbon and siamang) are located diagonally opposite upright, bipedal humans. (Colored points indicate individual samples; dark ellipses, 90% confidence interval of the mean; light ellipses, 90% confidence interval of the sample. Adapted from Young *et al.* 2015.) Courtesy of Lotus Publishing.

Each species is plotted according to overall morphology of the scapula, and we see the brachiating specialists (siamang and gibbon) in the bottom left and the *Homo* species in the top right—almost as opposite one another as possible.

While these comparisons may seem quite theoretical, they have important functional and evolutionary implications. The paper concluded that brachiation was an off-shoot locomotor development from the African ape lineage—a specialization for the gibbon branch and not a direct part of the *Homo* heritage. Although that conclusion will undoubtedly be questioned by some, the functional implications are less easy to overrule.

The human scapula does not fall at one extreme or the other on the graph, which shows that we have a generalized scapula appropriate for a range of uses. The supraspinatus fossa is neither deep nor shallow, the blade is broad and orients laterally to allow forward-facing manipulation (such as tools). The wide span of the scapula gives a broader range of fascicular directions for finer control over a greater range of glenohumeral motion. Compare this to the gibbon scapula, whose musculature is focused up and out to support the arm as the body swings underneath it in a wide arc which requires little glenohumeral range.

The conclusion we can draw from this is that we are not evolved from brachiators nor are we "designed" to brachiate; however, we can brachiate if we want to because we are generalists. Our "design" allows us to manipulate, to throw, to hug, to hang, and to perform handstands. However, since we lack the specialized scapular alignment, focused muscle concentration and muscular strength of brachiators, we must launch ourselves into brachiating with care and appropriate training!

There are many benefits to getting out, being active and using our bodies in novel ways, and it may take a "return to your roots" story to motivate you. However, be aware there are concerns with suspending and not all of them are gravity related. Climbing and suspension are great exercises, but they are just that—exercises. Our skeletal alignment has evolved so that we are no longer aligned for brachiating and, likewise, our soft tissues have not adapted to a repeated overhead supporting role in everyday life. As with barefoot running, we should build up tolerance and strength for the new stresses involved in exercises requiring supporting ourselves with an overhead reach, and we should ensure adequate range of motion of the scapula to orient the glenoid fossa upwards and prevent glenohumeral impingement.

References

Bramble, D. and Lieberman, D. (2004) 'Endurance running and the evolution of Homo.' *Nature 432*, 7015, pp.345–352.

Böhme, M., Spassov, N., Fuss, J., Tröscher, A. *et al.* (2019) 'A new Miocene ape and locomotion in the ancestor of great apes and humans.' *Nature 575*, 7783, pp.489–493.

Crompton, R., Vereecke, E. and Thorpe, S. (2008) 'Locomotion and posture from the common hominoid ancestor to fully modern hominins, with special reference to the last common panin/hominin ancestor.' *Journal of Anatomy 212*, 4, pp.501–543.

Young, N., Capellini, T., Roach, N. and Alemseged, Z. (2015) 'Fossil hominin shoulders support an African ape-like last common ancestor of humans and chimpanzees.' *Proceedings of the National Academy of Sciences 112*, 38, pp.11829–11834.

How we are changing our anatomy

Andre Leroi-Gourhan (1911–1986) was a French paleoanthropologist who influenced many of the thought connections between bipedalism and movement evolution into linguistics. He proposed the idea of technical changes in the brain influenced the anatomy and vice versa. "Central to [his] hypothesis is the idea that the birth of language was enabled by a series of 'liberations', i.e. the releasing of mechanical constraints on the body architecture which had powerful cognitive consequences. This fits into his general theoretical framework whereby physiological adaptation (technical means) to a habitat drives brain development (organizational means) which in turn promotes further evolution of the body…

The chances of evolutionary development are seen to depend on how well a body structure lends itself to behavioral remodeling through the activity of a more developed brain. Thus, the brain commands evolution but it remains inescapably subject to the possibilities of selective adaptation that are open to the skeletal framework" (Copple 2003, p.54).

Fascia movement guidelines for human bodies

Create space Lengthening the system before strengthening so we are not enforcing a negative pattern.

Hydrate In simple terms, this is all about tissue hydration and helping ease the quality of movement. We can drink water, but to hydrate fascia we are discussing the stimulation of the hydrophilic fibers of the fascia. Lack of movement and things like chronic sitting can compress the fascial extracellular matrix (ECM) and prevent the interstitial space maintaining water.

Challenge Think of your major planes of motion (sagittal, frontal, and transverse) and mix it up and think of creating motions in the in-between areas of movement. Multi-vectors are a piece of this, but miss the movement dynamics that dancers and athletes in particular know are important for training. Namely, vary your speed and intensity as well.

Pulse and rebound Think of in terms of encouraging elastic recoil. A modern dancer, for example, is trained in swing and release actions. Momentum can be an effective way to use less energy in the muscular system in particular. If we save calories through a highly efficient stride, for example, we can go longer with less effort.

Generate gracefulness through coordination of the fascial system which means less effort is needed in either movement or standing postures. This can be conceptualized as the myofascial connections dynamically balancing to create a distribution of stress or strain.

Cultivate spatial awareness By training spatial awareness, we increase the body's proprioceptive fascial abilities. As awareness goes around, the felt sensation of the body grows (or perhaps just comes back into our scope); the importance of fascia as a sensory organization is important for both its orientation abilities and felt sensations.

Build resilience Resiliency is both physical and mental in being able to "bounce back" from stress, tension, or unexpected events and continue to function. Part of this is not holding patterns that no longer serve the body system after a trauma (again either physical or mental).

Pandiculate Laughing, yawning, etc., is a way to change the movement of the body. Take a yawn right now and although if you are in a crowded space, you may be suppressing your yawn, you are still getting sensation moving through your chest. If you have the free space to do so, take a "full" yawn, moving and reaching out into the space around you. Maybe you can feel the reach into the front of the pubis, or even into the entire front of the body.

Pandiculation involves the soft tissues and occurs in most animal species. Bertolucci (2011) proposed that the stretch yawning syndrome or SYS, which combines yawning with other body region pandiculation, may help the locomotor system, "to maintain the animal's ability to express coordinated and integrated movement by regularly restoring and resetting the structural and functional equilibrium of the myofascial system."

Why are there so many lateral rotators in the hips?

The abundance of lateral rotation in the legs has a lot to do with the way humans develop anatomically in movement. As the body develops and expands outwards, the knees turn inwards. Lateral rotators as a group of muscles are good for push off and movement like speed skating and more. However, chronic use of only the lateral rotation can lead to imbalances in the pelvic floor. While ballet emphasizes the lateral rotation there is no equivalent aesthetic for internal rotation.

The shape of our pelvis has a lot to do with this. The function of the hip abductors in pulling the hip away from the midline, is also to control hip adduction from occurring too quickly. However, there is still the medial rotation of the calcaneus as we walk. We can think of muscles as the controllers of movement, not only about its production. Fascia negotiates the forces around the body and form.

A bit of physics and fascial forces

When I was in college, I took a course on the physics of dolphins and whales. All the science of physics was explored in concepts like sound waves and motion. We had a final project applying motion to some of the concepts. I filmed an ice skater to study torque and motion on ice, basing a lot of my work on the book *The Physics of Dance* (Law 1986) which put the laws of gravity (and other concepts) onto ballet dancers who routinely try to work with and against the forces of nature. I was thrilled for the application to movement but didn't encounter much more terminology from physics until I dove deeper into fascial research. Let's take a look at some of terms being discussed today.

Myofascial force transmission

We are beginning to question "can fascia transmit force?" and the answer appears to be a strong "yes."

Peter Huijing (2009) made some of the initial fascial studies on myofascial force transmission, noting that 70% of muscular force is transmitted by the tendon, with the additional 30% being transmitted by the connective tissue around the muscle. If one takes the concept of biotensegrity to the body, we can think of fascia as acting as a strain distributor, as well as serving a role in lateral force transmission. This changes approaches in training and rehabilitation from injuries.

Hydraulic amplification

Amplification is all about more force output due to optimizing the force/length and force/velocity relationships. According to Willard *et al.* (2012) this concept can be applied to understand that the fascial paraspinal retinacular sheath (PRS) can help the paraspinal muscles support the lumbosacral spine.

Earls (2020) notes, "tensioning the fascial sheets increases the efficiency of the associated muscles, either in series or in parallel. This can be brought about in a number of ways: 1) Tensioning of the muscles embedded within the sheet. This is seen with the tensor fasciae latae and the gluteus maximus (both of which are encased within the fascia lata), the platysma (within the fascia colli superficialis) and the pectoralis minor (contained within the clavipectoral fascia); 2) Contraction of the muscles deep to the fascial layer. The contraction of the thigh muscles will tension the fascia lata from below, just as the erector spinae will tauten the posterior sheet of the thoracolumbar fascia; 3) Stretching and thereby elastically loading the tissue by the natural momentum of body movement. The swing of the arm will tension the thoracolumbar fascia, while the swing of the leg will tension the epimysia of the hip extensors."

According to Roberts and Azizi (2011), power amplification is brought about as a means of power production from the muscle to tendon to the entire body. As they note, "...the term 'amplification' is potentially misleading, in that familiar electronic power amplifiers work by adding energy to a power source. Elastic mechanisms in animals do not add energy to the system, but rather amplify power only in the sense that they release energy more rapidly than it is stored." So, what does this mean for us in simple terms of movement and mobility? Nothing is in isolation. The importance of the fascial bags tensioning and releasing gives another level to our training.

Ground reaction force

The force of gravity pushes down on the surface supporting a body. At the same time, a force known as the ground reaction force (GRF) is exerted by the ground in the opposite direction. As movers, the ground reaction force will vary in angle as we move and push off the ground. Of course, environment again matters as the frictional force of ground or surface will have a different effect on the body. A hard surface will still deform when we press against it, but striking a foot, or handstanding, on concrete is quite a different feel than when I sink my boots into a snowy trail in the middle of winter in New York. Gravity pulls the body down, but the vector of the GRF will vary with the angle of either a heel or the edge of a hand.

So it stands to reason that different engineered surfaces would have a different effect on ground reaction forces. In a study by Dixon *et al.* (2000), runners with a heel–toe running style performed trials on three surfaces: asphalt, rubber-modified asphalt, and an acrylic surface, all noted differences in impact absorption. While surface absorption was predictable, the results were not. Different runners created adaption to the surfaces and angles in diverse manners, with some utilizing more initial knee flexion while others did not. The takeaway? Running style and strategy demand more individual assessment rather than the assumption all bodies react the same to all surfaces. However, most people will find a surface like a sandy beach

a much different running experience as the grains of sand will disperse the ground reaction force differently than a hard pavement path.

Force damping

Force damping is holding back vibration in motion. Some occur via mechanical components, like the pad under my carpet or the shock absorber in my car. With regards to fascia, it is when the absorption of the force is performed first by the fascial tissues so that the muscle can act isometrically (optimizing force/length), then when it is stored in the tendon, the muscle can lengthen to release that energy (optimizing force/velocity again).

In fancy terminology, force damping is reduction of the amplitude of any oscillations created in movement. The body itself can begin to dampen movement in terms of creating areas of immobilization, such as a fascial restriction that may be preventing free movement. Elastic loading allows muscles to offload or dampen the strain with a slower eccentric contraction. The rapid elastic lengthening allows the muscle to remain in a semi isometric state and then eccentrically contract at a speed closer to its optimal force/velocity relationship.

If a musician strums a guitar string, for example, and then puts their hand across the bridge of the instrument, the strings and their tone are dampened. Likewise, the environmental space around a body may act as dampeners to the body. This is particularly evident in the cushioning in shoes, which dampen the signals to the body. Due to this, many runners in cushioned shoes heel strike and have a loss of the proprioception feedback.

Catapult mechanism and elastic recoil

For some time, science was at a loss at how to explain how kangaroos jump so fast and efficiently (Figure 2.5). Muscles alone do not explain the action. If the idea of the catapult mechanism is added into the equation, one can understand that

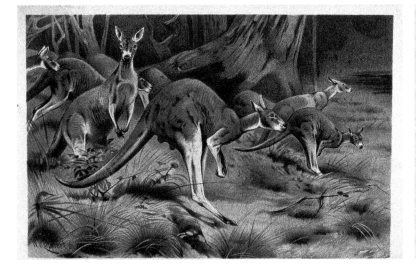

FIGURE 2.5 A group of red kangaroos on the move. Color reproduction of a painting by W. Kuhnert.

Credit: Wellcome Collection. Public Domain Mark.

the fascia and tendons are tensioning like elastic bands with a capacity for stored energy that is released, allowing the musculature not to be the most important feature of kinetically stored energy.

Lest we become too enamored with fascia alone, the muscle in a body system still needs to be strong enough to decelerate movement. This concept of muscle-tendon units is important, as in addition to creating elastic recoil, they have to transfer mechanical energy (Sawicki *et al.* 2009).

In working the deep fascial layer in manual or movement work, it is hard to say exactly if we should be thinking in terms of lengthening or shortening per se. Movement does appear to be a pathway to creating different possibilities for the body system. If I give the body more possibilities in the fascial system, my possibility for movement and, indeed, how I can express myself can expand.

As humans, we are designed to be energy efficient, but we are not designed to sit for long periods of time. Homeostatic regulation of body weight appears to rely on environmental input for feedback. As noted in a Swedish study (Jansson *et al.* 2018), "In this study, the body weight-reducing effect of increased loading was lost in mice depleted

of osteocytes. We propose that increased body weight activates a sensor dependent on osteocytes of the weight-bearing bones. This induces an afferent signal, which reduces body weight. These findings demonstrate a leptin-independent body weight homeostat ('gravitostat') that regulates fat mass." The takeaway here may be that if we become sedentary, our body isn't processing its own body weight and the osteocytes cannot sense the changes in load. It may make sense that the fascia is also not being loaded, and with a lack of feedback the body doesn't "know" what it weighs and it may "think" it weighs less than it does and overeat as a result. Even a chair may be providing false information in supporting one's body weight too comfortably. We can guess that perhaps even weight bearing, such as a long walk, could help bring the body back to itself by reminding it of its actual width and occupation of space.

Further thoughts on perception of load

As the modern body becomes more effortless in its movement and efficiency (Figure 2.6), an unchallenged environment may also be leading to our weight issues. In other words, if you don't move and have the feedback of load against the system, our bodies may be unable to have a realistic self-perception of healthy weight. Modern life has left us with easy access to sugar and fat, which our ancient ancestors craved when it was a scarcity. We are still wired to eat fats and sugar, leading to our ever-increasing waistlines as a cultural whole in "developed" countries with easy access to fast food. There is also another possible explanation to our increasing girth in modern life related to daily movement, or rather the lack thereof. We as humans are prone to perceiving ourselves as thinner than we are, which was explained in a 2018 study that showed humans have a bias toward perceiving their body size based on past and present experiences and combines, in essence, the two to create an illusion of smaller body size, often of our younger selves (Alexi *et al.* 2018). It's possible that fascia is important in the maintenance and perception of the self: "animals obey power law scaling both *within* individuals, in terms of the geometry and dynamics of their internal network structures, as well as *across* species, they, and therefore all of us, are living manifestations of self-similar fractals" (West 2017).

If fascia is seen as being both fractal and irregular in nature, it is important to discern why anything would be designed in a complex network, which shifts the point of equilibrium. These fractal areas of biology (Guimberteau and Armstrong 2015) exist in places including alveoli, vascular networks and more, noting that the body is rarely linear, but rather, "in the fascia we see an irregular, fractal, chaotic, non-linear system… In the course of our constant search for knowledge, we have had to gradually accept that nature does not function in straight lines, and that the law of proportionality of cause and effect, which refers to the relationship of two variables whose ratio is constant, could in fact be based on non-linear rules" (pp.175–176).

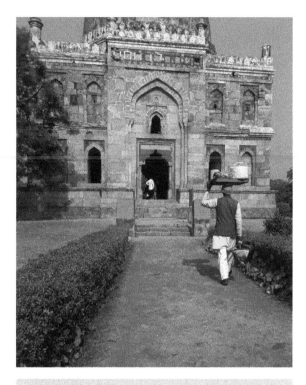

FIGURE 2.6 Load carrying. The body, when well-balanced in its tensegrity, can distribute stress and strain easily without significant increase in caloric intake.

Photo by Benjamin Feinstein (2019).

Is bone fascia?

Anatomically speaking, bone is a mineralized connective tissue, but so far it has not been formally accepted as fascia, just as fluids like blood and lymph can be classified as connective tissue but are also not considered fascia. However, the matrix of the bone is a combination of ground substance and collagen fibers, and the architecture of bone is responsive to structural stresses and created from trabeculae running in many directions. Some consider the periosteum, or outer coating of bone that connects to the myofascial anatomy, as a fascial layer, but not bone itself.

Depending on your high school science teacher, you may have taken a chicken bone and placed it in a vinegar (or hydrochloric) bath, which leaches out the minerals, rendering the bone pliable and malleable by dissolving the calcium salts. In the second, we could burn the bone in a hot furnace. The organic part (i.e. collagen) is removed so that the bone keeps its shape until touched, when it will turn into ash. In other words, the connective tissue component of bone gives both strength and elasticity, and the mineral salts the harder structure we typically think of in a non-living bone. If we consider the living body, collagen serves to help tensile strength, but it is the water composition that points to a healthy living bone. Both fascia and bone in the traditional definitions do act similarly in regards to Wolff's law and the concept of remodeling, which is critical in athletics and training. The basics of Wolff's law, simply stated, are that healthy bone will adapt to loads under which it is placed, building stronger under stress, and decreasing under light load. While bone is certainly structurally similar to fascia, we do have to draw the line at some point in our definitions, but we will give a nod of appreciation and further contemplation to this debate.

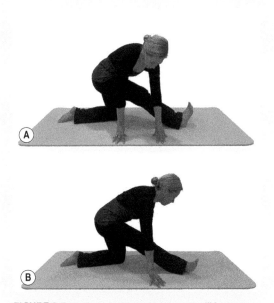

FIGURE 2.7 How we get to a movement will have a different effect on the fascial glide between muscular layers. In a) the "driver" is movement of the arms and torso to the right side of mat, while in b), the leg itself is laterally rotating.

movement will feel different. Both can be utilized to create slide and glide between the deep fascial layers. If one takes a leg in front (half split pose), if the upper torso is the driver in moving the arms to the outside of the leg, it will have a different sensation than if the leg itself is the driver, with the leg leading the movement in lateral rotation while the torso remains stationary.

Drivers

In looking at drivers in the body, what motivates a movement is as important as the myofascial connection affected. Take one leg in front in a half-split, runner's stretch variation (Figure 2.7a). In the first, allow your hands to come to the outside of the leg, with the arms acting as the driver of the movement. In the second, allow the leg to laterally rotate from the femur (Figure 2.7b). In this case the torso is fixed, and the rotation is coming from the leg itself. In both cases the lower leg myofascial connections are being affected (rolling through the three hamstrings in particular) but the initiation of

Life is about movement, and our evolution as humans has made us myofascially efficient walkers, but we live in modern environments that are often at odds with our evolutionary development. Understanding how our fascia functions in terms of our history and how movement, force and load distribution all play their parts, can help us to not only survive to the next generation but thrive in movement and life.

References

Alexi, J., Cleary, D., Dommisse, K., Palermo, R. *et al.* (2018) 'Past visual experiences weigh in on body size estimation.' *Scientific Reports 8*, 1, 215. https://doi.org/10.1038/s41598-017-18418-3

Ball, P. (2004) *The Self-Made Tapestry: Pattern Formation in Nature.* Repr. Oxford: Oxford University Press.

Beach, P. (2010) *Muscles and Meridians: The Manipulation of Shape.* Edinburgh, UK: Churchill Livingstone.

Bertolucci, L. F. (2011) 'Pandiculation: Nature's way of maintaining the functional integrity of the myofascial system?' *Journal of Bodywork and Movement Therapies 15*, 3, 268–280. https://doi.org/10.1016/j.jbmt.2010.12.006

Bramble, D. M. and Lieberman, D. E. (2004) 'Endurance running and the evolution of Homo.' *Nature 432*, 7015, 345–352. https://doi.org/10.1038/nature03052

Chen, T. L.-W., Agresta, C. E., Lipps, D. B., Provenzano, S. G. *et al.* (2019) 'Ultrasound elastographic assessment of plantar fascia in runners using rearfoot strike and forefoot strike.' *Journal of Biomechanics 89*, 65–71. https://doi.org/10.1016/j.jbiomech.2019.04.013

Copple, M. M. (2003) 'Gesture and Speech: André Leroi-Gourhan's theory of the co-evolution of manual and intellectual activities.' *Gesture 3*, 1, 47–94. https://www.jbe-platform.com/content/journals/10.1075/gest.3.1.04cop

Dixon, S. J., Collop, A. C. and Batt, M. E. (2000) 'Surface effects on ground reaction forces and lower extremity kinematics in running.' *Medicine & Science in Sports & Exercise 32*, 11, 1919–1926. https://doi.org/10.1097/00005768-200011000-00016

Earls, J. (2020) *Born to walk: Myofascial efficiency and the body in movement.* 2nd ed. Berkeley, CA: North Atlantic Books.

Eng, C. M., Arnold, A. S., Biewener, A. A. and Lieberman, D. E. (2015) 'The human iliotibial band is specialized for elastic energy storage compared with the chimp fascia lata.' *Journal of Experimental Biology 218*, 15, 2382–2393. https://doi.org/10.1242/jeb.117952

Grosso, F., Jones, R. L., Demetri, G. D., Judson, I. R. *et al.* (2007) 'Efficacy of trabectedin (ecteinascidin-743) in advanced pretreated myxoid liposarcomas: A retrospective study.' *The Lancet Oncology 8*, 7, 595–602. https://doi.org/10.1016/S1470-2045(07)70175-4

Guimberteau, J.-C. and Armstrong, C. (2015) *Architecture of Human Living Fascia: Cells and Extracellular Matrix as Revealed by Endoscopy.* Edinburgh: Handspring Publishing.

Huijing, P. A. (2009) 'Epimuscular myofascial force transmission: A historical review and implications for new research.' International Society of Biomechanics Muybridge award lecture, Taipei, 2007. *Journal of Biomechanics 42*, 1, 9–21. https://doi.org/10.1016/j.jbiomech.2008.09.027

Jansson, J.-O., Palsdottir, V., Hägg, D. A., Schéle, E. *et al.* (2018) 'Body weight homeostat that regulates fat mass independently of leptin in rats and mice.' *Proceedings of the National Academy of Sciences 115*, 2, 427–432. https://doi.org/10.1073/pnas.1715687114

Karageorghis, C. I. and Priest, D.-L. (2012) 'Music in the exercise domain: A review and synthesis (Part II).' *International Review of Sport and Exercise Psychology 5*, 1, 67–84. https://doi.org/10.1080/1750984X.2011.631027

Kemp, M. (2016) *Structural Intuitions: Seeing Shapes in Art and Science.* Charlottesville, VA: University of Virginia Press.

Kozma, E. E., Webb, N. M., Harcourt-Smith, W. E. H., Raichlen, D. A. *et al.* (2018) 'Hip extensor mechanics and the evolution of walking and climbing capabilities in humans, apes, and fossil hominins.' *Proceedings of the National Academy of Sciences 115*, 16, 4134–4139. https://doi.org/10.1073/pnas.1715120115

Law, K. (1986) *The Physics of Dance.* New York: Schirmer Books.

Lieberman, D. (2020) *Exercised: Why Something we Never Evolved to Do is Healthy and Rewarding.* New York: Pantheon Books.

Mauss, M. (1973) 'The techniques of the body.' Trans. B. Brewer. *Economy and Society, 2*, 70–88.

Mayor, A. (2011) *The First Fossil Hunters: Dinosaurs, Mammoths, and Myth in Greek and Roman Times.* Princeton, NJ: Princeton University Press.

Moore, C.-L. (2005) *Movement and Making Decisions: The Body–Mind Connection in the Workplace.* New York: Rosen Young Adult.

Myers, T. W. (2020) *Anatomy Trains: Myofascial Meridians for Manual Therapists and Movement Professionals* (4th ed.). London: Elsevier.

Roberts, T. J. and Azizi, E. (2011) 'Flexible mechanisms: The diverse roles of biological springs in vertebrate movement.' *Journal of Experimental Biology 214*, 3, 353–361. https://doi.org/10.1242/jeb.038588

Sawicki, G. S., Lewis, C. L. and Ferris, D. P. (2009) 'It pays to have a spring in your step.' *Exercise and Sport Sciences Reviews 37*, 3, 130–138. https://doi.org/10.1097/JES.0b013e31819c2df6

Shubin, N. (2009) *Your Inner Fish: A Journey Into the 3.5-Billion-Year History of the Human Body.* London: Vintage Books.

Sockol, M. D., Raichlen, D. A. and Pontzer, H. (2007) 'Chimpanzee locomotor energetics and the origin of human bipedalism.' *Proceedings of the National Academy of Sciences 104*, 30, 12265–12269. https://doi.org/10.1073/pnas.0703267104

Theofanopoulou, C., Gastaldon, S., O'Rourke, T., Samuels, B. D. *et al.* (2017) 'Self-domestication in *Homo sapiens*: Insights from comparative genomics.' *PLOS ONE 12*, 10, e0185306. https://doi.org/10.1371/journal.pone.0185306

Wainwright, S. A. (1988) *Axis and Circumference: The Cylindrical Shape of Plants and Animals.* Cambridge, MA: Harvard University Press.

Willard, F. H., Vleeming, A., Schuenke, M. D., Danneels, L. and Schleip, R. (2012) 'The thoracolumbar fascia: Anatomy, function and clinical considerations: The thoracolumbar fascia.' *Journal of Anatomy 221*, 6, 507–536. https://doi.org/10.1111/j.1469-7580.2012.01511.x

West, G. B. (2017) *Scale: The Universal Laws of Growth, Innovation, Sustainability, and the Pace of Life in Organisms, Cities, Economies, and Companies.* London; Penguin.

Further reading

Böhme, M., Spassov, N., Fuss, J., Tröscher, A. *et al.* (2019) 'A new Miocene ape and locomotion in the ancestor of great apes and humans.' *Nature 575*, 7783, 489–493. https://doi.org/10.1038/s41586-019-1731-0

Crompton, R. H., Vereecke, E. E. and Thorpe, S. K. S. (2008) 'Locomotion and posture from the common hominoid ancestor to fully modern hominins, with special reference to the last common panin/hominin ancestor.' *Journal of Anatomy 212*, 4, 501–543. https://doi.org/10.1111/j.1469-7580.2008.00870.x

Gordon, J. E. (2003) *Structures, or Why Things Don't Fall Down.* 2nd ed. Boston, MA: Da Capo Press.

Young, N. M., Capellini, T. D., Roach, N. T. and Alemseged, Z. (2015) 'Fossil hominin shoulders support an African ape-like last common ancestor of humans and chimpanzees.' *Proceedings of the National Academy of Sciences 112*, 38, 11829–11834. https://doi.org/10.1073/pnas.1511220112

Zanella, M., Vitriolo, A., Andirko, A., Martins, P. T. *et al.* (2019) 'Dosage analysis of the 7q11.23 Williams region identifies *BAZ1B* as a major human gene patterning the modern human face and underlying self-domestication.' *Science Advances 5*, 12, eaaw7908. https://doi.org/10.1126/sciadv.aaw7908

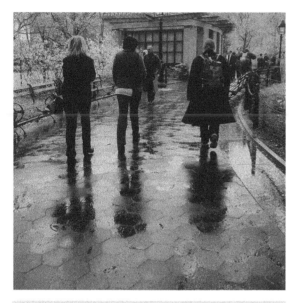

FIGURE 3.1 Walking, in simple terms, involves one foot in contact with the ground as a means of locomotion, usually to get from one place to another. We might label a pedestrian as a person who is walking, or as something rather commonplace as being pedestrian. Endurance (how far we can travel) and efficiency (how energy effective we are in getting there) are key components in studying gait. It is no surprise that movement is such a necessary part of human existence, but also a means to get to places, both literally and figuratively. Beyond walking, movement such as dance builds strength and efficiency but additionally works with emotional expression that in turn may impact how our myofascial system responds.

Walkers in New York City, photo by the author.

We do not grow absolutely or chronologically. We grow sometimes in one dimension, and not in another, unevenly. We grow partially. We are relative. We are mature in one realm, childish in another. The past, present, and future mingle and pull us backward, forward, or fix us in the present. We are made up of layers, cells, constellations.

Anaïs Nin

Ispent many years as a dance/movement therapist, working on expanding the possibilities in a body, both in movement and in mental states. When I started studying myofascial connections and tensegrity, this made sense to me. Fascia, slow to change compared to muscle, also holds patterns for long period of time. If we give more resiliency to this tissue, we can perhaps, in turn give more possibility to our expression in the world.

Our bodies connect our inner experience with how we sense the wider outer world (Figure 3.1). Life is emotional and that reaction is felt as a bodily sensation. The word "emotion" has its etymological roots in the Old French *esmovoir*, meaning to set in motion or shift feelings around. This may explain our strong relationship with emotions and physical sensations such as "butterflies in one's stomach" or awareness of the movement of heart palpations. We now are linking this to the interstitial receptors (that type of free nerve ending both sensing pain and touch) and the concept of interoception, which is all about sensing internal signals. Looking at myofascial connection and psychotherapeutic implications can explain some of our biologically based response patterns, but also give insight to treatment possibilities for body and mind. Coordination is a marker of a myofascial body moving well. Dance can be seen as having developed as a means of movement expression and practice for life actions.

Even the concept of pilgrimage, a long self-discovery journey along physical terrain, has appeared cross culturally and across different time periods. However, most expressive movement has traditionally developed closer to home as dance became a means to practice daily actions of work life and movement skills needed in everyday life and to develop them for optimal efficiency. It has also served as a creative expression of the human experience.

It is connected to us more directly than any other art form as the body remains the primary instrument of expression. Movement expression also helps develop the myofascial body both physically and emotionally. Rhythm is trained in any style of dance and works the easy quality of elastic recoil so constant muscular action isn't required. In working in myofascial balance, rhythm and coordination help the body gain a sense of tensile balance. Likewise in movement therapeutics, rhythmic synchrony in groups help to create a sense of belong to a larger system than the immediate self.

Noted biomechanist Daniel E. Lieberman wrote:

Dancing isn't running, but it's usually more fun and such a universal, valued form of human physical activity that we should consider it another gait akin to running. Indeed, while dancers sometimes use their legs like stilts as in a walk, most often they jump like runners from one foot to the other ... like long-distance running, dance can go on for hours, requiring stamina, skill, and strength. (2020)

Lieberman goes on to explain that any long periods of intensive exercise can produce a perceptional clarity (known as the runner's "high") whether in a trail run or an all-night dance gathering. This social aspect of dance (Figure 3.2) encourages side-to-side (lateral body) relationships in many cultures as well as being an opportunity to practice coordinated movements that help daily life skills.

The deeper need to stay emotionally healthy is also linked strongly to the body. The myofascial continuum helps with both spatial sense and emotional states and "is rich in interoceptors that are able to stimulate the areas of the brain that control the emotional state…" (Bordoni and Marelli 2017). In other words, if someone has a disorder in the myofascia, it may be reflected in the emotional state or vice-versa. While early research connecting myofascial tissues and emotion have been largely anecdotal, a recent study (Michalak *et al.* 2021)

was published in *Cognitive Therapy and Research* connecting major depressive disorder (MDD) with a reduced elasticity of myofascial tissue and increased stiffness suggesting, "the myofascial tissue might be part of a dysfunctional body–mind dynamic that maintains MDD." The motor patterns of a depressed individual (slumped body posture, forward head) lead to a self-perpetuating body pattern that creates more of the depressive state. This study represents a turning point in linking the body, fascia, and emotional state.

In body-based therapies, particularly in dance/movement therapy, the goal is "the psychotherapeutic use of movement to promote emotional, social, cognitive, and physical integration of the individual, for the purpose of improving health and wellbeing" (American Dance Therapy Association n.d.-a). By adding the understanding of new research in myofascia, the combination of this basic and universal form of expression can be a powerful tool in helping change the fascia tissue in response to how we process life. Life is unpredictable, so we have to be resilient—both in terms of anatomy as well as psychology.

Dance/movement therapy premises (American Dance Therapy Association n.d.-b)

- Movement is a language, our first language. Non-verbal and movement communication begins in utero and continues throughout the lifespan. Dance/movement therapists believe that non-verbal language is as important as verbal language and use both forms of communication in the therapeutic process.

- Mind, body, and spirit are interconnected.

- Movement can be functional, communicative, developmental, and expressive. Dance/movement therapists observe, assess, and intervene by looking at movement through these lenses, as it emerges in the therapeutic relationship in the therapeutic session.

- Movement is both an assessment tool and a primary mode of intervention.

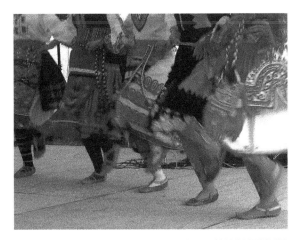

FIGURE 3.2 Folk dancers wearing traditional opanci shoes, originally designed for a rocky Balkan terrain. These dances cultivate myofascial efficiency, challenge balance, and increase social interaction through their lateral relationships in rhythmic movement.

Photo by the author.

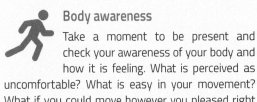

Body awareness

Take a moment to be present and check your awareness of your body and how it is feeling. What is perceived as uncomfortable? What is easy in your movement? What if you could move however you pleased right now, what would you do? Would it be a roar or a yawn?

Human beings, vegetables, or cosmic dust, we all dance to a mysterious tune, intoned in the distance by an invisible piper.

Albert Einstein

Dance/movement therapy—change the dance to change the myofascial body

When I was still in high school, my aunt gave me a copy of *Will You Won't You Join the Dance? A Dancer's Essay into the Treatment of Psychosis* by Trudi Schoop (1974), just as I was becoming interested in the body, both in its anatomical understanding and as a vehicle for expression. This would be the first of my introductions to pairing the body's emotional response as a visual pattern.

The primary principle of dance/movement therapy is the link between body and mind (Levy 1992, p.1). By affecting one, the other will shift and change as well. In other words, change the dance that one does with life, and the body and movement patterns will shift. By utilizing the tools of dance/movement therapy and its relatives in the related movement world, a new understanding can be reached of how to change our environment in order to help our movement. This, in turn, works toward the health of mind and spirit, beyond any bodily changes. As seen through new understanding in epigenetics, it is understood the absolutes are not the final answer and that gene expression may be turned on or off based on environmental and psychological factors.

Earlier pioneers in nonverbal communication, from Birdwhistle onwards, looked to how movement, particularly when codified into dance, becomes indicative of the inner emotional world. While Darwin (1872) is most famous for his pivotal work on evolution, he studied notes on the patients at the Wakefield asylum in England and concluded, "The movement of expression in the face and body … reveal the thoughts and intentions of others more truly than do words, which may be falsified" (p.364). This would be echoed years later by modern dance pioneer Martha Graham: "Movement never lies. It is a barometer telling the state of the soul's weather to all who can read it" (Graham in Carter and O'Shea 2010).

Likewise, Hall (1997) noted, "people in interactions move together in a kind of dance, but they are not aware of their synchronous movement and they do it without music or conscious orchestration" (p.72). The first dance/movement therapists came from the world of modern dance, intermixing their explorations of relationship to elements of space and emotion. As noted by Lauffenburger (2020):

Most uniquely, dance is the core of DMTP (dance/movement therapy/psychotherapy). Dance/movement therapists and our clients dance and/or move expressively together. No other creative arts, body-based, or verbal psychotherapy uses dance as its primary medium. Some therapies use movement, but movement is not the same as dance. DMTP includes movement but focuses on its expressive communication in order to access and engage parts of the self that no exercise, words, or repetitive actions can contact. (p.19)

Out of the modern dance movement there was Denishawn dance in the United States, Mary Wigman from Germany, and Martha Graham (also US) who were all beginning to break away from structured dance and looking more toward natural movement and expression that was gaining acceptance at the same time as the growth of psychotherapy. Graham followed Jungian psychotherapy, along with developing her modern dance company, whereas early dance/movement therapist and performer, Blanche Evan worked with the ideas of Alfred Adler. She believed people needed to take space for themselves and work in free movement (Evan and Benov 1991).

African American dancers in modern dance began to mix cultural and movement vocabulary from traditional African dance and American motifs. Choreographers such as Alvin Ailey created works like the seminal "Cry," featuring Judith Jamison, with movement incorporating pedestrian work actions and evoking church dances. This style of dance in terms of myofascial movement is also more dynamic in terms of fascial recoil and utilizes dynamics from shaping to strong directional movement.

While dance is inherently therapeutic, creating credentials in the formalized field developed over time. In 2009, the ADTA changed the status of its clinical therapists from a registry process to a board certification, allowing many therapists to obtain additional licensing in their respective states. This is still a rigorous process: dance/movement therapists have a minimum of a master's degree in the field with coursework from psychology to movement observation techniques. To practice as a board certified dance/movement therapist (BC-DMT), an additional 3640 hours of supervised work is required.

Group movement structure

In a group dance/movement therapy session (often structured around a circle), the general arc of the group goes through warm up, a way to both physically warm up the body, and to connect on a psychological level. As a theme begins to emerge from the nonverbal dance, the group therapist begins to clarify thematic material, but not dictate the meaning of the movement. The group, along with the therapist, begins to clarify the theme, and the movement also gains clarity, and either effort qualities may be developed, or a repetition of movement. During a cool-down, the time is focused on de-escalation and sharing time. The arts are expressive, and the verbal supportive piece of the group. It is important to support clients to develop their interoceptive abilities since their ability to deintensify experience is an important part of lowering emotional response to trauma.

Finally, there is a part that environment plays in shaping the experience of human movement. Ethnographers Alan Lomax, Irmgard Bartenieff, and Forrestine Pauley explored the concept of environmental space shaping movement in relationship to different folk dance styles in their choreometrics project (Bartenieff and Lewis 1980). Dance traditionally mirrored the cultural space where it was created. However, modern life has decreased the amount of space we explore, and the time we spend outdoors (Segran 2015), resulting in a loss of connection to the physicality of place.

Mirror neurons and mirroring

Mirror neurons have been widely discussed for their possible role in our brains as being responsive to executing an action oneself as well as observing others in movement actions. While there is ongoing debate as to the efficacy of these neurons, Acharya and Shukla (2012) note:

Mirror neurons are one of the most important discoveries in the last decade of neuroscience. These are a variety of visuospatial neurons, which indicate fundamentally about human social interaction. Essentially, mirror neurons respond to actions that we observe in others. The interesting part is that mirror neurons fire in the same way when we actually recreate that action ourselves. Apart from imitation, they are responsible for [a] myriad of other sophisticated human behavior and thought processes. Defects in the mirror neuron system are being linked to disorders like autism. (p.118)

In forms of dance/movement therapy, the first level of engaging nonverbally is often through mirroring the body posture of the other individual. This becomes a form of acknowledgement and body:

Mimicry involves duplicating the external shape of the movement without the emotional content that exists in the dynamics and in the subtle organization of the movement... Chace was aware that answering movement in similar forms dissipates the feeling of apartness... Empathy meant sharing the essence of all nonverbal expression resulting in what she called "direct communication." (Chaiklin and Schmais in Bernstein 1979, pp.26–27)

Kinesthetic empathy

What is kinesthetic empathy?

If I can imagine another person's movement, I can perhaps have insight into their felt experience in the world. The term kinesthetic empathy was coined by Miriam Roskin Berger (1989), who wrote:

our emotional reactions are not only determined in terms of kinesthetic recognition, but in terms of kinesthetic response as well. We assimilate what we perceive into our own present experience ... we may perceive emotional behavior in others and immediately experience it within our own bodies through kinesthetic empathy. (p.170)

This concept has been noted as a pivotal concept in understanding social interaction and communication in various fields from physical therapy to sport (Reynolds 2012).

Body conversation

Find a partner. Your role is to gain a sense of nonverbal body listening. In the first round, watch your partner move as you sit and observe. Your job is to be a silent witness. What do you observe? How do you feel? An appreciation of the emotional state of watching the other person move is part of the concept of kinesthetic empathy.

The Dances Unseen
Nada Khodlova
Are they really? Do they evaporate? Are they gone?

No! They are new pathways into and out of our expanding soul. They lay down new roads out and in. They can overwhelm us with their urgency, power, intensity, and travels to the unknown. They are the voices unknown in us, the wordless void of wounding, the womb spiral of grief let go to catch a star or become a constellation. They are you and they are everyone and everything. Please dance. Dance the unseen. The unknown. The unheard of. The stars are waiting.

The myofascial middle layer: fascia and feeling

Published work in complementary therapies is often non-clinical in nature, and even less has been done between fascia and cognitive work, but the field is growing. Joeri Calsius as an osteopath DO is working as a physical and psychotherapist in psychosomatic work, particularly engaging in fascial work of varied deep myofascial models in trauma. Doug Craig is adding in particular to the field of neuro and psychology in his writings and research in interoceptive movement. More recently, Abraham *et al.* (2020), published in *Complementary Therapies in Clinical Practice* their article "Integrating mental imagery and fascial tissue: A conceptualization for research into movement and cognition." As noted in their abstract, "mental imagery (MI) research has mainly focused to date on mechanisms of effect and performance gains associated with muscle and neural tissues." Their proposal is that MI could be used to work with fascial tissue and that, "MI has the potential to affect and be affected by fascial tissue" (Abraham *et al.* 2020, p.1).

If sports, movement, and therapeutically oriented movement therapies are to progress, the use of the fascial system in concept and movement cuing can help to further our ability to work toward a sense of creating the best health possible for our emotional state, which is tied in and intertwined with our psychological health.

Both our daily actions and our daily emotions are translated in patterns of the body, and held in the fascial system and essentially written in the structure of the body. The body can be celebrated as a gift with appreciation. If we have an issue with the body, emotional or physical, it is only a part of the larger identification of the self and the person in a larger community.

In Calsius (2020), the concept of the myofascial middle layer is presented as including adductors, pelvic floor, iliacus, psoas, diaphragm, and some of the neck and face muscles, echoing similarities to other deep myofascial anatomy, such as Myers's Deep Front Line. Admittedly, the author acknowledges overlaps with other systems. Note his explanation of the myofascial middle line (MML) as:

one of the first to be stimulated in subject development. Functions such as sucking, drinking and swallowing, but also breathing, screaming, crying, digesting, and excreting are not only our most basic functions, they are also our first attempts at processing the outside world. It is interesting to note that many psychosomatic and unexplainable complaints are related to these systems of functioning and regulation—and thus with the uroboric-pranic body and the MML. Just think of hyperventilation in case of panic, digestive complaints or irritable intestines, teeth grinding in case of stress and difficulties in the sexual arena. In other words, these functional systems within the MML appear to be very sensitive to tension and stress. (p.83–84)

Tension and stress are primitive reactions in the body, and in terms of psychotherapy, we can think of stress in both healthy and unhealthy reactions to life situations. In small forms, stress is a healthy reaction and helps us stay alert to the world around us. Under large amounts of stress, the mind is reactive to body sensations, and mental response can be disproportionate or continuous to a stress that may be in the past. When I worked with trauma after the 9/11 World Trade Center collapse, we would let clients know that stress often manifests in the extremes of physical reaction, i.e. one might find themselves sleeping too much or too little, eating large amounts or barely at all. Survival and sensory perception are our interpretations of both internal and external environmental cues.

When the stomach contracts and it is empty, the lack of fascial stretch reception tells the brain that it is hungry. The feeling or pulse between hunger and satiety go between the two halves of the autonomic nervous system. In eating disorders there is a disconnect between perception of what the body is needing nutritionally and the feeling of stretch reception. Those suffering from eating disorders are perhaps ignoring or overriding the fascial sensations in their body system. Perhaps creating more challenge to the fascial system (i.e. challenging the movement pattern) in addition to mindfulness techniques might disengage the body system. Many eating disorders have a root in needing to feel control in perception of self relative to the world around. Instead of controlling the environment (i.e. via food restriction and behaviors), perhaps challenging the system fascially in a new way while creating a deeper parasympathetic response in the

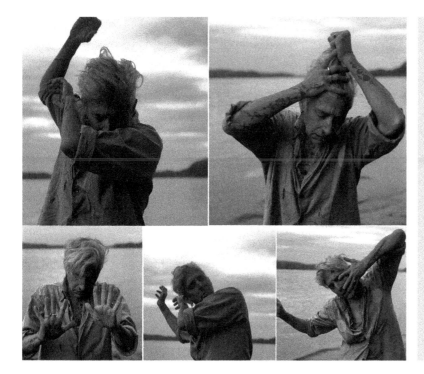

FIGURE 3.3 "While we know living in a human body is tough—what I know is that moving helps. I know that not everyone knows this, but why not? What stands in the way of noticing feelings, sensations, cravings, urges, breath, in other words, motion? We are designed to move; it is our birthright, our nature, our pleasure. We move for health, for connection to self, and perhaps that study of self is in the service of seeking wisdom. I practice lessons I learn from books, but it is my interoception, that inner awareness, that helps me to peer into the landscape within. This is what shapes me, day by day."
—Sondra Loring.

Photos by Kelly Kaam of Sondra Loring.

body might retune a system that has shifted away from noticing positive-self body sensations.

The experience of being human is difficult, but expression through the very body we inhabit can help with positive self-identity and coping (Figure 3.3) in our larger environments, physically, mentally, and emotionally.

Grief vs. growth and cultivation in movement

Sometimes what we so tenderly cultivate is damaged, and letting go for new growth is part of life on many levels. In our myofascial forms, we might hold onto patterns of grief, which immobilize movement and change the range of expressive qualities.

When I was working as a dance/movement therapist, I specialized in trauma work, first with Holocaust survivors, trauma survivors from inner cities, and then in my work post-9/11 after the World Trade Center Towers were hit. Many in the New York metropolitan area experienced re-triggered traumatic flashbacks from past experiences. In Figure 3.4, one client drew for me what she felt like. Noticed the collapsed chest.

In my own later training, this connected to the startle response and the higher level of fast twitch fibers in the front of the body that serve to engage quickly and protect the visceral and vulnerable organs in the front of the body.

The head, the exception to the flexing forward rule, goes into hyperextension of the upper cervical spine (in response to keeping the eyes forwards for danger). The pelvic and respiratory diaphragms have an easy relationship that can be compressed by any restriction of a ribcage. In other words, the lack of responsive movement, similar to the latest studies of major depressive disorder (MDD), may be part of the inability for both mental and physical resiliency.

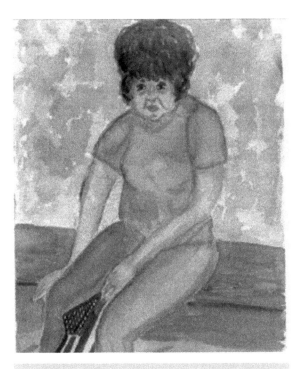

FIGURE 3.4 From author's personal collection. Image originally published in 'Being in the Body: Finding Reconnection after 9/11' (*DTAA Quarterly 3, 2*). The body shape reflects the emotional state.

More recently, I began to wonder at other fascial layers that might also be involved as connecting to a depressed rib cage, whether through grief or breathing issues. Like post-9/11, COVID has brought many of the same types of dual traumas, physical and mental, involving the position of the ribcage (Figure 3.4). In my past work as a dance/movement therapist, I would see clients with shoulders rounded in a protective posture that appeared to try to protect the heart and lungs from vulnerability in the front of the body. This may well have a fascial component in the suprapleural membrane (Figure 3.5).

Costovertebral fascia (other names for the same tissue include Sibson's fascia, cervicothoracic fascia, and suprapleural membrane) is a dense fascial layer. It has attachments to the inner border of

the rib and anterior costal cartilage, C7 transverse process (posteriorly), and with the mediastinal pleura. It also connects to the anterior scalene. This area is closely involved in functionality of the ribs and lateral flexion and rotation in the neck in addition to cradling the brachial plexus and subclavian artery. Sibson's fascia prevents compression on the neurovascular bundle. If our breathing is impacted through either physical or emotional stress, body positioning is likely to be impacted in both cases.

Appropriate touch

Using the appropriate touch is important in DMT work and somatics in general. Folk dance forms in particular utilize touch as part of connection, but often in current environments touch is lost, whether out of fear of lawsuits for sexually inappropriate behaviors or due to viral concerns such as COVID-19.

Somatics

In comparison to dance/movement therapy, "Somatics is the field which studies the *soma*: namely the body as perceived from within by first-person perception" (Hanna 1995, p.341). Dance, up until the performance driven ballet forms were created, was firmly rooted in the communal aspects of primarily line, circle, and couple dances. The individual rhythm was much less important than the overall community. It is interesting to note that the world of somatics has perhaps been populated more with male pioneers, as have the worlds of anatomy and architecture. The world of dance/movement therapy has its pioneers firmly rooted on the female side, with the obvious influences of male thinkers such as Rudolph Laban, whose movement analysis informed movement-related fields from Body/Mind, DMT, and somatics.

More recently, the field of physical literacy, led by pioneers such as Patrice Aubertin, has emerged and reintroduced the importance of early education

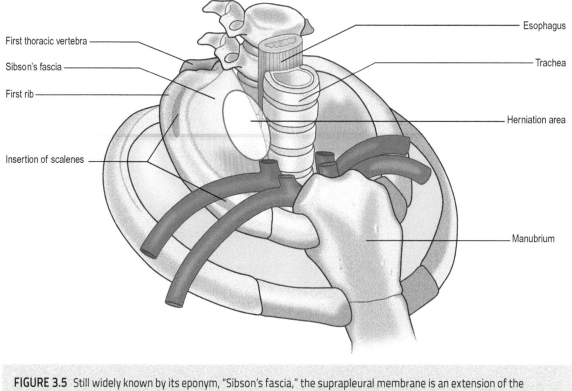

First thoracic vertebra

Sibson's fascia

First rib

Insertion of scalenes

Esophagus

Trachea

Herniation area

Manubrium

FIGURE 3.5 Still widely known by its eponym, "Sibson's fascia," the suprapleural membrane is an extension of the endothoracic fascia.

of movement for functional living and as a base for further recreational activity. As defined by Physical Health and Education Canada, "Individuals who are physically literate move with competence and confidence in a wide variety of physical activities in multiple environments that benefit the healthy development of the whole person" (Physical Health and Education Canada n.d.). In other words, to cultivate physical literacy, there is a need to work the building blocks of movement, rather than sports-specific training. Here again is a desire to create functional movement, instead of cultivating and rewarding individual athletic achievement. *Physical Literacy* also stresses a connection of movement to environment in four major areas: ground (basis for dance, sport, etc.),

water (all aquatic activities, snow, and ice/sliding sports) and aerial (gymnastics, aerial, and diving) (Balyi *et al.* 2005).

Ideokinesis

Originally developed as a somatic protocol to work with injured dancers while they were at rest, this approach was first conceived by Mabel Todd and developed by Lulu Sweigard, Erick Hawkins among many others, and then further developed more recently by Eric Franklin. In many of the approaches, visualization is utilized to suggest to the body a new way of being. This works on interoception in terms of the myofascial body and is a form of predictive coding, or self-fulfilling prophecy used for positive influence.

Many different strands of your past experience begin to weave together until gradually the new direction announces itself. Its voice is sure with the inevitability of the truth. When your life-decisions emerge in this way from the matrix of your experience, they warrant your trust and commitment. When you can choose in this way, you move gracefully within the deeper rhythm of your soul. The geography of your destiny is always clearer to the eye of your soul than to the intentions and needs of your surface mind. (O'Donohue 2002)

The paradox of Cassandra, or why our connected body matters

The paradox of Cassandra is a term used when someone's self-perception is out of sync with the views of others, resulting in psychological distress. It is a term that has been used in contexts from psychology to environmentalism, where the person speaking out isn't validated by those around them.

This concept comes from Greek mythology, where Cassandra was given the gift of prophecy, but cursed with no one being able to believe her forecasts. As the story goes, Cassandra was a young woman working at the Oracle of Delphi. One day, the young god Apollo visited the temple and was intrigued with her. As a son of the gods, he had great powers. He offered her the gift of prophecy if he could give her a kiss (we will leave the issue of "me too" amongst the Greek gods and goddesses for another time). She studied with him, but didn't return his affections, and he cursed her with the ability to predict the future while having the torture of both being treated with disbelief by everyone around her and being unable to change or have others consider her reality. In our modern age, we face the paradox of Cassandra often in situations where our felt perceptions of the body are out of sync with what is around us. We are often dulling our body and its felt perception. Hopefully, unlike Cassandra, we can break the cycle and change our body story.

Context and shape of the system

Context, from social to cultural, matters to the biological system. If we live in a society where certain ethnic groups encounter prejudice, access to the fascial skills that help the body system may be denied to those who could benefit the most. Breastfeeding mothers in Israel, for example, have been found to produce less milk under stress. The mind–body interaction is not an area of training for most doctors, and yet the connections between trauma and illness are high. Trauma often leads to more trauma. When I was working as a therapist post-9/11, the first cases we saw were those with past traumas, particularly body related. The first person I worked with was a Hungarian woman who had survived the concentration camps during the Holocaust. As she watched the Twin Towers burn, she had vivid flashbacks about smoke from incineration chambers she had witnessed. What we first did together was a czardas (Hungarian folk dance) to put a simple rhythm back into her body. As noted by biopsychosocial thinker Dr. Gabor Maté, "the more specialized doctors become, the more they know about a body part or organ and the less they tend to understand the human being in whom that part or organ resides…" (Maté 2011). In Maté's approach to compassionate injury, the therapist or doctor can look at why a person chose an addiction, for example, but instead of condemning the person or the addictive substance, one looks at what it did for them without judgement, and to reframe and understand where in the body things can be reframed. The idea is not to place judgment on a behavior but to give it understanding. In other words, provide context and shape to the situation.

In terms of the "me too" movement, there is still a blame culture where victims need to prove they haven't dressed inappropriately. The same is true for marginalized ethnic groups that have to be careful of the way they dress or hold themselves, lest they be mistaken for a criminal.

College campuses and workplaces still have posters aimed at women on how to avoid being assaulted, or advice on emergency numbers to contact if they have been, but rarely do we hear about campaigns aimed at would-be aggressors. Many of those victimized show a collapse in the front of the body, as if to hide the sexual organs deeper into body.

Early in my therapy career, I worked with inner city Baltimore kids at a "high needs" school, many of whom had been abused by the time they were in preschool. One 5-year-old brought a loaded gun to the school and swung it around. I don't believe he really had intent to harm, but he was following a movement pattern that he was part of, the pattern of movement from his home environment. He was able to be calmly disengaged from the gun through distraction about a game he enjoyed on the playground. Both swinging the gun and the playground game were practicing life actions through play and movement. We can do a lot in shaping children's experiences positively by having environment and movement sensations that are healthy.

Take care of the inner body by feeling outside of the body

For many, the inner body sensations are very overwhelming and are connective with past traumatic or perceived traumatic experiences. In the case of misperception, sometimes memory in an anxious person will create a felt sensation of past trauma that is reinforced by uncomfortable inner sensations. Often the trauma survivors, including sexually abused victims will be dissociative in their body reactions. Starting with external sensations (gravity, hard touch, resistance) is often powerful in organizing body literacy so work can begin internally. This is often labelled as exteroceptive awareness. This is why people in recreational or professional sports as well as movement disciplines from dance to mindfulness work in yoga practice and more often find breakthroughs in their ability to work into more balanced being in the body system. In dance/movement therapy this is often taught as ability to access different movement qualities, or efforts (in the Laban system, for example). In terms of myofascial systems, we could think of the ability to balance the lines. If someone is challenged emotionally, having more movement possibilities gives greater ability for richer expression.

References

Abraham, A., Franklin, E., Stecco, C. and Schleip, R. (2020) 'Integrating mental imagery and fascial tissue: A conceptualization for research into movement and cognition.' *Complementary Therapies in Clinical Practice 40*, 101193. https://doi.org/10.1016/j.ctcp.2020.101193

Acharya, S. and Shukla, S. (2012) 'Mirror neurons: Enigma of the metaphysical modular brain.' *Journal of Natural Science, Biology and Medicine 3*, 2, 118. https://doi.org/10.4103/0976-9668.101878

American Dance Therapy Association (n.d.-a) *Definition*. Accessed on 12/28/2019 at https://adta.org

American Dance Therapy Association (n.d.-b) *What Is Dance/Movement Therapy?* Accessed on 11/15/2021 at https://adta.memberclicks.net/what-is-dancemovement-therapy

Balyi, I., Way, R., Norris, S., Cardinal, C. and Higgs, C. (2005) *Canadian Sport for Life: The Role of Monitoring Growth in Long-term Athlete Development.* Ottawa: Canadian Sport Centres.

Berger, M. R. (1989) 'Bodily experience and expression of emotion.' In J. Fried, S. Katz, S. Kleinman and J. Naess (eds) *Toward a Body of Knowledge: A Collection of Early Writings.* Vol. 1. Columbia, MD: American Dance Therapy Association.

Bernstein, P. (ed.) (1979) *Eight Theoretical Approaches in Dance-movement Therapy.* Dubuque, IA: Kendall Hunt Publishing Company.

Bordoni, B. and Marelli, F. (2017) 'Emotions in motion: myofascial interoception.' *Complementary Medicine Research 24*, 2, 110–113. https://doi.org/10.1159/000464149

Calsius, J. (2020) *Treating the Psychosomatic Conflict: In Search of a Transdisciplinary Framework for the Integration of Bodywork in Psychotherapy.* Abingdon, UK: Routledge.

Carter, A. and O'Shea, J. (eds) (2010) *The Routledge Dance Studies Reader*. Abingdon, UK: Routledge.

Darwin, C. (1872) *The Expression of the Emotions in Man and Animals*. London: John Murray. https://doi.org/10.1037/10001-000

Evan, B. and Benov, R. G. (eds) (1991) *Collected Works by and about Blanche Evan, Unedited: Dancer, teacher, writer, dance/movement/word therapist*, January 28, 1909–December 24, 1982. New York, NY: Blanche Evan Dance Foundation.

Hall, E. T. (1997) *Beyond Culture*. New York, NY: Anchor Books.

Lauffenburger, S. K. (2020) '"Something more": the unique features of dance movement therapy/psychotherapy.' *American Journal of Dance Therapy* 42, 1, 16–32. https://doi.org/10.1007/s10465-020-09321-y

Levy, F. (1992) *Dance/Movement Therapy: A Healing Art*. Revised ed. Reston, VA: American Alliance for Health, Physical Education, Recreation and Dance (AAHPERD).

Lieberman, D. (2020) *Exercised: Why Something we Never Evolved to do is Healthy and Rewarding*. New York, NY: Pantheon Books.

Maté, G. (2011) *When the Body Says No: Exploring the Stress–disease Connection*. Hoboken, NJ: J. Wiley.

Michalak, J., Aranmolate, L., Bonn, A., Grandin, K. *et al.* (2021) 'Myofascial tissue and depression.' *Cognitive Therapy and Research*. https://doi.org/10.1007/s10608-021-10282-w

O'Donohue, J. (2002) *Eternal Echoes: Celtic Reflections on our Yearning to Belong*. New York, NY: Harper Perennial.

Physical Health and Education Canada (n.d.) *Physical Literacy*. Ottawa: PHE Canada. https://phecanada.ca/activate/physical-literacy

Reynolds, D. (ed.) (2012) *Kinesthetic empathy in creative and cultural practices*. Bristol: Intellect.

Schoop, T. (1974) *Won't You Join The Dance?: A Dancer's Essay into the Treatment of Psychosis*. Mountain View, CA: Mayfield Publishing Company.

Segran, E. (2015) 'Mayo Clinic launches ambitious study on how being indoors all the time affects us.' *Fast Company*, October 6, 2015. https://www.fastcompany.com/3051894/mayo-clinic-launches-ambitious-study-on-how-being-indoors-all-the-time

Further reading

Acarón, T. (2016) 'Shape-in(g) space: body, boundaries, and violence.' *Space and Culture*, 19, 2, 139–149. https://doi.org/10.1177/1206331215623208

Bartenieff, I. and Lewis, D. (1980) *Body Movement: Coping with the Environment*. Philadelphia, PA: Gordon and Breach Science Publishers.

Bloomgarden, A., Mennuti, R. and Cohen, E. (2003) 'Therapist self-disclosure: Implications for the therapeutic connection.' *The Renfrew Center Working Papers* 1.

Hemenway, P. (2005) *Divine Proportion: Phi in Art, Nature, and Science*. New York, NY: Sterling Publishing Co.

Ingber, D. E. (2008) 'Tensegrity and mechanotransduction.' *Journal of Bodywork and Movement Therapies* 12, 3, 198–200. https://doi.org/10.1016/j.jbmt.2008.04.038

Mallorquí-Bagué, N., Garfinkel, S. N., Engels, M., Eccles, J. A. *et al.* (2014) 'Neuroimaging and psychophysiological investigation of the link between anxiety, enhanced affective reactivity and interoception in people with joint hypermobility.' *Frontiers in Psychology* 5. https://doi.org/10.3389/fpsyg.2014.01162

van der Kolk, B. (n.d.) *How Trauma Lodges in the Body*. The On Being Project. Accessed on 12/29/2019 at https://onbeing.org/programs/bessel-van-der-kolk-how-trauma-lodges-in-the-body

When one tugs at a single thing in nature, he finds it attached to the rest of the world.

John Muir

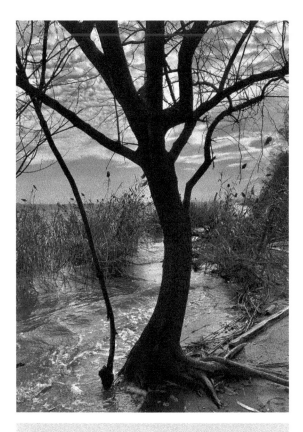

FIGURE 4.1 Trees respond to their genetic code, but also to the environmental space around them.

Photo by the author.

There are as many systems of body analysis as there are maps of the myofascial connections. Learning how to communicate in these different languages allows descriptive power for problem solving and strategies to work with the body. Models and maps are both useful constructs with some inherent challenges. We will unwind some of the different ways of seeing and how to work that within the concept of myofascia.

Whole body mapping

The shape of a life gets written into a body. When we look at a body donor in anatomy lab, I often tell students that what remains is like a seashell, shaped and curved by life, genetics, environment, ideas, values, and more. Even if I have a past medical history and "cause of death," I can't fully ever understand a person's own lived life experience, the pains or triumphs that have written themselves into the warp and weft of the body's myofascia, bones, and more. In looking at posture, we also risk imposing our own prejudices and opinions as well as reducing a person to a judgment rather than expressing compassion. In the best use, understanding ways of seeing a person can help unwrap a story and create a strategy for better movement.

People are infinitely more complicated than a cursory postural analysis of any sort can determine. Those twists and turns, like a tree responding to weather patterns and where it planted roots (Figure 4.1), are sometimes what make us interesting instead of problems to be corrected. There are not good or bad stances, but rather what works optimally. Finding the positive features in any person's shape is key. I often hear people ask me if I can give them verbal help about a client that has "an ACL tear" or "is suffering from a car accident." While this information has its place, it is not very useful in approaching an individual person and their reaction to the world. When we acknowledge three things that are going on well in the body and whole system, we are starting from the place of understanding what resources the client has.

Why do we need to describe the body system? How do we describe that body system in motion? If I gaze at a beautiful painting, or even at the landscape on my daily walk, I am taking in the whole picture as well as the individual components. Hemenway

Drawing the body—what shape and form do we take onto a piece of paper?

When we think of the shape of a person, what form does that take? It relies on the perceptions of what we can conceive and understand, and how the patterns at work in nature express themselves in different ways. Take a moment to use a blank piece of paper to draw a "body." No peeking at any atlases or notes, although you are free to reference your own body. Think of how you define the body's shape and form. What do you include in your drawing, what is left out?

Let's go by some common forms that the body is known for. If you draw a skeleton of the body, what do you remember and what do you leave out? What is your perspective for this exercise? If we are drawing a skeleton, how do you imagine that skeleton? In other words, are you choosing a general concept of a skeleton or a specific skeleton that has a gender orientation? Perspective is an interesting choice—do you draw it from the anterior, posterior, or (rarer still) a side or angled viewpoint? How do you think this may have been different at different points in history? Let's shift and take a moment to draw the muscular body. Again, what layer do you chose to depict? Or how do you conceive different levels of the body?

Finally, try drawing the fascial body. How do you choose to represent this form? Just like the muscle body, the fascial body is difficult to conceive. At what layer do you focus your attention? Do you link in your mind via connections or large septa?

(2005) notes, "Art is an experience of balance, of the relationship of its parts to the whole." These are two questions that typically arise in movement workshops that I have both taught and attended throughout the years. What practitioners of all stripes have typically "known" as intuition in working with another moving body can often be conveyed through a "way of seeing" or "movement reading" system. As humans, we have a strong need, no matter our holistic intents, to uniquely name things. This is of course useful for directions and finding places. One example is the US Postal Service Zone Improvement Plan (ZIP) codes. While this is a uniquely American term, of course other countries have postal codes or descriptions of place that help create a path to get a parcel from one place to another. If I want to describe a pattern that has happened, or predict and movement action to come, I need a way to describe that.

What you choose to read affects what you will be looking to see, of course. If I go to my doctor with an injury, I do need them to convey precise information on that injury to another professional. Sue Black, a forensic anatomist, notes:

Experts learn to read different parts of the body for their own purposes. A clinician will look to the soft tissue and organs for signs of disease and a clinical pathologist may examine biopsies of tumours or categorize changes in cells to establish the nature or progression of a pathology or condition. The forensic pathologist will focus on the cause and manner of the death while the forensic toxicologist analyses body fluids... (Black 2021)

For those of us in movement it is really not about an exact diagnosis, but rather the ability to ask smarter questions to unravel a story. For the artist, it is about spatial relationships. For the anatomist, it may be the naming of parts, to describe the internal and external geography.

In mapping the body, we can see twhat many of these body systems and ways of seeing are built around a concept or construct to frame the body and give it meaning. The movement analysis system of Laban is built around the shape of the isohedron. Anatomical language is built around planes of motion. A map is built around the geography of landforms and charts around bodies of water. We can "build" in both theory and living tissue a different understanding that can shift and change the way we relate to movement in the multitude of needs for us as humans, from sports performance, creative expression and negotiating daily life actions like walking and sitting at our computer desks.

I began my anatomy career as an art historian. Even in my master's degree, I used my early skill-set from visual assessment in one project where I recorded emotional reactions expressed after viewing works of art. I contrasted the state treatment-resistant schizophrenic population I worked with during an internship with "general" population responses. It didn't surprise me that the state hospital patients often perceived reactions of sadness or anger quite differently, and opposite from others. Anger and sadness were often confused. How they, in essence, read the posture of others was a mismatch of perception from others that often created challenges in communication and expression.

I have taken my skills into anatomical work as well, whether to problem solve through an artistic dissection, or to understand the posture and movement of my clients. There is really no such thing as "correct" posture, but there are without a doubt, ways that the body can be held, that amount to less caloric effort as well as easier ways of functioning. However, it would be incorrect to assume we should look a certain way. While resiliency is critical for all bodies, high level sports and different movement disciplines may have strengths in asymmetry, and of course, the body, anatomically, is not symmetrical in form. Our heart sits slightly to the left side of our chest, the liver high and on the right side (except in rare cases of situs inversus where organs appear on the opposite side, as in a mirror image from the large majority of humans). However, even in such cases, the body is asymmetrical.

Fascia is intimately connected with our body shape and with posture itself. As noted by Richter *et al.* (2019), "Posture tone and necessary adaptations to externally induced postured changes are provided by muscle spindles, Golgi's corpuscles in ligaments and capsules. Muscles play an active role in this process, while fasciae constitute a connecting element." Due to fascia's omnipresence in the body, it is highly responsive to environmental changes, whether in the physical sense of how the body is challenged or in a psychological state. Pressure will trigger more fiber to be laid down, essentially strapping down myofascial layers. Posturing, much of how we present ourselves out into the world, comes from years of how we have dealt with the world, emotionally and physically.

How do you stand? The Latin etymology for any form of standing has its cousin in the word for stability. However, the anatomical stance is not a natural place to be in for a long time. According to one definition, per Merriam-Webster (2021), stability is "the property of a body that causes it, when disturbed from a condition of equilibrium or steady motion to develop forces or movements that restore the original condition." The ability of the body to be responsive to the environment is admirable, but in the moving body we might want to take this one step further to being able to be even more responsive to the forces around.

Although many people will claim to have no knowledge or ability of a body interpretation system, we do look at our own and other people's postural patterns all the time in common language. We wonder if someone is able to "stand on their own two feet" (seen as strong) or to be able to "shoulder" a problem (seen as being able to take on the emotional weight of a situation). We interpret behaviors all the time and key into other people's patterns and movements.

Posture is often seen as static, but body analysis of any kind needs to take into consideration the dynamic body. If posture is static, how does the body work well dynamically in movement? This has an important part both in the emotional body as well in a sports specific practice. Patterns that are working well can be developed, but in both sports and an easy experience in the emotional body, there is an importance in being able to utilize a pattern when needed, but also to be able to access a different pattern as necessary.

In my years working as a therapist we often looked at movement patterns and the ability to access different patterns as needed. Any strong emotion, postitive or negative, can alter the body system and the ability to access appropriate emotional response when needed. The fascial system changes slowly, and because of those slow changes, the concept of time in training is important. Patterns are disrupted either through slow sustained movement, or a repetition of movement changes. In other words, your body changes can affect your psychological changes and vice versa. Let's relate it back to our metaphoric meal. Just as we eat a variety of foods in our diet in order to function at our optimal level, we need the same sort of nutritional variety in our myofascial movement. Variation in movement and in nutrition is just as important as quantity. If I run the same path, or lift at the same weight machine daily, I won't have the resilience needed for the unexpected strains on the system.

Athletes often strive for that extra millisecond shaved off a performance record, and most of us want to move easier throughout life. For many of my own students and clients, we talk about wanting to do more of their favorite activities with less effort. This is efficiency. The desired result comes about with less waste, whether metabolic or in any other sense.

When we are looking at an anatomical dissection, we are always making choices of what to take away in order to see another structure, or system. Something is always obscured to see something else. In a similar manner, if we have a plan for movement, we can know our end goal and figure out the most efficient means of getting there, making choices. For example, when I kayak, I have a plan for going from point A to point B. How I get there depends on a lot of factors, from tide, current, wind, weather conditions, and my skill in paddling, as well as additional factors such as the boat I chose to use. We begin our life outside the womb on an inhalation and exit our final time on earth with an exhalation. If we know the general framework, we can plan our approach as best we can, knowing the factors we have some control over. There is room for a lot of improvisation and individual creativity within a system.

There is the caveat, however, that while some absolutes are known, there are a lot of curveballs thrown into the mix. Resilience is needed for both body and mind as life is about the unpredictable. Each and every time I'm in dissection lab I have seen some anatomical variation that is not the "normal." There is so much that goes well in the body, but even our anatomical oddities are often the body's creative way to deal with the life it has gone through. What we see in the donors on the table are the remains of their life lived, much in the same way we look at a seashell and see the remains of the life carved into the body system. The actual life (apart from an active microbiome) is no longer present and, of course, the motivation of movement has left, even as we might be able to see the artifacts of the movement quality of that body system.

The variations always astound students. I know for myself that I continue to be fascinated by dissection because each and every body on the dissection table is as diverse as each and every body we meet on the street. Why should this be a surprise? Somehow, we have grown so used to standardized textbooks and images of the body that the model of one becomes the avatar of all. Skeletons that are studied in a classroom are often taken as an absolute for the shape and architecture of the body, but we see the variations in lab of ribcages shaped by asthma, a bone broken and healed, the enormous variations in the pelvis. Fascia likewise can vary tremendously.

About a year ago, while scrolling through a social media page for movement teachers, I came across a question essentially asking, "Studying anatomy, is it useful, necessary or completely unnecessary?" If you have this book in your hand, I'm imagining you have a strong interest in applying anatomy to the body, but in this this forum I was fascinated to watch the dialogue unfold from the cries of "absolutely" to "not at all," as well as the occasional "it depends," implying that context matters. Audience and understanding matter to how we should engage in discussion. If I am discussing movement with other scientists or even a client, having a deeper vocabulary and visual knowledge can enrich the picture and give us more possibilities. However, language can be alienating. Think of how you explain your knowledge to a client or doctor. Can you keep the description accurate without being condescending or patronizing? Does your language convey the quality of movement as well? Also, it may be a lovely thing to name the myofascial connections in the foot, but if I can't use that knowledge to fix plantar fascia pain, it won't matter to me as a client or someone who wants to run the trail.

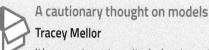

A cautionary thought on models

Tracey Mellor

It's easy to get excited about models, but in my opinion, models should come with a warning or caution that they are not reality.

Models are at best simplifications of complicated concepts, communicating a novel idea in a familiar or visual form.

Think of a tube (subway, metro) poster at the station. The poster has been created by a graphic designer using color and pictures to represent the destination, direction, and order of stations. Compared with a road map it will bear only a passing resemblance to reality.

Models have always been used to help explain how the body moves. As technology and research techniques advance, it is inevitable that models of concepts we have grown up with and relied upon will be improved upon, replaced, surpassed, or even disproved. Some models have been used for centuries, perhaps because there has been no reason to question them. Some models are more fleeting before being surpassed by a new idea. The speed of change often follows the speed of new technology, a gaining of momentum in an area of interest, a spark of genius, political intervention, or dare I say, commercial returns.

Whole careers or reputations can be wiped out when a new model is published. The evangelical fervor of the new model's promoters coming head to head with a conservative old guard. But who is right? Is there a right or wrong? Can a model ever be declared right and, if it is, should it be called a law?

Surely there can be space for more than one model to explain movement. In the world of the movement teacher or therapist which model should they use? In reality, what usually happens is that they will use the most appropriate for that client based upon their experience and the situation. After all, what is more important: the rightness of the model or the outcome of its application?

How to assess the body like an art historian

Only by art can we get outside ourselves, instead of seeing only one world, our own, we see it under multiple forms.

Marcel Proust

Analysis of art and science has similar features and can help develop a similar skill set. Art historians spend hours sitting in front of paintings, sculptures, and other works of art, often drawing on and assessing essential elements of that work in relationship to the larger context of the artist's life or historical relevance. Based on my own background, these questions are some of the most essential I have found to both art and movement analysis.

What do you see?

An assessment can be a neutral listing of a work, for example, I can describe an artist print in the following manner:

The work is a woodcut depicting a snowy February scene. The entire image is in black and white. Light pours in from the right side of the image, illuminating a pine tree. Broad, thick strokes create a sense of groundness to the scene.

In the body it may be a description of the injury, pattern, or relationship.

What do you feel?

In art analysis we consider how the work impacts the viewer. Shape, pattern, motif, and colors can influence the expression of emotion. In a body analysis, first impression is important and often accurate to the overall expression of the body, i.e. does this body look confident? Efficient? Exhausted? It can also give the therapist or trainer ideas if this is a client that brings energy to their work.

What is its context?

In the body there is also often judgement on different cultural differences in movement patterns as well as what is considered culturally appropriate spatial use.

What category would you place this under?

In art history, categories can be utilized for styles of art or periods of work within an artist's work.

Likewise in the body, we might be looking at a particular time period in this person's history (i.e. a pregnancy which might be affecting the body's laxity).

What is it trying to convey?

Art is often a commentary, a way of storytelling or invoking conversation. In the body, the most obvious "conversation" may not be the most important. For example, a raised shoulder might be related to a pain in the front of the body.

How does time affect the perspective of this work?

In art history there is the perspective of the relationship of a piece of work to the great elements of history surrounding its creation and validation (or lack thereof). In the body, time and life lived is reflected in the current state and the story that the body is trying to tell is often readily apparent.

The meander map

This meander map (Figure 4.2) was created by the cartographer Harold Fisk in 1944 and shows the paths of the Mississippi over time. As a kayaker I know this concept of river changes and how, despite the best efforts of Army Corps of Engineers to keep the boundaries of land and water exact, they shift and change. The general flow of a river may continue, but the exact contours it shapes change over time creating variations on a theme.

Waves are disturbances (vibrational) that travel through a medium. Interestingly, a wave where the oscillation direction is perpendicular to the path on which it is travelling is called transverse (e.g. water and light waves), whereas in longitudinal waves, the oscillation is parallel to the wave's direction (e.g. sound and ultrasound waves). Here again, we are conceptualizing directionality. In the case of a river there is little impedance, or stopping of the flow (i.e. in simple terms, resistance). The Mississippi flows generally south and has changed course due to avulsion of where deposits of sediment cause the water to find a more direct path. The Hudson River where I kayak is tidal, meaning there are long-period waves that move up and down in response to forces. High tide is when water is at its highest advance into a shoreline, and low tide is the retreat to the lowest level. In the case of the Hudson River, that is in response to the rise and fall of the water at the mouth of the river.

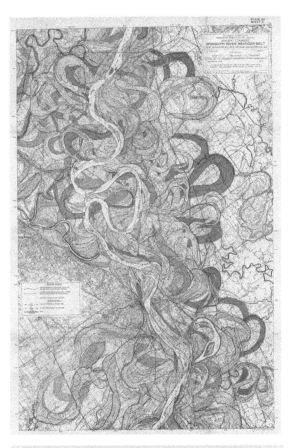

FIGURE 4.2 A meander map has movement and can resemble a shift of myofascial lines. Use the "How to Assess the Body like an Art Historian" guidelines to look at this picture again. *Meander Map of the Mississippi River*, Harold Fisk, 1944. (https://publicdomainreview.org).

How does this relate to fascia? General patterns due to DNA, environment, or even the route of the myofascial connections may influence the shape of the body. However, the meander map reminds us that we also continue to shift and change, and our watery myofascial medium is carving new pathways all the time.

Historically, Albinus negated asymmetry in the human body:

Crest and grooves of the bones, holes for nerves and blood vessels were systematically obliterated or relocated if they did not fit symmetrically and the corresponding notion of beauty and balance. In line with this, he also strived for a congruence between left and right, asking Wandelaar to draw only one half of a bone and copy the other half after folding the paper. By this procedure, Albinus paradoxically eliminated vital structures for the sake of symmetry—in his view a symbol of vitality—and sacrificed the vitality of form to the wholly dominating consistency of the pencil strokes. (Hildebrand 2005, p.561)

Pattern recognition

Pattern recognition includes cognate fields such as image processing, computer vision, analysis, and neural networks. A journal with the same name was established over 50 years ago in response to rapidly changing concepts in computer science, and the concept is now used in classifying objects based on key features through algorithms. According to Myers:

Pattern recognition in posture and movement is a central skill to what we could call "spatial medicine", the study of how we develop, how we stand, handle loads, move through our environment and occupy space—as well as how we perceive our bodily selves. (Myers 2020, p.1)

The diverse experts in movement fields can add to our pattern recognition in the body. In utilizing myofascial constructs, one can recognize the involvement of different lines or in effort qualities and then work through strategies for integration. Pattern recognition also deals with temporal dimensions and the concept of what is the desired goal and how we get there, as well as the important idea of the way to accomplish this action. We can see the body in many different conceptual ways from a building, to a machine, to the tensegral model that will be discussed in these pages more in relationship to fascia. In the years to come, there will doubtless be additional ways not only to conceptualize the body but also to think about pattern recognition (Figure 4.3).

History of plumb and governing lines

The plumb line comes from the lead weight that was hung on the end of a string and left to hang down from the gravitational pull of the earth, determining verticality. Architecture has the concept of "regulating lines," which have a proportional sense of balance between proportional items. The grid line often drops a plumb line through the body and in relationship to gravity. These grids, still used in many practices as a means of looking at body reading, miss the three-dimensional spatial relationship that has been critical to newer systems of body reading.

So where did this idea come from? Anatomist Christian Wilhelm Braune (along with his student Otto Fischer) took the military posture and dropped a plumb line as a measure of superlative posture (Braune and Fischer 1987). Braune could easily be written off as a quick side note in our study of anatomy, fascia, and movement, but Braune was also a dissector who furthered the studies of frozen cadavers (which preserves more of the fascial tissues). He co-authored another book with Fischer entitled *Der Gang des Menschen 1885–1904* (later translated as *The Human Gait*) which remains an important precursor to modern gait analysis.

We are not looking for "perfect" posture but rather, a real posture that is functional for the body system. While no motor nerves go to the fascia, we can think of the brain and movement in conversation with the brain listening to your fascia via the receptors

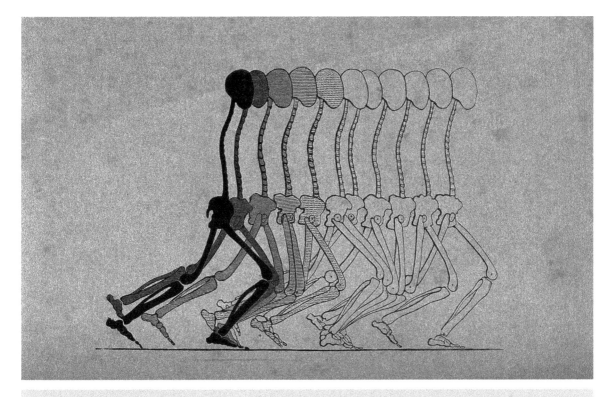

FIGURE 4.3 Our eyes look for patterns, both in static movement as well as in movement sequences, like a gait pattern.

Credit: A skeleton in motion. Lithograph, 18—. Wellcome Collection. Public Domain Mark.

as a listening device, and then "talking" to the muscles as a response. Also, an elite athlete often has a functional asymmetry that may, in fact, help their performance. Shape itself is written even right down to the bones. In the case of a body like mine, with a slight scoliosis, the asymmetry shows up in the face as well. Shape in a body can be about self-perception, reflective of environment and genetic factors, and definitely about the shape of the fascia system, which holds onto patterns.

If we look at people against a grid, we are missing the full shape of things, pun intended. If we looked at movement from Newton (for every action there is an equal and opposite reaction) just a moment ago, we are now moving into the idea of a more Einsteinian approach based on relativity. Relativity is everything. Changing shape, in terms of even moving from one foot to another, requires a force change and stability issue. If we continue with the idea of the body as a tensegral structure (with the theoretical caveat again that it is still a theoretical model), we look at the body posture as a nested tensegrity system.

Any compensation pattern starts as thought turning into gesture, habit, and then a pattern that develops into the tissue. Most of these really begin as neurological patterns. Fascial patterns follow the nervous system. There is a critical idea to takeaway in movement and anatomy. Movement is constantly reshaping anatomy. As Hedley (in Dalton 2011) notes:

When movement is called for, tissues dissolve and reorient accordingly. Where stillness reigns, the physical, material support for stillness is assembled. What you do is what you get. Nature is at our service in this regard. We supply the intention, consciously or unconsciously, on purpose or by accident, and nature supplies the form whereby that intention is made manifest. (p.69)

The book *Muscles: Testing and Function with Posture and Pain* (Kendall *et al.* 2005), now in its fifth edition, is another way of categorizing body types from "ideal" to "kyphosis lordosis" and several more. Utilized by many physical therapists and more, it is a quick reference for muscles that may be tight or weak. The goal is restoring alignment that creates efficiency in the body and "muscle balance." While it does not address myofascial posture, it does continue to have a similar concept of one part of the body affecting another.

In Aristides (2018), the author notes:

A great drawing always starts with an emotional response to your subject. Look past the details and likeness and, instead, focus on your subject's hidden essential patterns and structures. Often, this is no more than a single repeating line direction, or just a few dynamic angles, but the result is like a storyline that summarizes a whole book. You can actually draw these lines in your image, or just keep them in your mind, allowing them to subtly influence your drawing as it develops.

Where fascia holds form

If we think of what in the body holds form, we can look toward the fascial net or web like a giant open-weave blanket in the body. If it is pulled aggressively, it may deform. A snag can create need for repair. Stitch it up too quickly and the tight fibers will pull together but create an area of weakness in the surrounding fabric. Negate an injury, and a hole might enlarge and create an area of weakness around the tighter, overstitched fibers. Fascia also creates strength and stability in other places like the cross fibers of the sacral lumbar fascia (Figure 4.4).

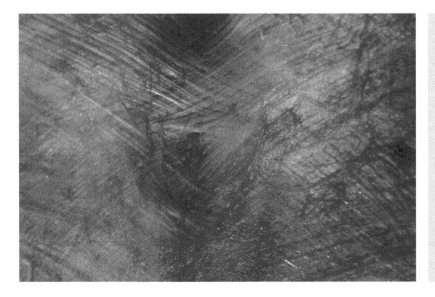

FIGURE 4.4 Cross fibers sacral lumbar fascia.

Photo by Lydia Mann, KNMLabs (author's dissection).

Movement and rest

In conceptualizing the body in motion, we have to keep in mind that it does at times need to rest in order to be ready for more activity or expression. As noted by Beach (2010):

Movement is the coherent changing of shape—some shapes we assume are more fundamental than others. Like the notes that underlie music, I suggest that some postures, particularly floor-based postures of repose, tune out bodies... We need to consider both sides of the coin, that is, both rest and movement...

Interestingly, rest for most of us does not involve standing in anatomic position, so is there value in assessing the resting body in terms of looking at a holistic view of body patterns?

Langer's lines: what are they important for?

Langer's lines (also known as cleavage lines) (Figure 4.5a) are lines that appear in dermis, parallel to collagen fibers. These lines are all about shape and are reminiscent of the patterning in wood (Figure 4.5b). These lines were named after the Australian anatomist, Karl Langer, who punctured the skin in cadavers, noticing an ellipsoidal shape in the holes that were made, and that the connections of these made ring like lines. They are sometimes studied by surgeons for the directionality of the lines that are best for surgical incisions to create minimal tension in wound healing. In other words,

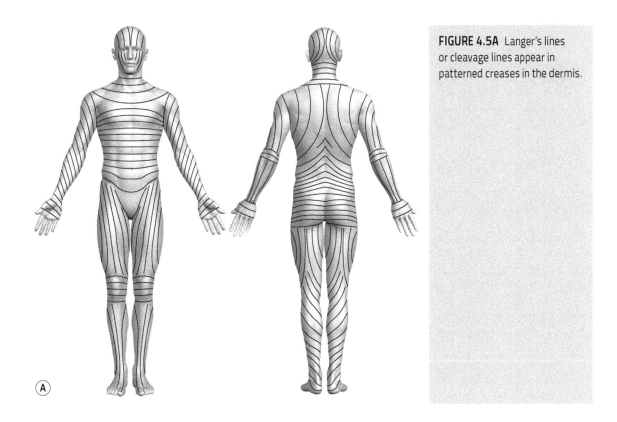

FIGURE 4.5A Langer's lines or cleavage lines appear in patterned creases in the dermis.

these topographical lines can affect cosmetic and functional outcome for patients if their surgeon has an eye toward keeping incisions parallel to these lines (Lemperie 2020).

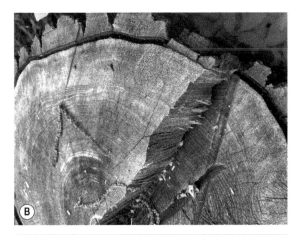

FIGURE 4.5B The grain of wood shows a similar pattern to Langer's Lines in the body. Every year, the layer (called cambium) just under the bark surface divides. Tree rings are related to the vascular changes in a tree's system from year to year. While Langer's Lines are on one layer of the body, stronger areas of fascia do sometimes appear like tree rings in adipose tissue, perhaps serving as a reinforcement layer during periods of weight gain, loss, or other trauma.

Photo by the author.

Body communication

In any system of body assessment, we must also recognize that our concept of knowledge may not match with someone else's self-perception of body reality and this mismatch may lead to prejudice which may be cultural, gender-identity focused. In a living body, we are always in motion; although many systems of body assessment are static, for our purposes we are interested in how the posture of the body works in motion.

On a basic level, take the sacroiliac (SI) joint which needs to have some degree of freedom, but also a great deal of stabilization. It functions well in the standing position over the seated position and assessment must be considered in both actions.

Laban and the concept of efforts

Laban Movement Analysis (LMA) and Bartenieff work

Laban Movement Analysis (LMA) is a theoretical system for explaining movement qualities and is used both for interpretation of movement, notation of performance in movement, and documentation in fields like dance/movement therapy but also with actors, musicians, choreographers, business consultants, athletes, and more. This system was named after Rudolf von Laban (1879–1958) who looked toward geometry as a means of explaining how people move, work, and express themselves in space (Figure 4.6).

While Laban and Buckminster Fuller were contemporaries, it is unclear if they ever overlapped or were aware of each other's ideas. However, the times seemed to have encouraged a parallel development.

This is important for several reasons. In the movement world, the concepts from Laban's work, and later into Bartenieff and others, helped to conceptualize space and movement expression. Buckminister Fuller, of course, overlapped into the science world, impacting the thought process in cell biologist Donald Ingber, Nobel Prize physicist Frank Wilczek, and into the world of tensegrity and fascia. Shapes and geometric forms have interested humans for centuries. Although similar sets of shapes have been found earlier, Euclid in 300 BCE outlined (in *Elements of Geometry*) what are known as the five "Platonic Solids" which are found throughout nature and art, including the isohedron used by Laban in his movement theories (Figure 4.6). More recently, scientists gave a nod to his contribution in naming Buckminster-fullerene (a molecule named after the geodesic dome architect that we know for his work on tensegrity). Likewise, you may have encountered the same form in the children's toy of magnetic Buckyballs.

A brief look into the movement of Laban

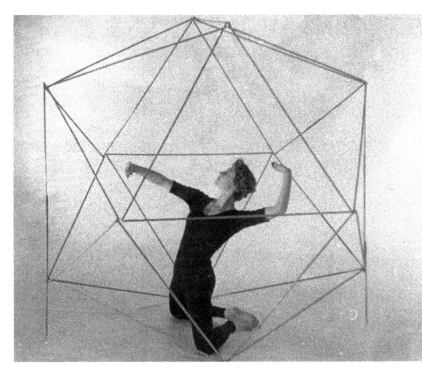

FIGURE 4.6 *Body: What* is moving? This is where we find connection—internal connections and awareness of interoception. *Effort: How* is it moving? This is the space to find the dynamic expression of the body. *Space: Where* is it moving? Develop presence in the world, in particular in how the body interacts with the larger environment. *Shape: Why* is the body moving in this way? Woman in center of geodesic structure, n.d. (L/F/4/88). From the Rudolf Laban Archive, University of Surrey, © University of Surrey.

Effort
Mary M. Copple

Dynamicity is inherent to every human movement. As movement sequences unfold in the space around the body that Rudolf Laban ([1966] 2011) called the kinesphere, their dynamic qualities unfold in what he called the dynamosphere and characterize the mover's inner attitude or mood "by the choice of dynamic stresses" (p.27) apparent in their rhythms. Laban regards "dynamospheric currents" to be "the primary factor in the actual generating of our movements; that is, the generating of visible spatial unfoldings and definite directional sequences with which they form a unity. In reality they are entirely inseparable from each other" (p.36). Effort (Laban and Lawrence 1947) is the term that he used to describe and analyze this

"origin and inner aspect" (Laban [1950] 1988, p.21) of human movement.

So how can effort be related to tensegrity? Whereas R. Buckminster Fuller used tensegrity principles to design self-stabilizing structures that do not use the articulatory potential of their joints to move from place to place, the tensegrity of the human architecture has evolved to do just that. We are built to move, to locomote; our bones (compression elements) are articulated by ligaments, muscles, and fascia (tensile elements). From an evolutionary perspective, whether running or walking instigated a decisive turning point in our anatomical history (Bramble and Lieberman 2004), it can be argued that we achieved upright stance and formed our bodily structure through mobility: operating within the earth's gravitational field entails physiological adaptation to habitats, which drives our brain development, which in turn promotes further evolution of the body (Leroi-Gourhan 1964).

Compared to other animals, whose movements are predominantly instinctive, we are more able to become conscious of and to shape the pattern of our effort habits:

> humans [...] can establish complicated networks of changing effort qualities, representing manifold ways of releasing inherent nervous energy. Man has the capacity to comprehend the nature of the qualities, and to recognise the rhythms and the structures of their sequences. (Laban [1950] 1988, p.12; cf. ibid. p.68). (See Moore 2014, pp. 65–87, for an overview of Laban's taxonomy of effort qualities with suggestions for creative movement explorations.)

Hence, the dynamic stability achieved by the body moving in its kinesphere relies on this capacity to regulate the articulation of the joints through our dynamospheric choices: "The impulse given to our nerves and muscles which move the joints of our limbs originates in inner efforts" (Laban 1948, p.26).

Like Fuller (1958, in Krausse and Lichtenstein 2001, p.232), Laban perceived the tensegral interplay of energetic forces in a wire wheel:

> The representation of a wheel by a circle gives its outer form as it is seen from the outside, so to speak. The representation of the wheel by the spokes shows us the inner tension forces which keep the wheel rim apart. The wheel is seen from within here. (Laban 1920, p.31, translation by Copple)

Without the tension members (spokes), the compression members (hub and rim) would not be held apart; the structure ensuring its function would collapse. The interrelationship between the tension members and the compression members underlies the tensegrity of the structure. The interrelationship of body parts in motion is evidently at the core of a central concept running through all of Laban's written works: *Spannung* (tension). As we create pathways between the hub of our bodies and the rim of our *kinespheres*, a "cohesive tension" (Bartenieff 1974, p.38) bonds them with effort qualities that we can perceive: "The individual parts of every movement, every gesture are: body tensions united with the arousal of feelings" (Laban 1926, p.67, translation by Copple).

References

Bartenieff, I. (1974) 'Space, effort, and the brain.' *Main Currents of Modern Thought 31*, 1, 37–40.

Bramble, D. M. and Lieberman, D. E. (2004) 'Endurance running and the evolution of *Homo*.' *Nature 432*, 345–352. doi.org/10.1038/nature03052

Krausse, J. and Lichtenstein, C. (eds) (2001) *Your Private Sky: R. Buckminster Fuller. Discourse*. Zürich: Lars Müller.

Laban, R. (1920) *Die Welt des Tänzers*. Stuttgart: Walter Seifert.

Laban, R. (1926) *Gymnastik und Tanz*. 2nd ed. Oldenburg: Gerhard Stalling.

Laban, R. (1948) *Modern Educational Dance*. London: MacDonald and Evans.

Laban, R. [1950] (1988) *The Mastery of Movement*. Plymouth: Northcote House.

Laban, R. [1966] (2011) *Choreutics*. Annotated and edited by Lisa Ullmann. Manuscript ca. 1938. Alton, UK: Dance Books.

Laban, R. and Lawrence, F. C. (1947) *Effort*. London: MacDonald and Evans.

Leroi-Gourhan, André (1964) *Le Geste et la Parole*: Vol. 1: *Technique et Langage*. Vol. 2: *La Mémoire et les Rythmes*. Paris: Éditions Albin Michel.

Moore, C. L. (2014) *Meaning in Motion: Introducing Laban Movement Analysis*. Denver, CO: MoveScape Center.

Further reading

Bartenieff, I. (1970) 'The roots of Laban theory: aesthetics and beyond.' In Bartenieff, I., M. Davis and F. Paulay (eds) *Four Adaptations of Effort Theory in Research and Teaching.* New York: Dance Notation Bureau, pp.1–27.

Buckminster Fuller, R. [1958] (2001) *Tensegrity.* In Krausse, J. and Lichtenstein, C. (eds). *Your Private Sky: R. Buckminster Fuller. Discourse.* Zürich: Lars Müller, pp.229–241.

Copple, M. M. (2003) 'Gesture and speech, André Leroi-Gourhan's theory of the co-evolution of manual and intellectual activities.' *Gesture 3*, 1, pp.47–94. doi.org/10.1075/gest.3.1.04cop

Hackney, P. (2002) *Making Connections. Total Body Integration through Bartenieff Fundamentals.* New York, London: Routledge.

Leroi-Gourhan, André (1993) *Gesture and Speech* (tr. Anna Bostock Berger). Cambridge MA: October Books, MIT Press.

Maletic, V. (1987) *Body – Space – Expression. The Development of Rudolf Laban's Movement and Dance Concepts.* Berlin: Mouton de Gruyter.

Moore, C.-L. (2005) *Movement and Making Decisions. The Body–Mind Connection in the Workplace.* New York: Rosen Book Works.

Moore, C.-L. (2009) *The Harmonic Structure of Movement, Music, and Dance according to Rudolf Laban. An Examination of His Unpublished Writings and Drawings.* New York: Edwin Mellen.

Moore, C.-L. (2014) *Meaning in Motion: Introducing Laban Movement Analysis.* Denver, CO: MoveScape Center.

Function in motion

Where there is form and function, there is collagen

Dr. Rebecca Pratt, PhD

One of fascia's primary responsibilities is to connect systems so that the body works as a whole. The major fiber in fascia is collagen. Collagen is one of three principal fiber types found in fascia. In fact, collagen is the most abundant type of connective tissue fiber. Because collagen is a ubiquitous protein it is intimately involved in providing the scaffolding for our entire body. The orientation of collagen bundles assists in providing tensile strength along various force vectors, whether in one linear direction or force from multiple directions. Because the body responds as a unit, minute alterations to fiber direction can be extremely dynamic. For example, a high density of collagen aligned in parallel, with minute ground substance and cells, will provide strength along the one direction that matches the fiber direction but less tensile strength against any other force vector (dense regular connective tissue). Take for instance the anterior cruciate ligament (ACL) of the knee. The fibers of the ACL match the angles maintained at the knee by the femur and tibia. The strength of the ACL can withstand the transmission of force and weight from the pelvis to the lower limb and inhibit translation of the tibia anterior to the knee. However, when force is directed at the knee from an angle or when the direction of movement is quickly corrected, the ACL is slightly less strong.

The range of movement our body permits is vast, therefore we need an infinite continuum of collagen bundle patterns in other areas of our body to provide strength and limit mobility when force vectors come from a multitude of directions. A large number of collagen bundles arranged at various angles to each other suspended in ground substance can support various tensions (stretch, sheer, etc.). Dense irregular connective tissue, for example meridians, is the body's response to these dynamic needs. Take for instance postural yoga. The dense connective tissue deep to our skin and enveloping all of our muscles must move with us as we change from one pose to the next, shift our weight, bend, and flex. If all of our collagen was always bundled together along one axis mountain pose would be easy, but

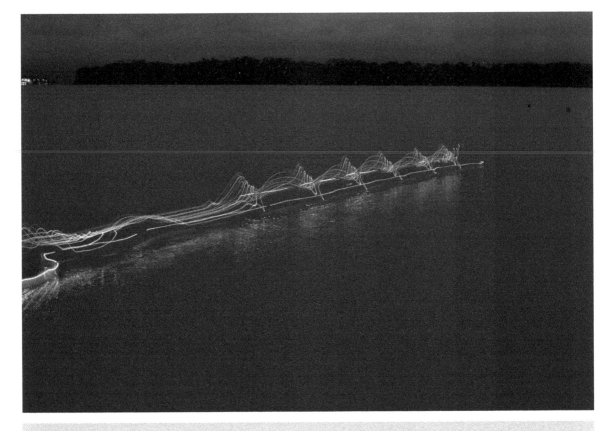

FIGURE 4.7 The author kayaking in a time-lapse photo (lights attached to the kayak and paddle).

Photo by Barry Knittle.

not others. Because fascia is a *continuum*, there are regions in our body where the collagen fiber density is region-specific. Manipulation of collagen bundle orientation as well as collagen density can therefore have a profound effect on structure and function. Increase the amount of collagen where fascia normally supports free movement of fluid, and you get adhesions, tightness, and limited mobility. Decrease collagen density where strength is required, and you may reduce tensile strength and or diminish muscle power. Because function and structure are inherently related, our collagen will adapt over time to our healthy and unhealthy habits.

Trace-forms and rhythmic patterns

Another piece in Laban's work is the concept of trace-forms which is again based on the idea of how the body moves through space. As noted in Sutil (2013):

The outer forms of kinespheric actions constitute what Laban calls trace-forms, *that is, points linked up into a line of pathway that is the trajectory made by a moving body as its transveres kinespheric space... trace-forms are best understood in terms of metrical rhythm.*

The body creates patterns, which create rhythms, like a musical score.

A few years ago, while winding up a paddle, the photographer Barry Knittle approached the kayak company I paddle for, wanting to create a time-lapse of a kayaker's stroke by placing lights strapped onto the paddle toward the blade on each side (Figure 4.7). While I consider myself a midlevel paddler, I was pleased to see that with a relatively short start, I could fairly quickly fall into a relatively even wave of pattern. So how do we apply this to myofascia? Waves and pattern are a piece of this just as in the meander map. In a trace-form we are looking at the pattern of the overall movement and examining it for a sense of easiness and coordination.

What the heck is balance anyways?

Balance is not about symmetry, but there is an importance in creating a sense of ease in the body, where functionally we are utilizing the least amount of effort and energy to move.

There is a difference between the body that is chronically stuck in a few patterns of movement and one that can have both different dynamics and directions available to it. This is what we are largely looking for: a body balance of the tensegral lines of tension.

However, since we are dealing in a book with the topic of movement, the concept of balance in action has to be addressed slightly differently. As noted in Coates and Demers (2019):

The idea of sigi *"sitting," in the Bamana language of West Africa, lies at the foundation of many traditional West African dances. The knees are bent, as if the dancer is about to sit, with the feet still in parallel, approximately hip-width apart. The torso leans slightly forward, the spine long, as the pelvis shifts back to accommodate...* Sigi *signifies an everyday action, sitting, even as it enables a readiness for the rhythmic play. (pp.12–13)*

Changing the body once we understand its shape

In movement or manual work, we look for the client/student to bring the desire for change into the system. Through creating more possibilities for different movement, the range of possibili-

Walk a mile in my shoes... taking body patterns in your stride

Walking is an immediate way many of us see our students or clients enter a space or room. Those who are non-ambulatory also can be observed in the way that they negotiate space.

Try this group exercise for a class to step into another body pattern. Ask a volunteer to walk around in their normal pattern. Before starting off, make sure to acknowledge some positive aspects of their movement. The rest of the group follows until the volunteer is pulled aside to watch the rest of the group in action. If there is a pattern, we then assume there may be a common theme to what the group is observing, whether or not they can articulate it yet clearly or be mimicking a sound in the rhythm of the walk.

I often take this a step (pun intended) further by taking this into a sports action, such as running, or even a baseball pitch. Again, what a movement group can observe often is a profound mirror to gain insight into patterns.

ties increases as well. Or in more basic terms, the greater number of possibilities that exists helps create more in life. Next, we see if there is a way for the system to change and change the pattern. One big exception is changing pattern too drastically, particularly with elite athletes while they are still in an active season. New patterns must have time to integrate into the body system, so we must give that time and space for the body to change.

Larkam (in Schleip *et al*. 2021) notes that understanding fascially oriented movement can help in tactile cues for a client...

by applying precise vectors at the depth of the superficial fascia layer, conveying myofascial direction in space can be given... Tactile cues are to be used judiciously, to inform or encourage rather than to force or overwhelm. In fascia oriented Pilates training, the client is the active agent who has the responsibility of shaping the movement rather than the role of a passive recipient of instructor actions. (p.486)

All of our work in assessment is pointless if we can't make a useful application to how to continue the work in daily movement.

Movement toward health

There is a belief that people move toward health and wellness wherever possible, but often patients and clients are stuck physically and mentally. The general movement may be a desire toward health and wellness, but often there are things that drive the body toward getting stuck, and patterns worn into place. As we will discuss in the chapter on yoga, the concept of patterns can be articulated as samskaras. Similar to a fascial pattern of scar tissue, that samskara can wear deeply into a groove that can be more difficult to overcome the longer the pattern has been in place.

Movements like lifting one's arms overhead become a pattern (Figure 4.8) that we often don't consciously think about, but is shaped by a mix of genetics, circumstances, and learned movement behaviors.

There are many different ways to "see" and interpret the body. It is important to understand these all as constructs and tools that help us get from one place to another. As our knowledge continues to expand, and our ways of visualizing movement grow more sophisticated, new tools will be developed. Perhaps you as the reader will be inspired to dive deeper into some of those mentioned … or create your own.

Myofascia and linear lines

Any of the myofascial connections that have been put forth help to map out strategies more effectively and efficiently. Looking at why one area of the body connects to another myofascially can allow one to plan a route of topographical map of connection between anatomical landmarks. This becomes more about the body as a whole, and less about the pieces. There has been pushback lately in the online movement community about the fascial "lines," as the claim is that the body is, of course, spiral and curves in nature, and not straight. Let's open this to a bit of conversation on natural design. If I grab a piece of the fabric from my pants, and then grab another point and pull about, a line results from the tension I put into the fabric.

In Western cultures, we may additionally have a preference toward linear thought as it is reinforced in the architecture around us. The concept of carpentered environments was developed by Segall *et al.* (1963) and suggested that we see rectangles and straight lines as the predominant art aesthetic, which could affect perception and interpretation of some three-dimensional objects for those group up in these places. Perhaps our love of metaphor of the body in terms of linear terminology is partially tied to our perceptions that come from this environment.

Dinner conversation and sound bites

Any system of thought is stripping language into essential points to make sense of who we are and how we can apply our treatment strategies. Think of our dinner conversation with our friends. Dinner conversations often begin with an introduction of oneself, but if you forget to engage your dinner guests, they will feel unimportant in the conversation.

We often introduce ourselves, and then ask our dinner friends a question. "What do you do?" is often a common default but a poor means to find out something meaningful about our guests. More interesting is to ask what they are excited or passionate about. When you see your dinner guest engaged, the reaction is often physical, whether a widening of the eyes or excited gesturing.

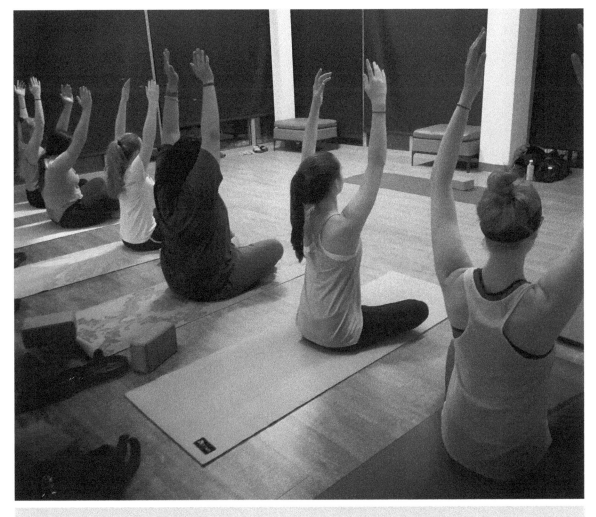

FIGURE 4.8 Arms uplifted. Lifting the arms is negotiated differently in each of these students.

Photo by the author.

References

Aristides, J. (2018) *Beginning Drawing Atelier: An Instructional Sketchbook*. New York, NY: Monacelli Studio.

Black, S. (2021) *Written in Bone: Hidden Stories in What we Leave Behind*. New York, NY: Arcade Publishing.

Braune, W. and Fischer, O. (1987) *The Human Gait*. Berlin/Heidelberg: Springer.

Coates, E. and Demers, S. (2019) *Physics and Dance*. Newhaven, CT: Yale University Press.

Dalton, E. (2011) *Dynamic Body: Exploring Form, Expanding Function*. Oklahoma City, OK: Freedom From Pain Institute.

Hemenway, P. (2005) *Divine Proportion: Phi in Art, Nature, and Science*. New York, NY: Sterling Publishing Co.

Hildebrand, R. (2005) 'Attic perfection in anatomy: Bernhard Siegfried Albinus (1697–1770) and Samuel Thomas Soemmerring (1755–1830).' *Annals of Anatomy-Anatomischer Anzeiger 187*, 5–6, 555–573.

Kendall, F. P. McCreary, E. K., Provance, P. G., Rodgers, M. M. and Romani, W. A. (eds) (2005) *Muscles: Testing and Function with Posture and Pain*. Philadelphia, PA: Lippincott, Williams and Wilkins.

Merriam-Webster.com Dictionary. (2021) *"Stability."* Accessed on December 12, 2021 at https://www.merriam-webster.com/dictionary/stability

Myers, T. W. (2020) *Anatomy Trains: Myofascial Meridians for Manual Therapists and Movement Professionals* (4th ed.). London: Elsevier.

Richter, P., Hebgen, E. and Richter, P. (2019) *Trigger Points and Muscle Chains*. Stuttgart: Thieme.

Schleip, R., Wilke, J. and Findley, T. (eds) (2021) *Fascia in Sport and Movement*. Edinburgh: Handspring Publishing.

Sutil, N. S. (2013) 'Rudolf Laban and topological movement: a videographic analysis.' *Space and Culture 16*, 2, 173–193. https://doi.org/10.1177/1206331213475776

Further reading

Beach, P. (2010) *Muscles and Meridians: The Manipulation of Shape*. Edinburgh: Churchill Livingstone.

Braune, W. and Fischer, O. (2012) *On the Centre of Gravity of the Human Body: As Related to the Equipment of the German Infantry Soldier*. Berlin/Heidelberg: Springer Science and Business Media.

Lemperle, G. (2020) 'Prevention of hyper- and hypotrophic scars through surgical incisions in the direction of the "main folding lines" of the skin.' *Plastic and Aesthetic Research 70*, 40. https://doi.org/10.20517/2347-9264.2020.14

Rodman, P. S. and McHenry, H. M. (1980) 'Bioenergetics and the Origin of Hominid Bipedalism.' *American Journal of Physical Anthropology 52*, 1, 103–106. https://doi.org/10.1002/ajpa.1330520113

Stecco, C., Pirri, C., Fede, C., Fan, C. *et al.* (2019) 'Dermatome and fasciatome.' *Clinical Anatomy 32*, 7, 896–902. https://doi.org/10.1002/ca.23408

Tversky, B. G. (2019) *Mind in Motion: How Action Shapes Thought*. New York, NY: Basic Books.

Yosifon, D. and Stearns, P. N. (1998) 'The rise and fall of American posture.' *The American Historical Review 103*, 4, 1057. https://doi.org/10.2307/2651198

The relation between what we see and what we know is never settled. Each evening we see the sun set. We know that the earth is turning away from it. Yet the knowledge, the explanation, never quite fits the sight.

John Berger, *Ways of Seeing* (1973)

How do we organize the body? When I teach my university students, we go through the anatomical planes of motion for two reasons. First, if we are going to share that common language with other professions, we need to communicate that clearly through a language spoken in diverse areas such as sports, dance, and physical therapy. Several of our movement therapy languages, such as Laban, are also built on the concept of utilizing these planes. Ultrasound images, x-rays, and more also key into to the basic orientation from these commonly utilized anatomical terms. Second, the major planes of motion can be a starting dialogue for the ways we motivate in space (Figure 5.1) and how we reference movement in relationship to our body position (Figure 5.2). Flexion and extension in the sagittal plane are often the start of athletic warm-ups all over the world, building into coronal plane motions and the twists of transverse plane. Training the body efficiently with the myofascia involves adding everywhere in between. When I first learned how to play jazz piano, I had to do a lot that was improvised off a common key or time signature. Working with the myofascial body is a lot like working in a collaborative jazz group. To sound good, you need to have learned the rules well enough to break them. So we are going to give a nod to some of the directional rules with the knowledge that we can improvise later.

We are now well established in the knowledge that fascia is made of loose connective tissue and fibrous components, and both respond differently to load and movement, which is a critical concept for the moving body.

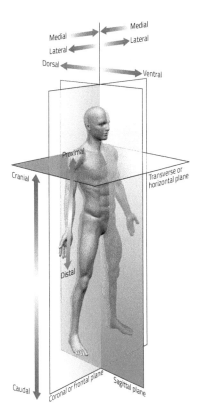

FIGURE 5.1 Planes of the body. Planes are surfaces about connection. Any points on any plane can connect together in a straight line. While training myofascia, we want to avoid movement along predictable planes of motion because life is rarely expressed in predictable ways. However, the major directions still give us a framework to discuss with other professionals and as a starting place to name movement. The anatomical language is one type of map of the body. The base of these words comes from Latin and Greek. While it has a predisposition to the Classical Western world, we will still look at these words for their description in many movement and anatomical settings with the recognition of cultural bias. Planes of movement are a construct which can provide useful points of reference. Like directional points on a compass, these planes of movement can be a point of orientation.

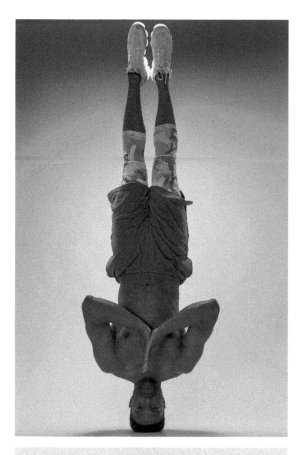

FIGURE 5.2 Turning the body upside down requires language that can help in proper orientation of the body. If I am referring to the something toward the top of the body, I might be tempted to explain through directionality such as up or down, but that doesn't describe a body accurately, particularly if that body changes its relationship to the environment around it. For example, if a body is in a headstand, "up" may very well be a descriptive of the feet. For this reason, a description of the body in terms of caudal (tail) or cranial (head) becomes more accurate in describing actions. Technically, we can look at any creature for the obvious head to tail anatomy (mouth to anus) that forms the basic end points and connect them with an imaginary drawn line that becomes what we call the anteroposterior axis, also defined as rostrocaudal, craniocaudal, or cephalocaudal.

Photo courtesy of Nile Bratcher.

In our experience on earth, we exist in space without seeing magnetic directionality until we use a tool, like a compass, that utilizes a pointer that finds alignment with the Earth's horizontal magnetic field.

The body exists in three-dimensional space perhaps as a tensegral form; an idea explored by architect Buckminster Fuller, but also explored in a parallel movement universe by thinkers like Rudolph Laban, who created an isohedron to map out the elements of movement vocabulary in weight, time, effort, and flow to newer models that we will explore with those working in fascial fitness and movement and re-conceptualizing the movement vocabulary. As we live in an environment that is self-reflective of the culture and challenges of where some of these vocabularies emerged, we will explore some of the historical context of human movement vis-á-vis the environment it came from and the takeaways to keep or dismiss.

In recent anatomical history, the body has been conceptualized and divided into individualized muscles, which act like mechanical levers and pulleys. The classical kinesiological model sees the skeleton as a frame, with the muscles as the movers of that puppet-like frame. A lot of this thought process can be traced to the ideas of Sir Isaac Newton (1642–1726), whose concepts of the body in relationship to gravity have made an impact into the fields of biomechanics including kinematics and kinetics. However, by connecting the body in larger way, we start to have a framework for conceptualizing how the bottom of the foot might relate to the hamstrings via its myofascial connection or how the utilization of dynamic stretching with soft elastic bounces at the end range of available motion can create deeper available motion (Muller and Schleip, in Schleip 2012).

You cannot step in the same river twice… everything flows and nothing stays.

Heraclitus

Circular resonant breathing in multiple planes

Breathing techniques have had a resurgence thanks to the popularization of yoga breathwork (pranayama), especially as a means to work into deep relaxation or mindfulness techniques made more common through figures like Dr. Andrew Weil and Jon Kabat-Zinn and recently with James Nestor (2020).

One of Nestor's described techniques is resonant (coherent) breathing which is "a calming practice that places the heart, lungs, and circulation into a state of coherence, where the systems of the body are working at peak efficiency." Described as an inhale for 5.5 seconds, and then a continued exhale for another 5.5 seconds, it creates a patterned cycle of easy breathing.

For my own clients, I'm always interested in how we can mix up the body in different dimensions, a key feature of resiliency for the fascial tissues. In a variation of this classic exercise, I have my clients begin the cycle, as described, in a comfortable seated position. Try several rounds of this for yourself.

If you haven't already, observe if you visualized the circle always cycling in one direction. Can you change the direction that the circle makes in your mind? Now, try to shift the focus to visualizing the movement of that breathing circle into the sagittal plane. Reverse the direction here as well. For many, this actually will increase the awareness of creating depth from front to back in the body as, anatomically, we have a narrow front to back ribcage as bipeds as opposed to quadrupeds that have a deep front to back ribcage.

Try now to visualize the same in the transverse plane in both directions. As the three major planes become easier to negotiate, see if you can create breathing in diagonals and in other directions to explore how the shift in focus will shift the effect in breathing awareness.

The lancelet fish and the points of body

Metamerism and segmentation

Another way to parse the body is through metamerism and segmentation, which have clinical and theoretical relevance to the body system. In vertebral anatomy, from our previously mentioned lancelet (Figure 5.3) onwards, a "segment" is the area that a spinal nerve innervates.

These segmental nerves innervate sections of the body, namely muscle (myotome), skeletal (sclerotome), visceral (enterotome), skin/surface (dermatome) and fascia (fasciatome).

Dermatomes are another map of the body, connecting areas of skin to their corresponding spinal nerve. There are 31 spinal nerves connecting to 30 dermatomes (C1 has no associated dermatome). There are some variations between dermatome mapping, which is often depicted in broad rainbow strips of color to indicate the innervated mapped area of tissue.

Mapping in these different systems will have logical overlaps. In understanding felt sensations, it is worthwhile to spend time contemplating the

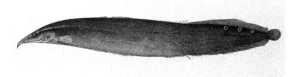

FIGURE 5.3 The lancelet (Amphioxus) is a part of the invertebrate subphylum Cephalochordata, the Chordata phylum, and has an interesting connection to the world of anatomy. It may seem out of place in a book on myofascial movement and anatomy, but this creature occupies an important place in understanding primitive vertebrate anatomy. In 1850, anatomists Ross and Voigt demonstrated that in early development of vertebrates, the nerve branches divide into three distinct groupings that supply dorsal, ventral, and lateral areas.

Credit: Fish "Kanichi," no. 14. Wellcome Collection. Attribution 4.0 International (CC BY 4.0).

nerve mapping. Indeed, the concept of fasciatomes has not made its way into either mainstream medical nomenclature, or the introductory anatomy book; however, the term is found in a paper by Stecco *et al.* (2019), in which the authors noted the differences between dermatomes and fasciatomes,

basing their approach to the literature on nerve root stimulation and comparing dermatomeric and myomeric maps. The former represents the portion of tissue composed of skin, hypodermis, and superficial fascia supplied by all the cutaneous branches of an individual spinal nerve; the latter includes the portion of deep fascia supplied by the same nerve root and organized according to force lines to emphasize the main directions of movement. The dermatome is important for esteroception, whereas the fasciatome is important for proprioception.

That last line is most critical in our interest in movement. Whereas the dermatomes help us identify sensations on the external body, the fasciatome is tied into our perception of where we exist in space.

The etymology of meridian has interesting origins in Old French (*meridien*) and Latin (*meridianus*) both implying north/south directionality as well as a sense of time (i.e. noon, midday). Utilized to describe geography of the larger world, the term also is applied regularly to people. The first well-developed meridians in the body, however, were not European in origin, but rather from the east (namely Japan and China) (Figure 5.4), which mapped pathways for the flow of life force and energy in a living body. The balancing of these different meridians and their associated organs are believed to bring the body into a state of health. This idea of working related areas of the body for treatment was largely missing from Western body work until recently. Looking to map connections myofascially, Thomas Myers developed a system of outlining longitudinal connections (Figure 5.5) to strategize working with the body more holistically. There are some overlaps from Myers's system to eastern meridians, which have been noted in his book (2020). My guess is that some of the similarities are due to places that fascia plays important connections. The shape of these systems is quite comparable and intelligently mapped.

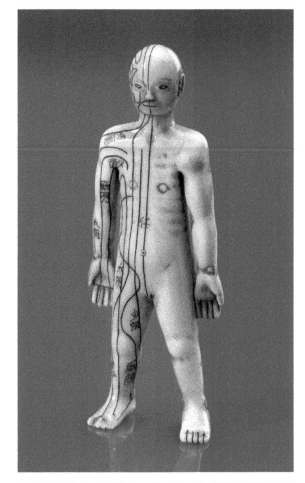

FIGURE 5.4 Major meridians of the Eastern systems. The major meridians predated modern fascial lines, and many have studied their similarities and overlaps. Upon looking at these lines, one can draw parallels and see similarities in shape and form. The Japanese meridians are largely utilized in palpation and assessment techniques. In Chinese medicine there are 12 standard meridians divided into groups of Yin and Yang and considered channel networks. While they lack scientific proof of existence, the recent literature on acupuncture benefits and fascia point to the possibility fascia fibers respond to the twist and stretch of acupuncture needles.

Credit: Wellcome Collection. Ivory anatomical figure, Japan, 1800–1920. Science Museum, London. Attribution 4.0 International (CC BY 4.0).

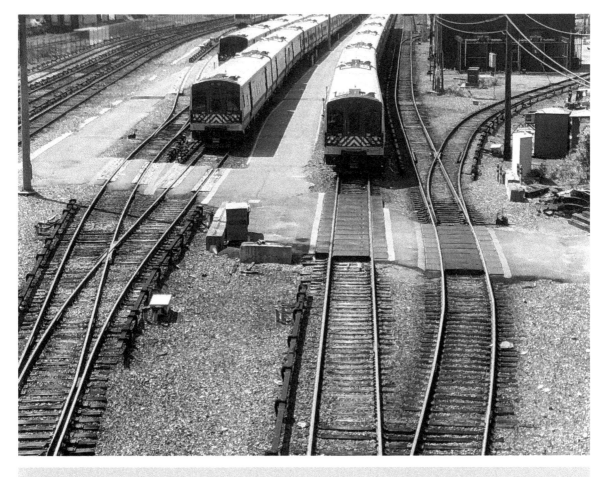

FIGURE 5.5 Thomas Myers pictured his connections (Anatomy Trains®) as a system of train lines, with directionality and pull, as well as places where there are "switches" where the anatomy can divide between pathways. The 12 "myofascial meridians" are connections of defined fascia and muscle with characteristics unique to each line.

Photo by the author.

Myers's (2020) book can be referenced directly for a better understanding the AT maps, as can the authors of the other maps and continuities that are referenced throughout this book. We use all of these systems, from the traditional anatomical planes of motion to myofascial maps as a starting point for any journey in the body.

To this point, years ago, I did intensive kayak guide training in eastern Canada's Bay of Fundy with some of the largest tidal changes in the world.

I was part of a small group that learned to read charts, tide tables, and utilize compasses with Bruce Smith, one of the best kayak guides in the world. None of this information fully came together until I tested my paddle strokes and rescue skills in the water itself. I also took time to carefully observe Bruce's paddle stroke, and how he watched the clouds, or the shifting water, noting that these were also clues like the hard skills in navigation. Our systems and patterns are useful for organizing thought and strategy, but we must continue to navigate the water and walk the pathways with the caveat that our body systems, and the larger environment around us are bigger than the individual connected pieces.

The plantar fascia and the moving body

The foot is quite fascial in nature and is important to our movement. The plantar fascia (technically the plantar aponeurosis) is a roughly triangular-shaped, strong structure running from the toes to the calcaneus and helps with the transfer of elastic energy. When we feel the bottom of our feet and then bring the big toe back in dorsiflexion, we feel the fascia tightening against the plantar. Originating on the medial side of the calcaneus, it also helps to invert the subtalar joint. This creates what is known as a rigid lever and related to this is the idea of the windlass mechanism.

In the push-off phase of the foot we use the energy transfer from the plantar fascia. If we look back at our body as tensegral form, when we tension through part of the foot we are demanding a rigidity in the forefoot through stability. Plantar fascia is sensory nerve rich, just like the rest of our fascial system. As we know, the sensory nerves help to give us body awareness of where we are in space, particularly when we are walking and active (dynamic movement) as well as in static moment, which we know can cause difficulties for those with plantar fascia issues. This is actually known as a reverse windlass mechanism and is important in dynamic stabilization.

Collagen fibers are often arranged longitudinally. This is the case with the plantar fascia, which transmits force from the forefoot to the back of the foot, continuing to transmit force upwards. A study on plantar fascia anatomy and its relationship with the Achilles tendon and paratenon (loose connective tissue that allows the tendon to glide smoothly) looked, in part, to see if there was permanent deformation after fascia stretching (Stecco *et al.* 2013). The fascia was found to not be plastic, but responsive each and every time it was stretched. This means the tendon responds very similarly and that a fascia structure is difficult to change.

Fascia pulled will decrimp and be stretched longer until a point at which it will tear. If we are playing tennis, we are pretensioning the anterior fascia and also activating muscles. When the ball is hit, the front of the body contracts. The more elastic the fascia is, the more efficient the energy return will be. Additionally, fascia (such as a crural fascia) has a strong anisotropy, which means it responds differently depending on the directional forces. In other words, in certain directions, fascia stiffens in response to a need for force.

The fascia is both longitudinal and horizontal in stabilizing the foot. The skin on the bottom of the foot (as well as the palm of the hand) is more tightly adhered to the fascial layer right underneath. The blending of the plantar fascia to the calcaneal/Achilles tendon is the next connection.

This connection is often difficult to prove in traditional dissection labs as the treated embalmed tissue will dry out, making the connection look less significant. In addition, the aging process will decrease the fat pad on the back of the heel. As in much of the body, the effect of aging is a process of drying out.

Plantar fasciitis pain is often the most painful on the plantar medial calcaneal tubercle and is felt on the medial heel. Usually pain in the medial side of the foot itself is more commonly felt when a microtear has happened in the middle of plantar fascia through an explosive dynamic movement where the elastic recoil wasn't able to take it. For myself, I believe I got my own foot pain from standing long hours teaching in workshops barefoot and simultaneously aggressively ramping up a running program without proper foot strength. The loss of elasticity diminished even more while I had to recover. Essentially, the next phase is happening as the scarring tissue is being laid down with a predominance of collagen type 3. The thickening of this type of layer of fascia can mean degeneration and stress over time. Degenerated tissue is weak tissue. Sometimes, heel spurs develop (Figure 5.6), where the periosteum comes away from the bone underneath and new bone builds into that space. It can be a point of irritation for nerves, or it may be just an adaption without added pain, and literal reshaping of the body in response to an issue.

When I could start to recover, I actually began to ramp up my walking again to be able to regain the fluidity in my foot. My flexibility was already high, so dorsiflexion in the toes, ankle did not gain more range of motion. Traditional treatment such as night splints (holding the foot in that dorsiflexion) did little. Myofascial release with an emphasis on the dorsiflexion of the toe isolated to encourage the windlass mechanism was useful, as well as release specifically in the gastrocnemius, continuing up the line of the Anatomy Trains® Superficial Back Line.

In general, in regards to footwear, less cushioning is better... probably. The harder surface will help to train the muscle as well as the elastic response in the fascia itself. Many of the traditional treatments involve things like orthotics. Just like braces for teeth, this works with the concept of trying to retrain the soft tissue. However, orthotics serve little use if they aren't changed as the body starts to

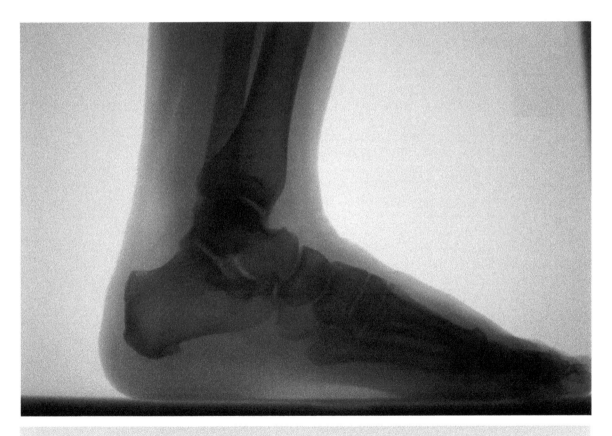

FIGURE 5.6 We see the "echo" of the fascial tissues in looking at heel spur (the small point pulling inwards) and how fascia reshapes bone. Both overuse and underuse can play a role in such issues. Bone spurs are pulled into form as the periosteum gets pulled away from the bone, and the body immediately wants to fill in the empty space, so the bone-making cells (osteoblasts—think of the letter "b" for building while the "c" in osteoclasts is for "cleaning" up) come in and fill in the space. Usually, this pairs with plantar fasciitis but it does not necessarily result in pain. In fact, heel spurs only cause pain in about 5% of those who are x-rayed.

Image courtesy of the author.

adapt and change. For temporary relief of plantar fascia, cushioning can provide rest and recovery while the tissue heals. Eventually, strength and training need to happen.

The modern shoe is designed, and perhaps overdesigned when it comes to "helping" the foot. There are many stories among athletic trainers about the lack of significant running injuries until shoes began to be overengineered, albeit with good intentions but poor results. One such example is "toe spring," which is where the box of a shoe is curved upwards. At first this sounds like a great idea to encourage the windlass mechanism and to encourage a lengthening through the whole of the back tensioning, but as we have come to observe, the body craves a state of equilibrium. Toe springs hold the toe in extension instead of allowing them to rest in neutral during other phases of natural gait. During the push-off phase, the foot acts more like a lever, and the toe goes into extension and then relaxes. Padding, arch supports, and heel lifts may feel good in the short term but can set the foot up for issues. Of course, going too rapidly to "natural" footwear can be detrimental. Most shoes have a bit of heel lift, so going to a minimal shoe right away can set the heel up for Achilles tendinosis or tears if training is too quick. There is a tendency to assume that the body needs "comfortable" soft surfaces, but actually we are designed to be challenged in a healthy way to stay adaptive for change.

Plantar fascial tears tend to build up scar tissue in the place of the original tear, but this can create additional concerns. Related can be issues like Baxter's nerve entrapment, which runs right underneath the plantar aponeurosis. In this case, the trapped nerve needs freedom in order to feel comfortable under the surface of the plantar fascia. In flat or pronated feet, tarsal tunnel syndrome can be another entrapment issue, similar to carpal tunnel syndrome.

Cheng *et al.* (2008) noted that plantar fascia tension helps the body go forwards at the release of the push-off phase. Dorsiflexing the big toe "may have a positive effect on treating plantar fasciitis by providing proper guidance for collagen regeneration" (p.845). Additionally, nonlinear modelling of the plantar fascia created higher stress along the fibers in the fascia.

A simple test

Working any one area of the body can affect another. Myers (2020) has outlined what he has called "A Simple Test." As noted:

A forward bend with the knees straight links and challenges all the tracks and stations of the Anatomy Trains® Superficial Back Line. Work in one area, e.g. the plantar fascia, can affect motion and length anywhere and everywhere along the line. After work on the right plantar surface, the right arm hangs lower. (p.32)

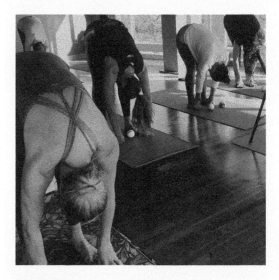

FIGURE 5.7 A forward fold can be used as both assessment and treatment in working "A Simple Test." While changes in forward folds are seen by stimulating connected areas of myofascia, this test may be affecting neuromuscular response as well as connective tissues.

Photo by the author.

Test a client or yourself by taking a forward fold pre-warm up of any sort (Figure 5.7). Notice where any tension is felt throughout the back of the body. Take a ball under one foot only and begin to roll. Any ball can work. Personally, I like the pinky balls (bought at five-and-dime stores) or blue racquetballs, for this. Tennis balls and golf balls may be a bit more aggressive, but harder isn't necessarily better. In moving along the surface of the plantar fascia, slow shearing for several minutes will be more effective than a quick roll. Test the forward fold again, and also take the movement into walking to see if the pattern is felt differently in the gait.

We can take this from the other end as well. I worked for many years with autistic children who are often toe walkers with a tight superficial back line. One of the treatments given to this highly sensitive group was hair tinglers, which work the galea aponeurotica. Try giving yourself a scalp massage, again, for several minutes and again forward fold to see if there is a deeper release.

We may or may not be fully affecting the myofascia as much as working on the neurological response.

Myofascial alignment and real-life movement

James Earls

Much has been written about myofascial continuities over the last 20 years but work still remains to explore their functions in real-life movement. The fact that different continuities and chains have been mapped by a number of different authors (Vleeming, Tittel, Méziere, Myers) illustrates the lack of consensus on how to organize the interpretation of anatomy. The work of Vleeming grew from a predominately biomechanical model, Tittel analyzed sporting performance, Méziere mapped functional muscle chains, and Myers mapped, in the first instance at least, from a structural point of view. This has led to some confusion in the understanding and interpretation of the myofascial continuities.

A useful way to address some of this confusion is to look at function. Rather than analyzing an immobile anatomy or the fantasy of consistently open-chain movement supplied by most anatomy texts, can we extrapolate from universal movement patterns to

anatomy? To rephrase Dobzhansky's famous quote ("Nothing makes sense in biology except in the light of evolution"), can we think along similar lines and say that "Nothing in anatomy makes sense except in the light of *function*?"

Interest in Myers's Anatomy Trains® (AT) model blossomed partly from the ease with which its mapping system could be superimposed onto controlled movement modalities such as yoga and Pilates. However, it is unlikely that myofascial continuities exist for the smooth performance of, or as a result of, repeated Sun Salutations or footwork on the Reformer. We must instead look to functional anatomy to see where myofascial continuity might play a role. However, it becomes much more difficult to analyze and explain due to the complexity of how force transfers through the moving body. The reality of natural movement requires us to hold the "maps" loosely, be guided by the body's actual movement/reaction, and not impose our expectations onto it. Within this text we will contain our exploration to the anterior and predominately sagittal plane Superficial Front Line (SFL), but much of the analysis mentioned below could be applied to any other line and movement plane.

A major hindrance to understanding real-life movement is its multi-dimensional nature performed with varying degrees of momentum. During movement classes, a number of variables are often removed—there is less movement "noise" during a held or repeated stretch or movement, especially when performed predominantly in one plane of movement. For example, when performing a full-body extension such as Dart or Cobra, we can see and feel the sagittal plane engagement without any interference from the other planes of movement. Exercise-based movements are most often performed in expectation of specific reactions and are commonly contained in this way to ensure safety or efficacy.

The controlled environment of movement class is quite unlike natural movement, which rarely takes place in one plane of motion and is often complicated by variety of force inputs. As we saw in my previous breakout box (Chapter 2), movement patterns and anatomy are entwined, and each species has its own common movement patterns. The one movement considered most significant for the evolution of *Homo sapiens* is that of upright walking[1] and it makes sense that the common walking pattern is visible within our anatomy.

A typical (ideal?) position for most of us is the almost full-body extension achieved prior to toe-off. When we freeze that moment, the outline of the SFL becomes quite apparent. The filter of the AT model appears to help us visualize and identify the overall lines of strain in the body during complex movements (see Figure 5.breakout.1).

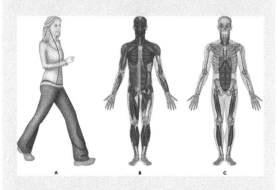

FIGURE 5.BREAKOUT.1 Freezing the body in the moment before toe-off reveals the extension pattern though the whole body (a). By matching the vector of tissue strain with the sagittally-aligned tissues (b and c), we perceive the line of the Superficial Front Line. However, the degree of myofascial continuity and force transfer of the SFL is challenged within the literature (Wilke *et al.* 2016). The reality is that the complexity of this apparently simple movement will necessitate a response on many layers of tissue.

Image courtesy of Lotus Publishing.

However, although we see and often feel the extension pattern described above, it is not necessarily evidence for the SFL as a myofascial continuity. The most commonly quoted concern about the AT model is that the body is continuous and separated only by trauma or sharp blades. Critics often cite the fact that any shape can be carved from the body during dissection. One response to these critiques is that we must first look at the reality of how the body moves and let that guide our interpretation of the anatomy, not the other way around. Arguing from the anatomy has been endemic and mostly without conclusion. If we begin by accepting the integrated wholeness of the body and then observe how it moves, we can let the reality of common movement patterns assist our understanding of anatomy. Although the fascial continuity of the SFL is strongly challenged (Wilke *et al.* 2016), the idea of the AT lines can give a lens to visualize the lines of stress within the moving body. However, it is important to keep in mind that the AT classification is a simplification of the reality.

To understand the anatomy of real-world move-ment we must see the form in terms of long-chain movement. Thankfully the concepts of tensegrity/ biotensegrity explored elsewhere in this text give us a language for the human form we see during normal movement. If we look at the full-body ex-tension created at the toe-off phase of gait[2] we see a shape that is similar to that of Dart and Cobra but in a different orientation to gravity, which means that the body's shape has been created through a very different arrangement of forces.

In walking we progress from hip flexion to extension as we move forward over the foot to achieve the toe-off position, and the momentum

---

[1] While there has been much discussion over the role of endurance running in the evolution to *Homo sapiens*, it is generally accepted that walking arrived first. Detailed discussion can be found in Pontzer 2017.

[2] I use the term "toe-off" in preference to the common "push-off" as I argue we have the choice to actively *push* or to release energy captured and momentarily stored in the stretched tissues as we walk—they are different events.

involved has to be controlled by the tissues anterior to the hip joint. Without controlled, decelerated extension we would fall over, and the deceleration provides a range of benefits as it strains the anterior tissues to provide a "free" energy source for the imminent forward swing. Along with some contributions from muscle tissue, the negative work (deceleration of extension) is partially performed by the elastic tissues of the hip joint, which then contribute significantly to the positive work (acceleration of flexion) during initial swing (Silder *et al.* 2007; Whittington *et al.* 2008).

The passive elastic structures named in the studies include the skin, ligaments, and joint capsule—all elements commonly omitted from standard listings of "continuities." I mention this because it emphasizes the need to stop compartmentalizing the anatomy of movement. If we look at the extended position again, it should be no surprise that all the tissues crossing the extended joints should have some degree of stretch.

It is not only hip extension that requires deceleration, as our upright gait also requires spinal extension as it progresses toward toe-off. When discussing the upper portion of the Superficial Front Line, Wilke (2016) points out the lack of fascial continuity between the rectus abdominis and sternocleidomastoid, the structures that would be involved in controlling the spinal extension. Discontinuity of the fascia is not necessarily an issue for the moving body, a fact Myers applies in his analysis of the lower portion of his SFL. He proposes bone as a mechanical link—the pelvis is used to couple mechanical transfer between the rectus femoris and rectus abdominis. Perhaps, in the same way, the sternum can provide the same service in the upper portion?

Force transfer through bone was studied earlier by Vleeming and his team when measuring tissue continuity between the sacrotuberous ligament and biceps femoris (van Wingerden *et al.* 1993), part of what Myers later called the Superficial Back Line. The study showed the continuity to be

variable, but, regardless of continuity or not, force was still transferred between the two myofascial structures in both anatomically neutral and hip flexed positions. Vleeming's team's conclusion was that force may be transferred by the ischial tuberosity's natural elasticity.

Given that tissues on multiple layers are involved in any movement and that myofascial continuity is not necessary to transfer force, discussions over continuity or its lack may be a distraction from appreciating the reality of movement. The question of myofascial continuity is only one of anatomical analysis, it is not a problem of function, a fact illustrated by the movement practitioner's experience and sense of connection through this line of strain when exploring extension patterns.

We gain deeper insight into anatomy through appreciation of movement patterns. Anatomical shape is organized on two major levels—that of inheritance of overall body pattern (phylogeny, see my breakout box in Chapter 2), and through the individual's movement during life (ontogeny). There is a two-way relationship between function and anatomy. The fact that movement is difficult to comprehend from the current study of anatomy is demonstrated within the many texts available. An appreciation of shape and movement and their interrelationship is a better starting place to understand anatomy.

The analysis of movement highlights the problem associated with any system—there is a complex interplay of variables and factors. For example, to achieve the extended hip position and capture kinetic energy in preparation for the limb's forward swing after toe-off, there must be enough speed within the gait. Whittington *et al.* (2008) showed higher speeds increased the workload of the passive elastic structures. Efficiency and ability of the elastic tissues to capture and return such energy is also affected by numerous factors including age, tissue architecture, and timing.

Clearly there is no simple formula to optimize use of elastic tissues, especially as other joints ranges are also necessary to allow the body to progress into the extended position. Any reductions in knee extension, ankle, or toe mobility and spinal extension will inhibit hip extension during gait (for further exploration see Earls 2020). Just as elastic tissue loading is velocity dependent (Whittington *et al.* 2006), it is also range dependent—if we inhibit extension, we reduce tissue strain, reduce passive elastic strain and we lose its contribution to the positive work during swing. We can, of course, compensate for the loss of elastic energy by increasing the work done by active muscular contraction, but at what long-term cost to tissue health?

Understanding real-life function requires a 3D mental picture of anatomy and is not restricted to single muscles, planes, or lines. This understanding should encourage us to widen our therapeutic vision and investigate the ability to attain full body shapes rather than simply assessing individual joint ranges. We need a truly holistic and functional vision of the body to see how its tissues adapt and strain under the application of gravity, ground reaction force and momentum. Individual joint ranges are important, but our life is lived in long-chain movement for much of the time. The ability to achieve toe-off position requires an interrelated chain of toe extension, foot stability, ankle mobility, knee, hip, and spinal extension. This position allows us to load the many tissues that efficiently assist swinging our leg forward. But this position requires healthy myofascia, healthy joints, healthy motor control strategies, and a healthy walking speed. If any one of these is compromised, it may affect any or all the others. There will not be one solution to every issue.

References

Earls, J. (2020) *Born to Walk.* Berkeley, CA: North Atlantic Books.

Pontzer, H. (2017) 'Economy and endurance in human evolution.' *Current Biology 27,* 12, R613–R621.

Silder, A., Whittington, B., Heiderscheit, B. and Thelen, D. (2007) 'Identification of passive elastic joint moment–angle relationships in the lower extremity.' *Journal of Biomechanics 40,* 12, 2628–2635.

van Wingerden, J., Vleeming, A., Snijders, C. and Stoeckart, R. (1993) 'A functional-anatomical approach to the spine-pelvis mechanism: interaction between the biceps femoris muscle and the sacrotuberous ligament.' *European Spine Journal 2,* 3, 140–144.

Whittington, B., Silder, A., Heiderscheit, B. and Thelen, D. (2008) 'The contribution of passive-elastic mechanisms to lower extremity joint kinetics during human walking.' *Gait and Posture 27,* 4, 628–634.

Wilke, J., Krause, F., Vogt, L. and Banzer, W. (2016) 'What is evidence-based about myofascial chains: a systematic review.' *Archives of Physical Medicine and Rehabilitation, 97,* 3, 454–461.

Front to back

We've already discussed how the front of the body is quite sensitive to trauma, emotionally and physically, due to its vulnerability in bipedalism. Unlike quadruped mammals that protect both sexual organs and access to the front body (visceral, etc.), we have vulnerability. If we look at the relationship between front to back continuities in tandem, we are looking at the relationship of movement issues in the sagittal plan of motion, also called the wheel plane. The front of the body is exposed anatomically, so the fast twitch fibers serve to pull the body into protection and keep the eyes forward to scan for danger. When the body is balanced along its primary and secondary curves, back connections of myofascia work easily. It keeps us from falling forward as well. However, if the hips are in front of the ankle, the body has to engage and work harder through connections like the gastrocnemius and soleus. As a mediator of movement, Myers's

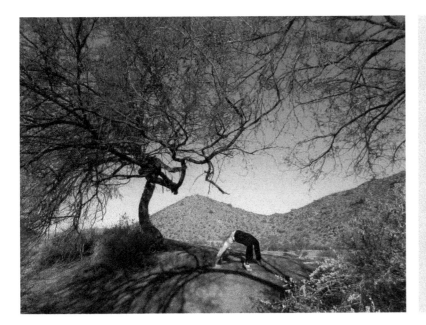

FIGURE 5.8 Lengthening of the front myofascial body and arm connections. The front of the body is quite sensitive to trauma, emotionally and physically, due to its vulnerability in bipedalism. Unlike quadruped mammals that protect both sexual organs and access to the front body (viscera, etc.), we have vulnerability in this area. Deep opening in this area coordinates several areas of anatomy.

Photo by the author.

Superficial Front Line is thought to stabilize or exaggerate the lumbar curve of the spine while limiting or exaggerating flexion in the thoracic spine (Figure 5.8).

Lateral and side body connections

The lateral myofascial connections in multiple systems from Wancura-Kampik's segmental anatomy (Figure 5.9) to Myers's Lateral Line continue to have an important relationship with how we move. Fish, snakes, and other creatures motivate by moving their lateral line in order to negotiate their way through space in a serpentine movement. In contrast, we stabilize the sides of the body in order to motivate and move forwards. The movement of the lateral line helps in lateral flexion, but also in stabilization.

Skating actions (think speed skating and similar side-to-side exercises) works in pre-tensioning the body through the raised arm (Figure 5.10a,b) and also requires stability in the entire side of the body. Any breaks in coordination may have a related area of tension or injury, such as where the IT band provides lateral support to the knee (Figure 5.11).

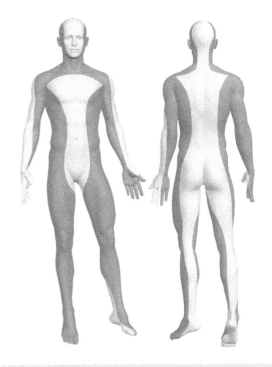

FIGURE 5.9 Image of side-to-side relationships can be seen in the work after Wancura-Kampik. In this version, the lateral connected anatomy includes a continuity to the arms.

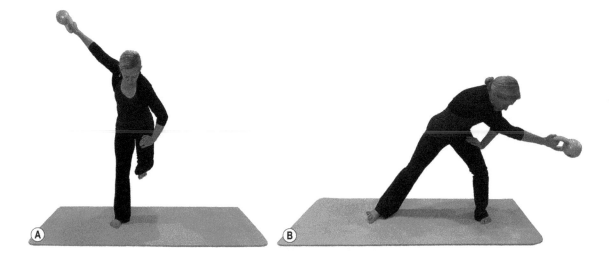

FIGURE 5.10 A kettlebell swing with a lifted leg in the pretensioning phase works a combination of the lateral connections in the body.

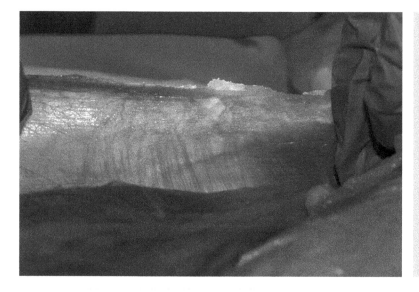

FIGURE 5.11 The iliotibial (IT) band doesn't exist in babies. It is pulled into form when we begin to walk. Resembling packing tape with its horizontal and vertical fibers, it provides structural stability for the knee.

Photo by Lydia Mann, KNM Labs (author's dissection).

Lateral line neck release—sideways figure eights

I have been fascinated with the simultaneous yes/no head gesture, sometimes known a "head bobble" which is common in many South Asian cultures (Storti 2021). Moving in the coronal plane, I found that when I worked a similar action, I could feel a dance between the sternocleidomastoid and the splenius alternating. I also found it interesting to bring a sense of balance into the top of the lateral myofascial sides of the neck, an area that chronically has issues.

It may be doing even more in coordinating all three movement planes in relationship to the semicircular canals (SSCs) which work with the suboccipitals in stabilizing vision through coordinated movement in the head and neck. As noted by Earls (2020):

> The SCCs are an essential part of the vestibular system for balance and orientation. As part of the inner ear, the three fluid-filled canals are oriented to the sagittal, frontal, and transverse planes...when movement occurs in one of the planes, it causes the canal to move further than the endolymph fluid that is contained within and creates relative motion between the two. The relative movement stimulates stereocilia within the ampulla, which then signal the brain regarding direction and amount of movement. (p.106)

How to do a similar action. Imagine an infinity symbol or a side-lying figure eight and draw it with the tip of the nose while keeping the action smooth and continuous, as if you are gently spilling water out from your ears. After working on one side, switch to the other side with the same action. Try to lead gently with the tip of the chin as an alternative.

Stick Mobility
Dennis Dunphy

The lateral tissue line which vertically extends from the side of your foot up to the side of the neck is often neglected in training protocols. Unfortunately, this can lead to deficiencies that can prevent you from acquiring the tissue quality and neuromuscular control that's needed in your daily activities. The lateral line is the linchpin that connects and supports your anterior and posterior chains, so restricted range of motion can be detrimental to your body's overall performance. The Lateral Bow and Arrow is one of Stick Mobility's signature movements that isometrically lengthens to overcome those constraints often observed in movements and resting posture.

Using a strong and flexible stick (Figure 5.breakout.2) allows you to add energy to the kinetic chain to build strength in the lengthened position. Flexibility enhancement (stretching) requires neuromuscular control, which is the missing element in passive stretching practices. We want you to own your range of motion, not just rent the space. Adding isometrics to your mobility work will engage your body like never before and allow you to make the changes that you're seeking, quicker. The Lateral Bow and Arrow helps work lateral flexion, an important but often missing component in movement warm-ups.

Begin with a shoulder-width stance and place the stick at either the 3 or 9 o'clock position. The bottom of the stick should be approximately 8–10 inches from your mid-foot. You need to ensure that your hips remain square during the entire movement to address the lateral tissues. Any rotation of the hips will move the line of pull to either the front or back. The hand nearest the stick is placed around the midpoint and the opposite hand reaches over and grabs the stick near the top. Both of your palms should be facing forward. Begin the movement by pushing your hips away from the stick and then use the bottom hand to actively push the stick in the opposite direction. Both legs and top arm need to be straight with no knee or elbow flexion to ensure optimal access to the targeted line. Your head should also be tilted as the lateral tissue line runs up into the side of the neck. Lastly, be sure to breathe to enhance your new range of motion. If you can't breathe in a position, then you don't own that position yet.

You can integrate this into your warm-up by dynamically holding for multiple short reps of 3–6 seconds to prep your body for moving external loads. Finish your workout by holding the position for longer periods of time to help down-regulate your systems. This will feel amazing, and your brain and body will thank you for finding this missing element.

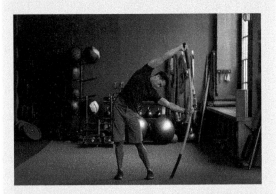

FIGURE 5.BREAKOUT.2 Photo courtesy of Stick Mobility.

Parts of lateral line connections are seen historically, particularly in the lower limbs (Figure 5.12). The interest in the iliotibial band (IT), and its widening relationship to the muscles around it is likely of continuing interest for walking and gait patterns. Imbalances in sidedness of the IT can contribute to asymmetry in the pelvis and knee.

Theories help us further map the body, but they are only useful if they give us ideas that lead to strategies that help better ourselves, our clients and our loved ones. Movement is a multi-directional event that is fuller than just "front," "back," and

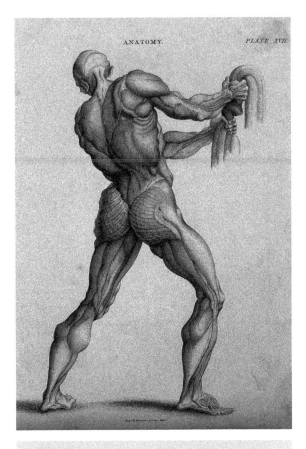

FIGURE 5.12 An écorché is a painting or drawing of the human body with the skin removed to show the muscles underneath. These drawings were sometimes standalone works of art but were really meant as a figure study exercise to understand the body underneath the clothing that might appear in a final work of art. While the anatomy is focused on the muscles, more of the myofascial connections can sometimes be seen. Here, pieces of Myers's Lateral Line are quite apparent on the right leg (gluteus maximus, tensor fasciae latae, iliotibial band, peroneals [fibularii]).

Credit: An écorché pulling down on a rope, seen from the back. Line engraving by Kirkwood & Sons, after W. Cowper, 1813. Wellcome Collection. Public Domain Mark.

"sides." However, starting with these major areas gives us several theoretical myofascial connections and ideas as long as we can acknowledge that many maps are square while the world is round.

My GPS often gets me to my destination, but I will still override it on occasion because I know a short cut or a path where the view is better.

References

Berger, J. (ed.) (1973) *Ways of Seeing*. New York, NY: Viking Press.

Cheng, H.-Y. K., Lin, C.-L., Wang, H.-W. and Chou, S.-W. (2008) 'Finite element analysis of plantar fascia under stretch—the relative contribution of windlass mechanism and Achilles tendon force.' *Journal of Biomechanics 41*, 9, 1937–1944.

Earls, J. (2020) *Born to Walk: Myofascial Efficiency and the Body in Movement*. Berkeley, CA: North Atlantic Books.

Myers, T. W. (2020) *Anatomy Trains: Myofascial Meridians for Manual Therapists and Movement Professionals* (4th ed.). London: Elsevier.

Nestor, J. (2020) *Breath: The New Science of a Lost Art*. New York, NY: Riverhead Books.

Schleip, R. (ed.) (2012) *Fascia: The Tensional Network of the Human Body: The Science and Clinical Applications in Manual and Movement Therapy*. Edinburgh: Churchill Livingstone.

Stecco, C., Corradin, M., Macchi, V., Morra, A. *et al.* (2013) 'Plantar fascia anatomy and its relationship with Achilles tendon and paratenon.' *Journal of Anatomy 223*, 6, 665–676. https://doi.org/10.1111/joa.12111

Stecco, C., Pirri, C., Fede, C., Fan, C. *et al.* (2019) 'Dermatome and fasciatome.' *Clinical Anatomy 32*, 7, 896–902. https://doi.org/10.1002/ca.23408

Storti, C. (2021) *The Art of Crossing Cultures*. Boston, MA: Intercultural Press.

Further reading

Beach, P. (2010) *Muscles and Meridians: The Manipulation of Shape*. Edinburgh: Churchill Livingstone.

Bolgla, L. A. and Malone, T. R. (2004) 'Plantar fasciitis and the windlass mechanism: A biomechanical link to clinical practice.' *Journal of Athletic Training 39*, 1, 77.

Cook, T. A. (1979) *The Curves of Life: Being an Account of Spiral Formations and their Application to Growth in Nature, to Science and to Art; with special reference to the manuscripts of Leonardo Da Vinci*. Mineola, NY: Dover Books.

Thayer, B. (n.d.) 'Vitruvius on Architecture—Book III.' *Marcus Vitruvius Pollio: De Architectura, Book III*. Accessed on 12/28/2019 at https://penelope.uchicago.edu/Thayer/E/Roman/Texts/Vitruvius/3*.html

Van Boerum, D. H. and Sangeorzan, B. J. (2003) 'Biomechanics and pathophysiology of flat foot.' *Foot and Ankle Clinics 8*, 3, 419–430.

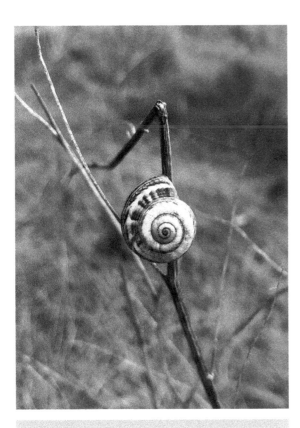

FIGURE 6.1 Spirals found in nature. Shells are logarithmic spirals in shape.

Photo by the author.

that we find in lab are often twisting and spiraling in growth patterns. Disease has movement, as does normal life functioning. Fascia itself, on the level of the spiraled collagen fibers, also shows this pattern (Scarr 2018).

This movement has inspired scientists for hundreds of years, from René Descartes mapping out a logarithmic spiral in 1638 to Theodore Andrea Cook's *The Curves of Life* ([1914] 1979). Cook referenced earlier scientists such as Professor Pettigrew who "showed that the propeller of a steamship exhibits the same functions as the fin of a fish, the wing of a bird, or the limbs of quadruped; and that in the whole range of animal locomotion these functions are most exquisitely displayed in flight." We continue this in our bipedal, contralateral walk, and the efficiency in many sports actions. Spirals encourage movement.

The spiral crosses cultures and history as a visual symbol as well as motif in many folk dances across the world. The labyrinth is a spiral path that circles inwards and outwards, enabling us to pass the same point over and again but from a different perspective each time. To walk and then stand in the center of a spiral or labyrinth has been a psycho-spiritual exercise for centering the consciousness. The Hopi Native Americans use labyrinths as a representation and awakening of the spirit, and as a tool in walking meditations. If one thinks of the pattern of the seasons in relationship to the arc of a lifetime, the pattern is a spiral with a repetition of seasons but viewed from a vantage point of the years.

Spirals are a key feature in our development. During the eighth week in utero, the lower limb is twisted from front to back, bringing a spiral into movement. This rotation brings the dorsal surface to the front (think of the back of your foot which is the front of your body). Dorsiflexion is, of course, bringing the back surfaces of the talar joint

It is worth pausing for a moment to reflect on how common spirals are in the body system as well as in our greater universe. They are prevalent in nature as well as in myofascial connections in the body. Think for a moment of all of the spirals you can name, including fiddleheads, shells (Figure 6.1), a flower folding inward at night, and the helical pattern in DNA. When I teach anatomy, I invite students to feel the shape of bones—there is a subtle curve and twist of the spiral pattern, mimicking our developmental dances as well. Even the tumors

axis together. Any rotation or general twist in our transverse plane will have a response of supination and pronation in the ankle.

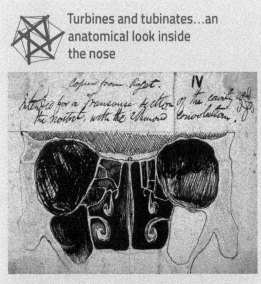

Turbines and tubinates...an anatomical look inside the nose

FIGURE 6.2 Dissection of the skull and nasal cavities. Pen and ink drawing, copied by J.C. Whishaw, ca. 1852. Wellcome Collection. Public Domain Mark.

When I kayak on the east coast of Canada, I have always been amazed to see that the fishing weirs are still designed in a spiral, taking advantage of the tidal changes in the ocean, and forcing the flow and directionality of the fish deeper into the inner portions. Found in cultures throughout the world including Asia, South America, and England, weirs are extremely effective in channeling fish and water. Spirals also have another advantage. Their shape allows for efficiency in movement in a small area.

Inside the skull are the turbinates (specifically the bony structures inside the nose that are covered with a type of soft tissue known as mucosa). The spiral shape (Figure 6.2) in this case helps to increase the surface area of air that is drawn into the body. The turbinates filter and keep out unwanted things (although a stray Lego block has

been known to lodge in a toddler's nose now and again) while channeling air. As noted in Nestor's *Breath* (2020), "the lower turbinates at the opening of the nostrils are covered in that pulsing erectile tissue, itself covered in mucous membrane, a nappy sheen of cells that moistens and warms breath to your body temperature while simultaneously filtering out particles and pollutants."

Technically, mucous membranes, including those of the stomach, urinary bladder, and lungs, are usually consistent in having a deep layer of connective tissue covered in a surface of epithelial cells. Most of these membranes secrete the mucopolysaccharide (known as mucin), the primary substance of mucus. Most erectile tissues are covered in fascia. Scarpa's fascia, covering the abdominal wall, continues in men with the external fascia of the Colles. Continuous with the perineal fascia is the deeper fascia commonly known as Buck's fascia. The ligaments are likewise fascial in nature, and perhaps importantly noting the sensory nature of sexual organs. Likewise, the clitoris is encased in a fascial layer with suspensory ligaments. As a sidenote, the superficial fascia in these areas, as well as the eyelid and ear, do not contain adipose but are highly viscoelastic (Eizenberg *et al.* 2007).

Returning to the turbinates and breathing, we all accept that if you are moving, your breathing will impact your performance.

> The spiraling shapes of muscles and bones bear witness to the living world of water and also to a purposeful aim toward mastery of the solid and are reminiscent of the way water flows in meanders and twisting surfaces in the interplay between resting in spheres and being drawn in an earthward direction.
>
> Theodor Schwenk (1978)

Spirals and loops in motion and stability

In the body, spirals and loops of any sort can serve functionally in both allowing rotation and movement, but also serving to stabilize the body,

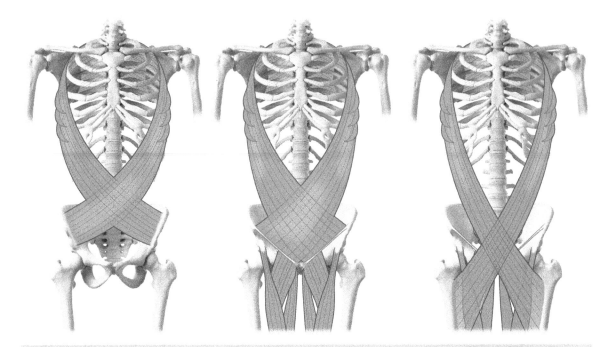

FIGURE 6.3 Muscles and fascial connections including rhomboids to serratus anterior muscles, as well as the more global shoulder girdle and abdominal interconnections. Illustrations after Porterfield and DeRosa (2004).

particularly where spirals overlap. In looking at the issues of back pain and postural concerns particularly related to the middle of the body, James A. Porterfield and Carl DeRosa outlined several different muscle slings and anatomical linkages which are noted via their fascial and ligamentous connections (Figure 6.3). Most myofascial spirals cross at some point, providing a support to the body through the crisscross of fiber directions, via the internal and external obliques, and in several continuing via serratus anterior and rhomboid connections such as in Myers's spiral line or the diagonal crisscross of Raymond Dart's concept that helped the body support itself upright.

Embrace your spirals
Rebekah Rotstein

My first cadaver dissection in 2007 opened my eyes to spirals. Nothing in the human body was linear as I had expected it to be, and everywhere I looked, I discovered curves and contours. It made me wonder: if this is in fact our structural makeup, wouldn't it make sense that our motions naturally follow those sinuous paths as well? In other words, shouldn't function follow form in this instance? The more I studied, the more I learned that indeed, human movement innately spirals, inspired by the orientation and shape of the joint surfaces. (And these surfaces in fact form through spiraling actions during embryological development!) Forces transmit through the joints resulting in helical motion. We see this in the arthrokinematics of the spine, which, along with ground reaction force, produce a visible spiral in the gait cycle as each joint responds to its neighboring joint from heel upward and outward. What we consider a sagittal plane activity is far from it when examined closely.

So how does this awareness affect the way we perceive movement, if we no longer consider walking a strictly linear activity? And what about other multiplanar movements like throwing a ball?

Can the shifted perception of movement also change the way we move, and perhaps improve the quality of that movement?

Embracing the notion of our innate spirals changes our embodiment from a more mechanical approach to a more fluid quality. The spiral evokes a sense of continuity. There are no clear breaks of the line of a spiral, no edges or corners. In fact, the spiral is a curvature of line (Figure 6.4).

Spirals are elegant and sinuous, not sharp or jagged. People often equate elegance with softness and delicacy. Yet in the context of movement, elegance can relate to quite the opposite. Think of a flamenco dancer—the elegant, sweeping movements are also stark and swift.

In the same manner, we can consider the spiral as the enabler of this efficiency of movement. After all, the helix is a fundamental component of biotensegrity. This model of structure and function explains the body as a self-supporting system that obtains its inherent stability from tension and compression forces, without fulcrums or levers. It's precisely this paradigm of force distribution where the entire structure is interconnected that supports and explains the significance of the spiral to integrated human movement.

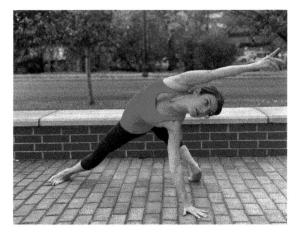

FIGURE 6.4 Spirals are part of our movement interactions in the world. Our myofascial body, especially torso and limbs, has an ability for rotation. Our cross-pattern locomotion (opposite arm/opposite leg) also encourages medial and lateral rotation. All of these spirals allow a wide range of movement and an easy cadence for walking long distances.

Photo courtesy of Rebekah Rotstein.

A helix is a smooth spatial curve within a contained structure like a tube. Corkscrews and spiral staircases (Figure 6.5) are examples of helixes, as well as the common strand of DNA. Collagen, our building block in fascia to bone, is constructed around spirals and, in particular, around the form of a helix. In addition to contractions, one of the main principles of choreographer Martha Graham's work was the concept of spiraling. In spiraling, one imagines the center of the body as a shaft with two axis points in the throat and the base of the spine. The external line of the spine starts from the hip and spirals to the upper shoulder on the opposite side. Much of the fall and recovery techniques in modern dance and rolls in Parkour involve spiraling to aid the distribution of strain. Even the

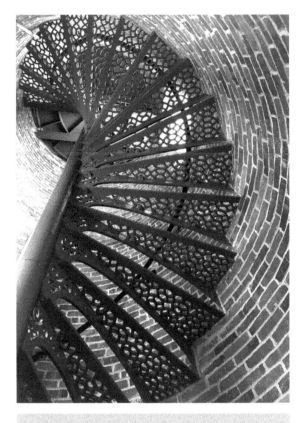

FIGURE 6.5 A spiral staircase in a cone tower is a helix.

martial arts technique of "sticky hands" involves rotating and spiraling an opponent to disable them without much effort.

Spirals are written into our shape, whether our DNA, spiraling myofascial connections, or much of our most economical and beautiful movement expressions. Spirals are efficient means to maximize space and how to move through it.

References

Cook, T. A. (1979) *The Curves of Life: Being an Account of Spiral Formations and their Application to Growth in Nature, to Science, and to Art with special reference to the manuscripts of Leonardo da Vinci.* Mineola, NY: Dover Publications.

Eizenberg, N. (2007) *An@tomedia.* New York: McGraw-Hill.

Nestor, J. (2020) *Breath: The New Science of a Lost Art.* London: Riverhead Books.

Scarr, G. (2018) *Biotensegrity: The Structural Basis of Life.* 2nd ed. Edinburgh: Handspring Publishing.

Schwenk, T. (1978) *Sensitive Chaos: The Creation of Flowing Forms in Water and Air* . New York: Shocken Books.

Further reading

Anatomy 101: The Windlass Mechanism and Great Toe Extension. (n.d.) Rayner & Smale. Accessed December 28, 2019 from www.raynersmale.com/blog/2017/9/5/anatomy-101-the-windlass-mechanism-great-toe-extension

Bolgla, L. A. and Malone, T. R. (2004) 'Plantar fasciitis and the windlass mechanism: A biomechanical link to clinical practice.' *Journal of Athletic Training 39*, 1, 77.

Caravaggi, P., Pataky, T., Goulermas, J. Y., Savage, R. and Crompton, R. (2009) 'A dynamic model of the windlass mechanism of the foot: Evidence for early stance phase preloading of the plantar aponeurosis.' *Journal of Experimental Biology 212*,15, 2491–2499.

Movement is what we are, not something we do.

Emilie Conrad, Founder of Continuum Movement®

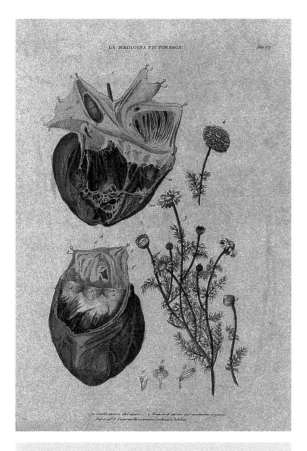

FIGURE 7.1 Anatomy and botany; top, human heart; bottom left, human heart; bottom right, chamomile flowers. Colored engraving, 1834–1837.

Credit: Wellcome Collection. Public Domain Mark.

How do you define core? Does it exist at all? And yet, we language "core" to connect to meanings such as "deep" and "profound." Many of our myofascial connections also embody this aspect and there are many similar overlaps in our human reactions to "core." Think of the metaphoric terminology of the French "coeur," or heart, which has similarities to the Middle English "core" like the center of a fruit like an apple core. "Core" can be the "heart" (Figure 7.1) or essence of a being, both metaphorically and physically. Go to any modern gym and classes abound with descriptions of "core power" and "core strength," but what does this mean? Even those with extensive backgrounds in movement are often unsure of an exact definition or will debate with colleagues in similar fields. When I ask mixed groups of movement professionals, most define the core as the "abs" and "support for the back." The Pilates world feels they have it a bit more defined. Ah the core—it is the "powerhouse." The concept of core came about as terminology in the 1990s and started getting explored more in scientific terms around the turn of the century. "Center" of the body has been around, though, early in our history, from the idea of central channel of sushumna in yoga to particular other styles of core.

Many concepts of core look at the containment of the abdominal cavity and, as such, the middle of the body in traditional terms includes muscles such as the transversus abdominis (TA), which has the action of pulling the front of the body into the midline. If you place your hands on your hips, most of the thin muscle fiber of transversus and the obliques sits underneath. The rectus abdominis of course, has its fiber direction vertically in the front of the body, but dives down deeply under the facial arcuate line. Without the ability to agree what we are discussing, the concept of "core" is meaningless, and we cannot place it spatially in the body.

Core, as noted by Bond (2007), is technically the organs contained in the fascial peritoneum bag, but also can be conceptualized as two core muscle girdles. The first girdle contains the transversus abdominis (TA), which, in front,

*blends into a layer of fascia that runs between the breast-
bone and the pubic bone. In back, its fibers attach to the
upper rim of the pelvis, the fascia of the lumbar spine, and
the insides surface of the lower ribs. (p.93)*

Responsible for stabilization when the appendicular body is moving, in activity such as walking, it
has difficulty properly engaging in those with back
pain. The outer corset is defined as including the
external obliques and while unable to stabilize
the same way since they don't connect to the spine,
they have an effect in downward pull on the rib cage
when tight which can restrict both breathing and
the free swing of the legs. However, finding the TA,
both experientially in the body or in dissection lab,
can be a challenge. Often, as I have assisted dissections, students will find the internal and external
obliques, but question where the TA muscles have
gone. Usually, we can find the horizontal fibers and
peel back a paper-thin layer that is often quite less
substantial than one might expect.

The National Academy of Sports Medicine
(NASM) defines "core" as "lumbo-pelvic hip complex" with the musculature of the core divided into
three areas: "local stabilization system," global stabilization system, and movement system. In the
concept of the local, muscles are primarily those
attaching directly to the vertebrae such as the lumbar multifidus, internal obliques, transversus
abdominis, pelvic floor, and diaphragm. "Global
stabilization system" takes into consideration stabilization between the spine and pelvis and includes
the adductors, rectus abdominis, psoas, quadratus lumborum, and external obliques. "Movement
system" is primarily for the spine or pelvis to
extremities and includes hip flexors, hamstrings,
quadriceps, and latissimus dorsi (Clark *et al.* 2018).

The spine, via the lamina and spinothalamic
pathway, is one pathway of interoception, which
is just behind the anterior longitudinal ligament.
The vagus nerve (which is the tenth cranial nerve)
is known as the wanderer and in its journey travels through the volume of the central portion of
the body cavities and passes through many fascial

spaces as well as organs. It is powerful because
it is such an extensive neural pathway that links
mind (brain), body (maybe feeling-wise situated
more deeply in our gut than we ever realized), and
the heart with its pericardial sac (traditionally the
soul of the body, and actually what the ancient
Egyptians believed was the center of the body).

As noted in Earls (2021), "The internal organs
are contained within layers of serous membranes
that allow independent movement between the
thoracoabdominal contents and the outer musculoskeletal locomotor system. The layered arrangement reduces external mechanical stress reaching
the visceral tissues" (p.119). Again, while holism
may rule the conceptual world, there is a practical
aspect of being built around sliding layers that helps
protect our most central self. Core doesn't need to
be hard, but rather a yielding and mobile center of
the body can make the entire body responsive.

Breathing

Breath is central to life and to movement, and the
shape of the core myofascial connections becomes
part of this. Even on its small surface, a cell needs
the exchange of matter from the outside to the
inside and this movement is all managed through
expansion and contraction. In the middle of this is
of course the diaphragm, with attachments to the
lumbar spine, the psoas major, as well as the quadratus lumborum and abdominal muscles. The human
diaphragm is like a giant jellyfish, responding to
the fluid nature of the internal body and moving
around 17,000 times a day. This myofascial combination of pericardial sac to diaphragm is at the very
center of a living, breathing body (Figure 7.2).

The shoulder muscles often get utilized as
accessory muscles of breathing. Think of an asth-
matic person, who will brace their arms against
a surface to help breathing during an attack, or
an elderly person who elevates their shoulders as
a means to help the breath. The rib cage is often
considered to be a basket more precisely than the
often named cage, with two significant myofascial

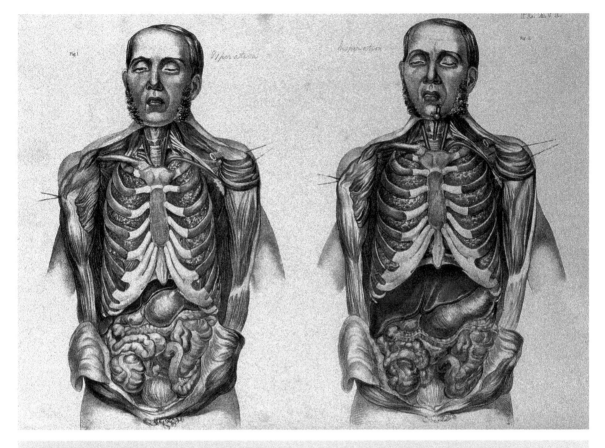

FIGURE 7.2 The body of a man with the trunk dissected: two figures showing the lungs after breathing out (left) and after breathing in (right, simulated by inflating the lungs). Colored lithograph by William Fairland, 1869. Attribution 4.0 International (CC BY 4.0).

suspensions: the scalenes at the top and the quadratus lumborum pulling down at the bottom. In a way, the lungs can also be considered part of this suspension. We also often see fascial adhesions limiting range of motion of the lungs against the rib cage.

Breathing and speech

Breathing gets tied in to the "myofascia middle" via the movement of the diaphragm. Although the lungs are not generally considered part of the core, the movement of the diaphragm contributes to many of the benefits of breathing including enhancing fascial glide, moving lymph and blood, and helping with stabilizing the spine.

The Arabic maqam is a tone that is also spatial in nature, with the root of the word meaning "placement." In terms of yoga, the "bija" sounds are like a type of ultrasound, creating a vibration in different parts of the body system. Additional concepts such as the chakras (Figure 7.3) work with esoteric anatomy as do the koshas, or layered sheaths of the body. Breathwork is a large part of classical as well as newer yoga therapeutic traditions.

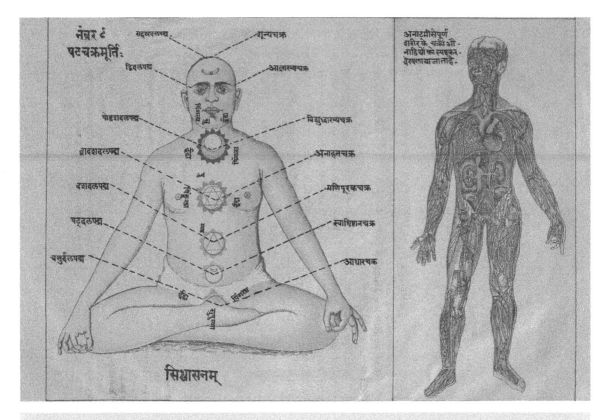

FIGURE 7.3 Illustration of the six chakras of tantric yoga in Sanskrit and Hindi. One of eight colored plates, drawing explicit parallels between the yogic view of chakras etc., and the medical/anatomical view of the body. Svamihamsasvarupakrtam Satcakranirupanactiram: bhasyasamalamkrtam bhasatikopetan ca = Shatchakra niroopana chittra with bhashya and bhasha containing the pictures of the different nerves and plexuses of the human body with their full description showing the easiest way to practice pranayam by the mental suspension of breath through meditation only; drawings by Shri Swami Hansa Swaroop. Author: Svami Hamsasvarupa. Sanskrit MS 391.

Credit: Two drawings: the easiest method to practice pranayama by. Wellcome Collection. Attribution 4.0 International (CC BY 4.0).

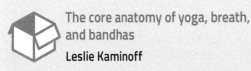

The core anatomy of yoga, breath, and bandhas

Leslie Kaminoff

When studying the anatomy of breath from the perspective of yoga practice, much attention is understandably given to the primary role of the respiratory diaphragm—yet for breath and movement to be fully integrated, the location and function of other muscular diaphragms must be taken into account. Of particular interest to yoga practitioners are the coordinated actions of the pelvic and vocal diaphragms in movement, posture, and breath technique.

All three diaphragms (pelvic, respiratory, and vocal) come together in yoga movements that are coordinated with inhaling and exhaling. In addition to giving more length and texture to the breath, valving actions in the glottal region (ujayyi)[1] create

---

1 Ujayyi derives from the Sanskrit ud, "to flow out" and jaya "victory or triumph."

a kind of back pressure throughout the abdominal and thoracic cavities. This pressure can protect the spine during the long, slow flexion and extension movements that occur in the breath-synchronized flowing practice of *vinyasa* (arrangement or placement), such as during sun salutations. In yogic terms, these coordinated actions of the diaphragms are referred to as *bandha* (binding, bonding, or tying).

Mula bandha, or root lock (*mula* meaning firmly fixed or root) is a lifting action produced in the pelvic floor muscles that also includes the lower fibers of the deep abdominal layers which creates an upward stabilization of the central tendon of the respiratory diaphragm. The corresponding upward shift in the abdominal contents created by mula bandha requires the circumference of the costal margin to make space by "flying upward" (uddiya). This lifting action is referred to as *uddiyana bandha* or flying upward lock. Mula bandha and uddiyana bandha are, in fact, the bottom and top of a singular gesture; uddiyana is the space toward which mula rises, mula is the support upon which uddiyana roots to rise. Because the rib cage acts as an integrated unit, lifting the lower ribs also lifts the upper ribs and sternum, and when that action is combined with cervical flexion, jalandhara bandha is activated. When all three bandhas are engaged, the practitioner is said to be performing "maha bandha," or "the great lock." Breathing with all three locks in place stabilizes most of the usual shape changes in the body cavities, and thus challenges the practitioner to find a deeper, more subtle space for breath movement deep within the core of the body. This space is referred to as sushumna in yoga's esoteric anatomies and is considered to be the ultimate destination for prana—life force.

In the highly influential teaching tradition of T. Krishnamacharya, an essential concept of practice involves what could be referred to as "vertical axis integration." This is the breath-centered, yogic version of core work. Krishnamacharya's techniques show how to correctly use the pelvic, thoracic, and vocal diaphragms in the work of breathing so that the practitioner experiences their inhaled breath as a movement descending from the head toward the epigastric region, and the exhaled breath as an ascending movement from the pelvic floor toward the epigastric region.

Yoga practitioners who have been influenced by these ideas are understandably enthusiastic when exposed to myofascial models that can help them to embody the cues and pathways of sensation with which they have become familiar through practice. For example, a common cue given in standing practice is to look for the origin of the diaphragm's support in the lifting of arches of the feet, which is often referred to as "pada (foot) bandha." When presented with an image of Albinus' famous etching of the anterior view of his "fourth order of muscles," which connects the myofascia supporting the foot's arches to the leg and pelvic floor, iliopsoas, diaphragm, and deep anterior neck musculature, many yoga enthusiasts experience a deep sense of recognition and validation, as these are pathways with which they have become very familiar through countless hours spent on their mats.

Concepts of body/mind core

In *Body Movement* (1980), Bartenieff and Lewis noted the "Central Inner Support" (Figure 7.4) as containing the iliopsoas, diaphragm, and the related quadratus lumborum as a link unit. Moreover, Bartenieff emphasized the use of vowels in the control of breath, which they subtitled, "inner space." As noted:

Movement rides on the flow of the breath. Frequently, students in their overconscientiousness about breathing or negation of breath will tend to hold the breath at one part of the phase—either the "in" or the "out." By doing this, they forego the many subtle inner changes that occur in different configurations of limbs, trunk, head. They also forego many subtleties in phrasing. (Bartenieff and Lewis 1980, p.232)

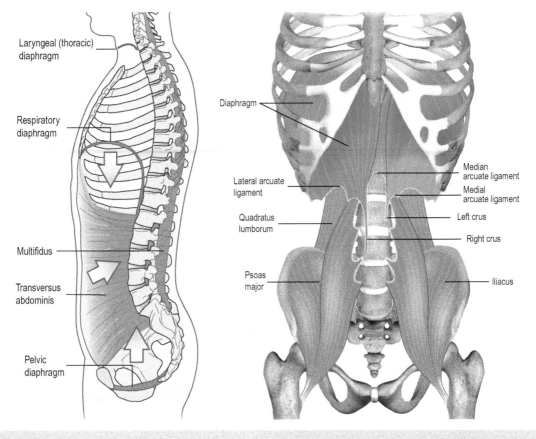

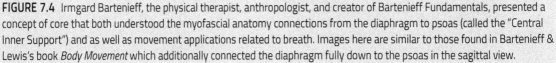

FIGURE 7.4 Irmgard Bartenieff, the physical therapist, anthropologist, and creator of Bartenieff Fundamentals, presented a concept of core that both understood the myofascial anatomy connections from the diaphragm to psoas (called the "Central Inner Support") and as well as movement applications related to breath. Images here are similar to those found in Bartenieff & Lewis's book *Body Movement* which additionally connected the diaphragm fully down to the psoas in the sagittal view.

Bartenieff further noted that sounds create different shape qualities in the body.

A number of Hindu or Buddhistic (particularly, Tantric Buddhism) meditation and inner concentration traditions involve inner and outer body shape changes by using definite vowels and sequences of vowels for support of different inner spaces—abdomen, chest, mouth. These sounds cause reverberations in different segments. (Bartenieff and Lewis 1980, p.232)

I read Bartenieff's book as part of my early training as a dance/movement therapist but had forgotten about this passage until years later, after studying yoga and chanting what is known as the "bija" sounds, essentially a vibrational chant that is meant to correspond with the seven major chakras along the spine. When chanting, they vibrate very clearly in different areas, which always made me wonder if they are a primitive (or highly sophisticated) form of ultrasound, or activation via another mechanism. Kalyani *et al.* (2011) focus on the concept that the vibration of Om may have the potential for vagus nerve stimulation. By using functional magnetic resonance imaging (fMRI), the researchers noted limbic deactivation, meriting further research.

Frank Wilczek, the winner of the Nobel Prize in physics and author of *A Beautiful Question* (2016), also offers his contribution in Core Theory. This whole idea builds upon the physics concept of "Standard Model" which, he notes, implies that it is waiting for the real thing to come along. He also notes, "'standard' connotes 'conventional' and hints at superior wisdom. But no such superior wisdom is available. In fact, I think— and mountains of evidence attest—that while the Core Theory will be supplemented, its core will persist" (Wilczek 2016, p.8). So, in a metaphoric and physical anatomical sense, whatever we define as "core" remains the strong center of the theory, universe, or body (Figure 7.5).

In understanding the concept of Core Theory in physics (which expands upon Einstein's theory of relativity), one also takes a look at the relationship of particles and forces, and of space and form. Wilczek wanted to discuss Core Theory in terms of what we know now.

What does this have to do with the form of fascia and the way we move it? According to Wilczek, "two obsessions are the hallmarks of Nature's artistic style:

Symmetry—a love of harmony, balance, and proportion

Economy—satisfaction in producing an abundance of effects from a very limited means" (Wilczek 2016, p.11).

In anatomy we know that the body is not symmetrical (just look at the asymmetry present in the digestive system) but looking for relational balance within the body for ease and health is important as well as what we term "myofascial efficiency."

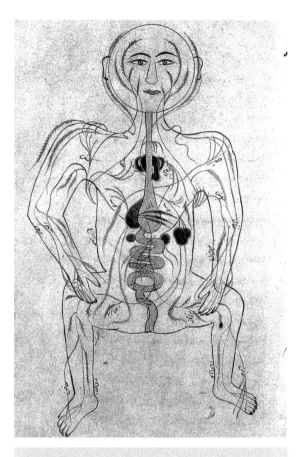

FIGURE 7.5 The center of the body can be conceptualized as fluid and air-filled sacs of fascia. Here, the artist has chosen to represent the body as largely symmetrical despite the asymmetry in the viscera, perhaps as a nod to much of Nature's expression of form and efficiency.

Credit: Human figure showing arteries and viscera, Persian, 18th C. Wellcome Collection. Attribution 4.0 International (CC BY 4.0).

The breathing body: lungs as core "packers"

The lungs are not typically defined as part of the core, but their intimate relationship to the pericardial sac, the diaphragm (Figure 7.6), and their fascial relationship are worth considering as another core line. This consists of the nasal passages and the lungs with their relationship to the pericardial sac, with an alternative route through the mouth, including the vocal cords. Tone and sounding have become interesting to those working in polyvagal theories, or in the ability to hold the breath without panic.

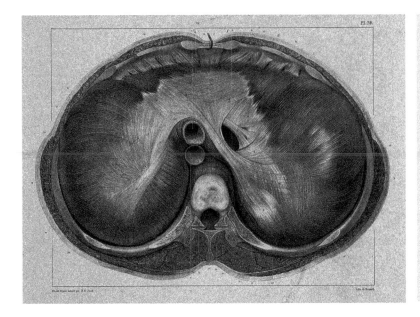

FIGURE 7.6 Horizontal dissection of the diaphragm, at the level of the 10th dorsal vertebra. Lithograph by N.H Jacob, 1831/1854.

Credit: Wellcome Collection. Public Domain Mark.

As noted by Bond (2007):

...it has been observed that the laxity of the jaw and inner corset often coincide, contributing to a vicious circle of inadequate core support and anxiety-producing breathing patterns. In such cases, the crura of the diaphragm may be recruited to stabilize the core, making matters worse. (p.159)

Breathing is an interesting area that has been explored by many in sports, including free diving. Free divers need to train to hold their breath for extremely long periods and remain calm during the time that they are under extremely deep water. The preparation for a free diver is to take long, slow inhales and slow exhales to reduce CO_2 in the system, and then they further do a technique called "packing," which is several short final inhales to fill the lungs.

Remember our spiral chapter and the turbinates that swirl the air? In an article published in *Nature* (Sobel *et al.* 1999), the effects of a known difference between the two nostrils due to a slight difference in the turbinates has been shown to create air switches between the two sides for still unknown reasons. However, the authors of this article proposed that the differences between the two nostrils seem to sensitize each to slightly different olfactory perceptions.

Don't just do something...be there

When we pause and take a moment, we can step out of our thought process. Close your eyes and let go of trying to control the breath in this moment. While we work many different breath techniques, we can unite in the shared experience of being human. Take in a deep breath and breathe out in any way that feels good to you. Allow the breath to be a shared experience of being in the body and connected to each and every one around you.

Many of us hum when we are thinking through something. While I haven't seen a gym machine for oropharyngeal exercise (Figure 7.7), the importance of sounding in relationship to the connections through the body may be a self-soothing way to access "core." Myofascially, it makes sense that representations of myofascial continuities are voluminous in nature, such as Myers's (2020) Deep Front Line which follows three different tracks in the center of the body, highlighting relationships from the feet to deep throat, and encircling diaphragm and pericardial connections (Figure 7.8).

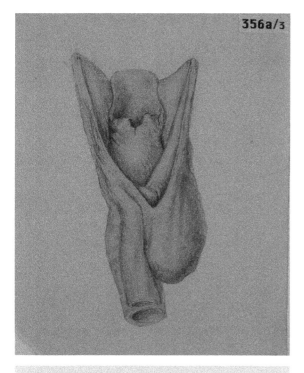

FIGURE 7.7 Pharyngeal pouch.

Credit: St Bartholomew's Hospital Archives and Museum. Attribution 4.0 International (CC BY 4.0).

The fascial female floor

The core of the body could be argued as containing both the strongest muscle in the body (the uterus) as well as the fastest muscles (the vocal cords). Sacro-uteral ligaments are connected to the SI joint. When the cervix swells it can pull on these ligaments fascially. The cervix can twist or pull in every monthly cycle for women.

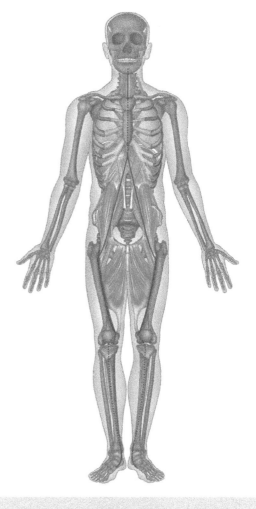

FIGURE 7.8 The inner core of our body, the Deep Front Line, which is also an interface between the musculoskeletal and visceral body. Image courtesy of David Lesondak and Handspring Publishing with kind permission from Thomas W. Myers.

Inner space

The concept of "inner space" is both defined as space "at or near the earth's surface and especially under the sea" as well as "one's inner self" (Merriam Webster 2020). This idea of how we defined both a metaphoric and physical core is still up for debate but seems to link in many systems with the idea of stability, both in relationship to movement as well as a psychological sense of being okay. Ida Rolf thought about an "inner line" of the body in the early work of Structural Integration. When the body is stabilized internally, it allows graceful and easy movement.

Balancing the Diaphragms
Julie Hammond and Fiona Palmer

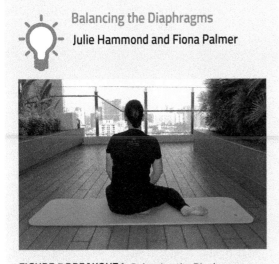

FIGURE 7.BREAKOUT.1 Balancing the Diaphragms.
Julie Hammond and Fiona Palmer are both ATSI teachers and SI practitioners and have a passion for anatomy. Balancing the Diaphragms is a collaboration based on a love of anatomy, dissection, and the desire to gain a more cohesive understanding of these areas and how they can support each other. Balancing the Diaphragms looks at the five diaphragms and one honorary sixth diaphragm, the foot's arch.

They both believe that there is always another rabbit hole to dive down, another question unanswered. Their focus is on collaboration and global connections in the body and collaboration and cooperation between health professionals for more effective client outcomes.

> A group becomes a team when each member is sure enough of himself and his contribution to praise the skills of others.
>
> Norman Shidle

Balancing the Diaphragms
Julie Hammond and Fiona Palmer

Adductor magnus/cleaning the ischiopubic ramus
This exercise (Figure 7.breakout.1) is one of the easiest to add to your class. Pelvic repositioning has been shown to help balance the tone of the pelvic diaphragm and can enhance the outcome of pelvic floor exercises. Done as an exploration exercise, it will often lead to a better starting point for pelvic diaphragm training. Clients have reported feeling more grounded, with a sense of more space and the ability to activate the pelvic diaphragm more easily. It can help to facilitate more fluid movement and stimulate the muscles.

Go into a deep, pain-free squat or knees wide four-point kneeling weight transfer forward and back exercise before the exercise, to test for freedom of movement. This will also allow you to compare changes after the exercise. You can also take the time to notice how your arches respond to the ground. Notice differences between the left and right sides of your body. What happens when you take a breath or engage and relax your pelvic diaphragm?

Use a chair and sit to the left edge with a prickle pod placed under the right ischiopubic ramus. Start the exercise by taking some deep breaths. When you feel the area on the pod ease a little, try some small anterior/posterior pelvic tilts. Aim to clean the bone and mobilize the soft tissue gently. You may increase this by adding some weight transfer from the right to the left foot to create a small semi-circle action of the ischiopubic ramus on the pod. Do the mobilization on one side, and then try your squat again. Have a walk and sense the position of the pelvis. This exercise is good for clients with a posterior or lateral tilt of the pelvis and creates adaptability in the pelvic diaphragm.

Deep lines

Historically, "core" myofascial anatomy has been depicted with an emphasis on the diaphragm/psoas relationship, including in "Tabulae sceleti et musculorum corporis humani" by Albinus (Figure 7.9), which shows a myofascial connections from the lower leg to the adductors,

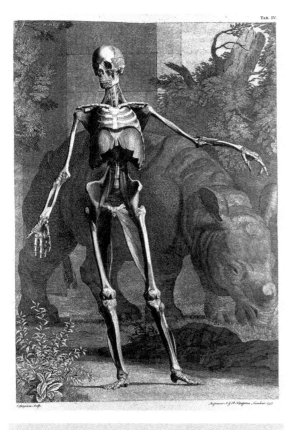

TAB. IV.

FIGURE 7.9 Tabulae sceleti et musculorum corporis humani, Bernhard Siegfried Albinus. Credit: Wellcome Collection. Attribution 4.0 International (CC BY 4.0).

has been pursuing the idea of a Deep Back Line, which is not part of the official AT canon. The Deep Front Line goes from the medial plantar fascia surface, following much of the initial route of the Superficial Back Line (gastrocnemius, to portions of the hamstring, continuing to the sacrotuberous ligament) but diverts and dives to the deep lamina of the thoracolumbar fascia via the suboccipitals to the dura mater, falx cerebri, and tentorium cerebelli to the inner cranium (Carmel 2014).

As noted in Gabler (2017):

Deep fascial elements of the Deep Front Line affect the organs and the breath, the Deep Back Line also affects the deep fascia of all the bones and joints along the spine, which also connect to the sympathetic and parasympathetic nervous system... [this line] could also be registering our reaction to trauma and stress—our startle reflex. (p.77)

Interestingly, the fascial continuities of the deep body have been studied in comparative anatomy as well, most notably in equines. Elbrønd and Schultz (2021) published a comparative study of myofascial anatomy between horses and humans, based on Myers's Anatomy Trains®. Interestingly, they concluded a

new line identified in this study, is a Deep Dorsal Line (DDL), which starts in the dorsal tail muscles. It comprises myofascial structures of the spinocostotransversal system from the tail to the head including the nuchal ligament. It connects to the dura mater and has a major role in controlling the motion and stabilization of Columna vertebralis.

continuing the deep psoas/diaphragm relationship and including some of the deep neck tissues. For the curious, the addition of the anatomically correct rhinoceros, named Clara, was both a nod to the interest in exotic animals (she toured Europe at this time), and to give scale to the figure, positioned in life-like gesture and in a landscape setting, as did others, such as Vesalius' depictions of his "de Humani Corporis Fabrica Libri Septem" with figures pictured against an Italian landscape.

More recently, Yaron Gal Carmel (an Anatomy Trains® teacher and structural integrator)

Both humans and horses have connection via the dura mater and its relevance for posture and form expression, but the front limb connections differ between horses and humans due to the differences in biped vs. quadruped anatomy.

Whether or not Carmel's Deep Back Line qualifies as a formal line, there appears to be a relevance in both humans and horses, at minimum, in looking at the connections of the dura mater for its relevance in posture and form expression.

Accessing the deep core—from the ground up
Dr. Emily Splichal, DPM, MS, CES

Feet, fascia, and functional movement

As the only contact point between the body and the ground, our feet play a very important role in how we stabilize and coordinate dynamic movement. From the moment our foot contacts the ground, powerful sensory stimulation triggers a series of interconnected motor responses designed to load and transfer the potential energy associated with foot strike.

The utilization of this impact force potential energy is directly related to the timing and coordination of our stabilization. The faster we can stabilize, the more efficient we will be at loading and transferring the energy.

When considering energy transfer and stabilization we need to think not of our feet in isolation but rather how their function relates to the rest of our body, namely to our center of mass or core. This association between our feet and core stabilization is established fascially through the Deep Front Line, as well as via co-contractions or muscle synergies which exist between the flexor hallucis longus and the posterior pelvic floor.

To activate and integrate the foot to core fascial stabilization patterns I recommend using the exercise short foot. First introduced by Dr. Vladimir Janda of the Czech Republic, short foot has been shown to be an effective intrinsic foot muscle exercise as well as a foot to core activation exercise.

When performing short foot exercise, it is important to remember the Deep Front Fascial Line and how the foot connects to the core muscles. Every contraction of the foot should be coordinated with a lift of the pelvic floor and an exhalation of the breath.

To perform short foot: Stand with feet in a split stance position with the knees slightly bent. Start by finding the front foot tripod which is under the 1st metatarsal, 5th metatarsal, and heel. Lift the toes, spread them out, and place them back down to the floor. To properly engage short foot, push the tips of the toes down to the ground like you are grounding or anchoring the toes. Hold for 5 seconds. Avoid curling the toes or rolling to the side of the foot. Allow the 1st metatarsal head and medial arch to lift. After you become familiar with the pushing of the digits down, start to find a lift of the pelvic floor during the foot activation. Try to feel the connection between the foot and core when holding the toes down.

Repeat on both sides, and eventually progressing to both feet at the same time.

This foot to core activation and integration via the Deep Front Line is one of the most important functional concepts for achieving optimal stability during dynamic movement. What seems a simple foot contraction actually lays the foundation through which all other fascial lines can then contract.

Horizational aspects to the central myofascial body—the lateral raphe

Lateral to the spine is the lateral raphe (meaning union of parts). It is a ridged structure of dense connective tissue formed by the bringing together of anterior and posterior lamina of the thoracolumbar fascia (Stecco and Hammer 2015, p.208). According to Stecco and Hammer, who favor the two-layered model, the lateral raphe's role is to redistribute the muscular tensions into both layers to avoid localized load on just one or two vertebrae. In terms of movement, these different layers (Figure 7.10) may be tightening in order to support the body due to other weaknesses.

As part of the Fascial Net Plastination project I conducted a fascia focused dissection of an abdominal cross section, which was repeated by the team in 2022, to highlight these horizonal fascial connections.

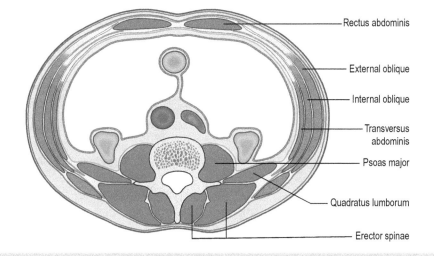

Labels:
- Rectus abdominis
- External oblique
- Internal oblique
- Transversus abdominis
- Psoas major
- Quadratus lumborum
- Erector spinae

FIGURE 7.10 Abdominal and thoracolumbar fascial layers after John Hall Grundy's *Human Structure and Shape*. Bringing together two layers (Stecco and Hammer 2015) of thoracolumbar aponeurosis is the lateral raphe (meaning a union of parts), creating a ridged structure created from 1) hypaxial muscles of QL (quadratus lumborum), psoas, rectus abdominis and transversus and 2) erector spinae (iliocostalis, longissimus, spinalis) and the transversospinal (multifidus, semispinalis, and rotators). Some define this structure as three layers, including transversus abdominis and the internal and external obliques, different in terms of histological features being different from the thoracolumbar fascia.

The dawn chorus

I am not a singer, but I hum when I'm thinking through a problem. Nor was I ever an "early bird," so to speak, but rather for most of my life I preferred catching my second wave of energy late and was often what one considers a "night owl." Perhaps biology dictates more of our habits and tendencies than we care to admit, but as I moved further and further away from my own adolescence and into adulthood, I got up earlier, but still only readily woke up with the dawn when I was on kayaking camping trips and much more closely attuned to the natural rhythms of daylight and darkness. All that changed recently, perhaps due to shifting hormones, a series of challenging personal events with family and work, or that minor inconvenience of a pandemic. I found that by waking at dawn I could easily squeeze in two to three hours of walking and be home before the rest of the house awoke and I'd need to be online.

I became interested in this phenomenon of the dawn chorus and began to wonder more about it. The singing of birds at dawn has a limited time frame seasonally. There are many reasons that those certain days of midsummer yield such sound in the eastern US. The time of year might be about defending territory or singing for an existing relationship and just as importantly, early morning gives the cooler air temperature to allow sound to travel well and far. When we sing, the mylohyoid is acting as a diaphragm in the same way as the pelvic floor. The fibers run horizontal and act as a barrier. Along with the geniohyoid, this mylohyoid creates the floor of the mouth in a similar way as the pubococcygeus and iliococcygeus form the pubic floor.

Ancient forms of singing and breathwork may indeed have tonal benefits in a variety of ways.

The myofascia in the center of the body has deep and strong connections which have been outlined by several thinkers. Some have seen our center as including the psoas on each side connecting our lower and upper limbs, as well as the fascial connections from the diaphragm to the pericardial sac surrounding the heart. More than simply tightening the abs, the myofascial structures supporting our bodies may give us new ideas, even extending to our feet, voice and more, as being connected in this dialogue.

References

Bartenieff, I. and Lewis, D. (1980) *Body Movement: Coping with the Environment*. Philadelphia, PA: Gordon and Breach Science Publishers.

Bond, M. (2007) *The New Rules of Posture: How to Sit, Stand, and Move in the Modern World*. Rochester, VT: Healing Arts Press.

Carmel, Y. G. (2014) 'The deep back line and a proposed alternate superficial back line.' *International Association of Structural Integrators Yearbook*. Severna Park, MD: International Association of Structural Integrators.

Clark, M., McGill, E., Lucett, S. and National Academy of Sports Medicine (eds) (2018) *NASM Essentials of Personal Fitness Training*. Burlington, MA: Jones and Bartlett Learning.

Earls, J. (2021) *Understanding the Human Foot: An Illustrated Guide to Form and Function for Practitioners*. West Sussex, UK: Lotus Publishing.

Elbrønd, V. S. and Schultz, R. M. (2021) 'Deep myofascial kinetic lines in horses, comparative dissection studies derived from humans.' *Open Journal of Veterinary Medicine 11*, 01, 14–40. https://doi.org/10.4236/ojvm.2021.111002

Gabler, K. M. (2017) *Your Body's Brilliant Design: A Revolutionary Approach to Relieving Chronic Pain*. New York, NY: Skyhorse Publishing.

Kalyani, B., Venkatasubramanian, G., Arasappa, R., Rao, N. et al. (2011) 'Neurohemodynamic correlates of "OM" chanting: A pilot functional magnetic resonance imaging study.' *International Journal of Yoga 4*, 1, 3. https://doi.org/10.4103/0973-6131.78171

Merriam-Webster. (n.d.) *Space*. Accessed on 03/28/2022 at www.merriam-webster.com/dictionary/space

Sobel, N., Khan, R. M., Saltman, A., Sullivan, E. V. and Gabrieli, J. D. E. (1999) 'The world smells different to each nostril.' *Nature 402*, 6757, 35–35. https://doi.org/10.1038/46944

Stecco, C. and Hammer, W. I. (2015) *Functional Atlas of The Human Fascial System*. London: Elsevier.

Wilczek, F. (2016) *A Beautiful Question: Finding Nature's Deep Design*. London: Penguin Press.

Further reading

Earls, J. (2020) *Born to Walk: Myofascial Efficiency and the Body in Movement*. Berkeley, CA: North Atlantic Books.

Häfner, K. (1994) *Lanz. 1: Firmenchronik, Dampfmaschinen, Benzinzugmaschinen, Verdampfer-Bulldogs: von 1859–1929*. Stuttgart: Franckh-Kosmos.

Myers, T. W. (2020) *Anatomy Trains: Myofascial Meridians for Manual Therapists and Movement Professionals* (4th ed.). London: Elsevier.

Richey, R. (n.d.) *Core Objectives: Making a Case for Progressive Core Training*. NASM. Accessed on 11/12/2021 at https://blog.nasm.org/progressive-core-training

Rolf, I. P. (1989) *Rolfing: Reestablishing the Natural Alignment and Structural Integration of the Human Body for Vitality and Well-being*. Rochester, VT: Healing Arts Press.

Rosenbaum, T. Y. (2007) 'REVIEWS: Pelvic floor involvement in male and female sexual dysfunction and the role of pelvic floor rehabilitation in treatment: a literature review.' *The Journal of Sexual Medicine 4*, 1, 4–13. https://doi.org/10.1111/j.1743-6109.2006.00393.x

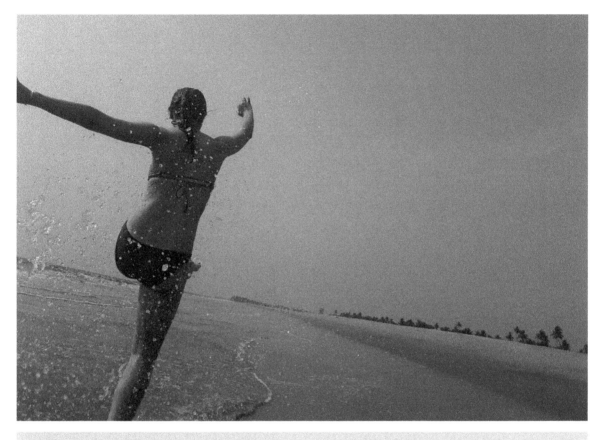

FIGURE 8.1 Cross body concepts and the fascia of the arms and legs take the body into dynamic action.

Photo courtesy of Benjamin Feinstein.

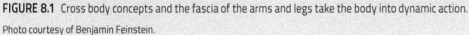

When I was very little, my family used to visit my grandparents in St. Louis. Their house sat adjacent to a railroad track and I would climb up the apple tree in the middle of their backyard to be able to wave at the trains that would come by. Climbing, jumping (Figure 8.1), and other sports actions, be they recreational, work, or athletic discipline, involve the arms, and often the connections from the arms to opposite legs or occasionally same side of the body (ipsilateral). A general concept in all of the myofascial slings in

relationship to movement is the idea that muscle and fascia working together produce a transfer of load. The directionality of this type of force can be thought of as a force vector.

In Diane Lee's book on *The Pelvic Girdle* (2011) she outlines four sling systems that assist this concept of load transfer through the lumbar/pelvic region. They are: anterior oblique sling (AOS), posterior oblique sling (POS), deep longitudinal sling (DLS), and the lateral sling (LS). Kurt Tittel's "muscle slings" look at the muscles that are in connection to functionally work together in movement and what he often notes as dynamic stabilization of central axial skeleton. The Functional Lines according to Anatomy Trains® (2021) (front, back, and ipsilateral) work in movement, connecting opposite limb to limb in the case of front to back lines, or same-side in ipsilateral. They are important in working in accelerating or decelerating the trunk in rotation as well as producing torque and power in movement.

Cross-patterned movement, counterlateral Xs, and functional lines

In all of these similar systems of connection, the idea of movement comes in connecting opposite appendicular limb to opposite appendicular limb (front and back) in most all walking, running, and athletic activities as well as occasionally recruiting through the same side (ipsilateral). These are the lines of motion and action, whether we are throwing a baseball pitch or dancing the tango with a partner. Since their tissues are superficial, their role in static patterns is minimal, although they do provide postural support in active yoga poses, for example.

The arms and legs have a parallel in their anatomical set-up in bone number, but from there the structures vary quite a bit. The ball and socket joint of the leg is meant for overall stability, useful in bipedalism, but the arm is meant for large range of motion and sits in a shallow socket, which can compromise lines showing clear connection. Quadrupeds keep their weight underneath them, with narrow rib cages. However, as we became bipedal, we broadened through our shoulders, bringing the arms wide out to the sides of the body.

In sports activity, arms and cross body connections can be involved in understanding healthier movement options, as well as explaining some of the common injuries seen in this part of the body. The continuation of the arms to the opposite appendicular limb (i.e. the opposite leg) as well as

the newer ipsilateral continuity, create the family of Functional Lines. The arm lines are important for their recognition of the larger tie-in to the central part of the body. While the arms are logically sequenced, in real life, the variations in connecting these myofascial meridians becomes more confusing with a concept called crossovers, essentially switches between the muscles being utilized.

Movement applications: tennis elbow

Although we are known as bipedal creatures, our past roots in brachiation still have remnants in our anatomy (Figure 8.2). Anyone who has had the pain of tennis elbow can attest to the extreme discomfort and challenge of this fascial injury. In healthy tissue, hyaluronan keeps everything sliding and gliding but in injury, inactivity, or immobilization, hyaluronan gets thick and as it densifies, it doesn't work as well in movement. Fascia biosynthesizes hyaluronan via fasciacytes and can respond well to shearing motions and are found predominantly in the epimysium (Stecco *et al.* 2018).

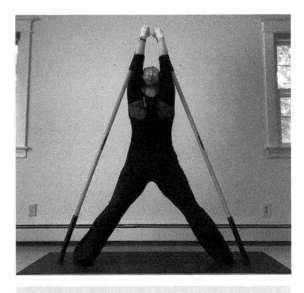

FIGURE 8.2 Stick Mobility.

Photo by the author.

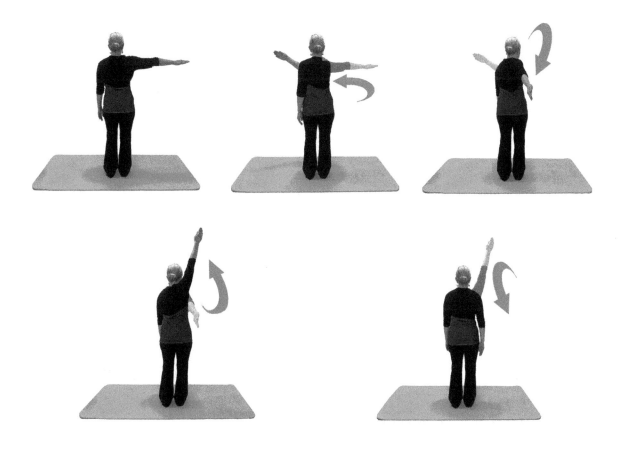

FIGURE 8.3 Arm swing—creating multi-dimensional volume and fascial resilience.

Pectoralis minor is sometimes used as an accessory breathing muscle when asthmatics use the arms to brace themselves during an asthma attack. Think of catching one's breath after exertion such as running to catch a bus. You will often see the arms braced on the hips or thighs to facilitate upper body stability for accessory breathing.

Building on the idea that we are closer in our anatomy to suspensory locomotion than full-out brachiation, we are still far away from utilizing the same movements as our tree-loving relatives. However, creating movement range of motion over time can lead to greater resiliency in the body for sports and daily activities.

Arm swing-creating multi-dimensional volume and fascial resilience

Based on a modern dance warm-up exercise, this arm sequence (Figure 8.3) brings the arms through their range of motion, while emphasizing activating myofascial connections in the arms to the central body.

Directions

Begin with your right arm out to the side and then swing across (frontal plane). Come around and back, making a circle in the sagittal plane.

Return to the beginning

All the concepts of fascial pre-loading and pre-tensioning can be added by bending the knees and taking little jumps throughout the sequence.

Throwing a ball via cross-body myofascial connections

Throwing a baseball (or other small ball) can demonstrate the work needed to take the arm lines into their functional extensions as cross-body myofascial connections. In working with wheelchair users, it is still important to try to connect contralaterally in order to throw a ball. Try it for yourself. Sit in a chair with your sacrum posteriorly tilted and leaning into the back surface of the chair. Try to throw the ball. Chances are strong that you will be throwing from just your arms and missing the myofascial connections. Now come to the front of your chair and think of utilizing the opposite side as part of the whole throwing connection. This is the basic principle in efficient kayaking as well (i.e. utilize the contralateral connections for efficiency versus fatiguing the arms). Functional connections are connections of movement and sport actions.

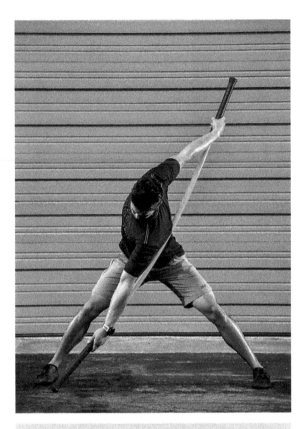

FIGURE 8.4 Feedback can come through tools, such as a stick, that help access the outer ranges of motion.

Photo courtesy of Stick Mobility.

Using feedback tools for myofascial training improvement

Dennis Dunphy, Co-Founder of Stick Mobility

An ingredient that is often missing in training programs that prevents someone from understanding and improving their movement(s), body awareness, and overall performance is *feedback* (Figure 8.4). Kinesthetic learning is a great way to help improve your movement. Using a tool like Stick Mobility will supercharge your proprioceptors by helping you feel and activate areas of your body that you weren't aware of. The act of pushing or pulling on the stick initiates the tensioning of the fascial line(s) that you're looking to stretch and/or strengthen. This allows the user to target specific tissues or lines that are inhibited along with targeting specific joint function(s).

We are often too passive regarding our approach to mobility work. Humans innately create tension along lines of tissue when yawning and stretching, which allows us to reach into an extended range of motion. Yet this is not a regular practice among most stretching protocols. By pushing and/or pulling on a stick, or other tools, we strengthen our tissues and improve neuromuscular control in these outer ranges of motion giving us more freedom to move.

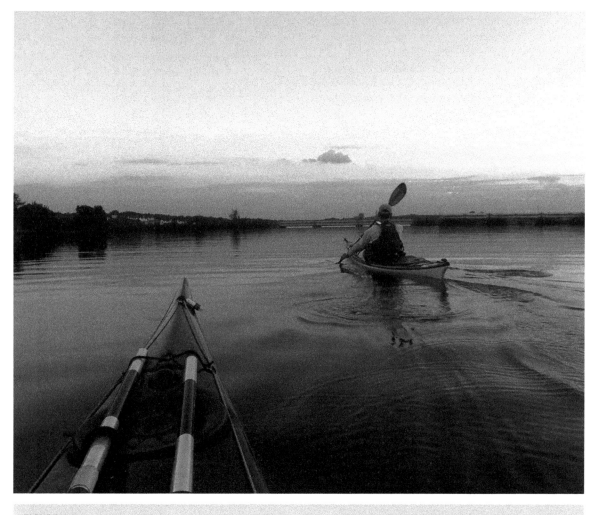

FIGURE 8.5 Kayaking.

Photo by the author.

The paddler's diamond and moving form into efficiency

The general feel of this action can be done on land in groups of four using a wooden dowel as a paddle. The "kayaker" sits in the middle with the legs in a kayaker's diamond (knees out) and ankles and toes dorsiflexed. Begin the paddling action and there isn't much power behind the movement. However, two people give support to the outside of the knees, and one can be at the base of the feet giving something to push against. Paddle again, and suddenly the action is translated through the Functional Lines and power, bringing the paddling action out of the arms and into a fuller body sensation.

As noted in in Myers (2020):

The paddling arm connects from the Deep Back Arm Line, pulling from the little finger side through to the BFL, and thus stabilized to the opposite leg. The upper arms push through the Deep Front Arm Line to the thumb, stabilizing via the FFL to the opposite thigh. If the knee is not fixed against the hull of the kayak, the push will be felt passing from foot to foot, almost in imitation of a walking movement. (p.144)

The push/pull of these lines is critical in any sport, but kayaking provides an example of the lifted arm pushing through the Front Functional Line (FFL), while the side of the paddle pulls via the Back Functional Line (BFL). Sea kayaks are built thin and narrow, with the paddler's knees in contact with the top or side of the hull.

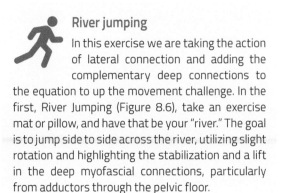

River jumping

In this exercise we are taking the action of lateral connection and adding the complementary deep connections to the equation to up the movement challenge. In the first, River Jumping (Figure 8.6), take an exercise mat or pillow, and have that be your "river." The goal is to jump side to side across the river, utilizing slight rotation and highlighting the stabilization and a lift in the deep myofascial connections, particularly from adductors through the pelvic floor.

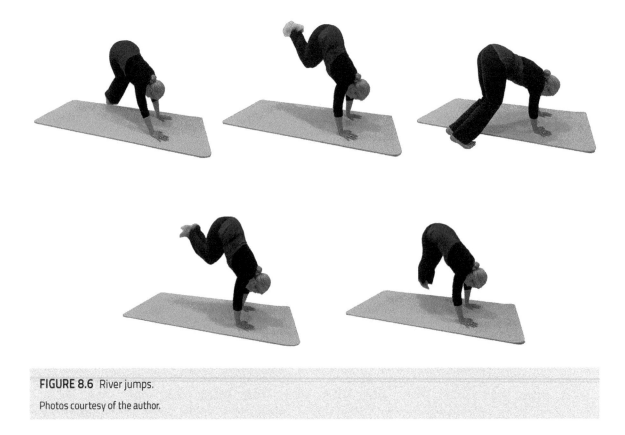

FIGURE 8.6 River jumps.

Photos courtesy of the author.

Optimizing a golf swing

Michael Jacobs, 50 Best Golf Teachers in America—Golf Digest, Top 100 Golf Teachers in America—Golf Magazine

Swinging a golf club is one of the most complicated movements of any sport. Throwing a ball and swinging a bat or racquet are closely aligned with the structure of the human body—and in fact take advantage of the physical traits humans possess. But a golf swing requires a full rotational movement of the torso coupled with extreme mobility within the shoulder complex—all while oriented toward a small object on the ground.

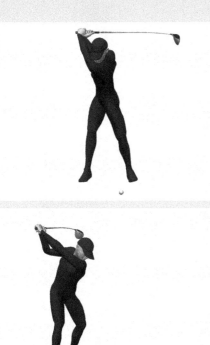

FIGURE 8.BREAKOUT.1–4 These pictures are all examples of the golfer's swing. The best golfers use whip-like action of the body with myofascial efficiency.

Photos courtesy of Michael Jacobs.

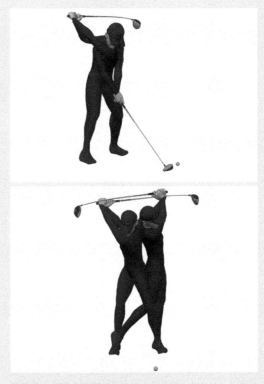

FIGURE 8.BREAKOUT.1–4 *Continued*

Our research has established that a golf club in the hands of a skilled player experiences more than 80 g of acceleration on its path down toward the ball, and that same player is imparting more than four horsepower to the club. To do this effectively and repeatedly, a player has to create a system that is essentially a human whip (Figures 8.breakout.1–4). Because a player is limited by his or her specific individual physical characteristics, the manner in which he or she creates that whip obviously must vary. But the world of performance training has mostly preferred to oversimplify the individual assessment phase, and it usually attempts to standardize every player's mechanical motion. This leaves great potential for practitioners who can combine the worlds of sport-specific technical instruction with body-specific spatial medicine concepts to truly personalize and optimize golf (and sport) learning and performance improvement.

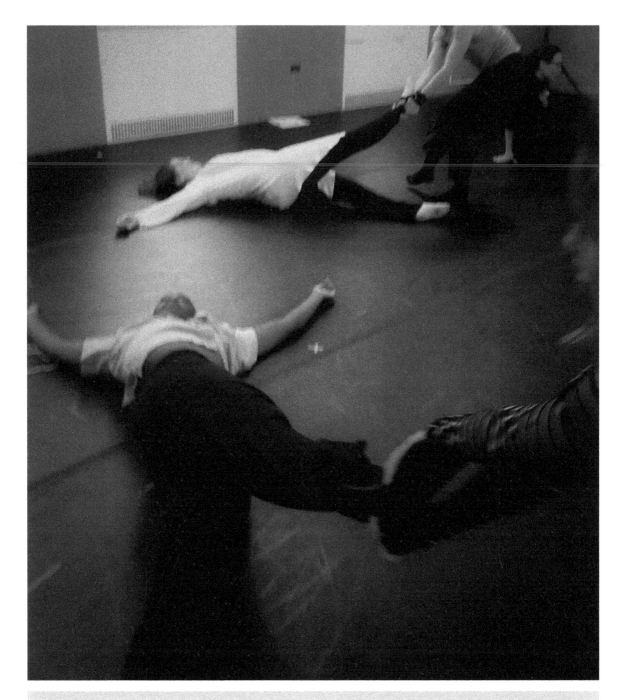

FIGURE 8.7 Cross body connections can be felt, such as in the Bartenieff Fundamental x movement in which a distal part of the body leads the movement in rolling over. We are essentially working with the myofascial net. This can be both treatment and assessment. Photo by the author.

Fascial continuities can be felt both contralaterally (opposite limb to opposite limb) and ipsilaterally (same side). When we tension the myofascial net of a friend (Figure 8.7), we can feel both freedoms and restrictions in the body.

An important component for strength, conditioning, and athletic performance

Holly Clemens, PhD, LMT, CSCS

Strength and conditioning coaches are always looking for training programs that can improve an athlete's performance across a wide range of both general and sport-specific skills while also reducing risk of injury. Traditionally, training programs have focused on resistance training exercises that emphasize muscular strength by using maximum load strategies. While traditional resistance training exercises do strengthen the muscular contractile elements, they don't provide the stimulus to optimize many properties of the fascial system such as myofascial force transmission, elastic recoil, and strain distribution.

There is now greater recognition regarding the significant role the fascial system plays in enhancing movement and sports performance. Research continues to evolve on fascia and its potential role in enhancing strength and power gains, athletic performance, injury prevention, and sports-related rehabilitation (Bond *et al.* 2019; Zugel *et al.* 2018). Much of the research on fascia has led more coaches to incorporate fascial training into their current strength and conditioning programs with an emphasis on training the global myofascial chains.

The myofascial chains play a large role in enhancing force transmission, power, speed, and myofascial efficiency in sport-specific movements such as hitting, pitching, throwing, catching, kicking, jumping, and running. Coaches can incorporate fascial training using the myofascial chains during dynamic warm-ups, as secondary exercises in training workouts, or as recovery movements in cool-downs.

While there are many myofascial chains that can be incorporated into an athlete's training program, the following progressions provide an example of how to incorporate the anterior and posterior diagonal chains (Wilke 2021). These chains are also referred to as the front and back functional lines (Myers 2020), the anterior and posterior oblique systems (Vleeming 1995), and the anterior and posterior spiral kinetic chains (Schwartz 2017). The anterior diagonal chain connects the lower limb to the contralateral upper limb through the ventral cavity while the posterior diagonal chain connects the lower limb to the contralateral upper limb through the dorsal cavity. These chains are important myofascial force generators, accelerators, and decelerators for sport-specific movements, such as throwing a football, kicking a soccer ball, and serving in tennis. The following movement progressions were inspired by A. P. Lindberg's Anatomy Trains® in Training.

Learning and sensing the diagonal chains
Have the athlete start in a staggered stance. For the anterior diagonal chain, have an athlete tie one end of an elastic band on the back leg near the adductor longus attachment of the femur, move the band anterior across the torso, then tie the other end of the band to the contralateral upper arm at the pectoralis major attachment of the humerus. For the posterior diagonal chain, have the athlete tie one end of another elastic band on the back leg at the vastus lateralis attachment of the femur, move the band posterior across the gluteus maximus, then tie the other end of the band to the contralateral arm at the latissimus dorsi attachment of the humerus. The bands may help the athlete develop a kinesthetic sense of the lower body to core to upper body myofascial connection and the relationship between the anterior and posterior diagonal chains.

To start, have the athlete press both feet into the ground, rotate the hips and torso toward the front stance leg and reach the arm diagonally up and back to finish the countermovement. During this slow wave-like motion, the athlete should see the anterior band lengthening, sense increasing pre-tension in the band, and develop a kinesthetic awareness of the anterior diagonal chain. The athlete may also sense less pre-tension in the band representing the posterior diagonal chain. At the peak of the countermovement, the athlete will press the feet into the ground, rotate the hips, torso, and arm forward and move the back leg diagonally forward, as in a stepping or kicking motion. The wave-like motion finishes with the arm reaching diagonally down toward the contralateral hip or leg. During this motion, the athlete should see and sense the band representing the anterior diagonal chain losing pre-tension and stiffness. At the same time, the athlete should sense the band representing the posterior diagonal chain pre-tensioning as it lengthens to aid in deceleration of the forward movement. Have the athlete continue practicing the sequence using slow wave-like motions from start to finish.

Progression 1

Once the athlete can perform the unloaded, slow, wave-like movement sequence proficiently, have the athlete progress to an unloaded rhythmic, dynamic movement sequence. The emphasis is on the proximal initiation of the feet, hips, and torso followed by a distal delay of the contralateral arm at the peak of the countermovement. This distal delay will pre-tension the fascia even more to help create a dynamic whip-like movement. The additional pre-tension and whip-like movement makes use of the elastic storage and recoil properties of fascia. Progressing to this more dynamic whip-like movement prepares the athlete for sport skills that occur in "real-time" and helps the athlete understand how the anterior and posterior diagonal chains complement one another during acceleration and deceleration.

Progression 2

The athlete can progress the movement sequence by introducing load. The added load will help enhance proprioceptive refinement, provide additional pre-load, and improve the strength and resiliency of myofascial tissue. Have the athlete start with a low

load in one hand, such as a dumbbell, and initiate the slow wave-like movement sequence, eventually progressing to the more rhythmical, dynamic sequence (Figure 8.breakout.5). The orange band represents the anterior diagonal chain, and the blue band represents the posterior diagonal chain.

To add additional variety, have the athlete micro-progress using various speeds, rhythms, loads, angles of pull, and even different myofascial chains. These variations will help enhance not only fascial resiliency, but also the athlete's kinesthetic intelligence as they learn how to change and adapt timing and rhythm into their sport-specific movements.

It may be valuable to remind coaches and athletes that the fascial system takes time to adapt, and conditioning results are accumulated slowly, over a period of 6–24 months. Coaches and athletes also need to be aware that 24 hours after heavy exercise

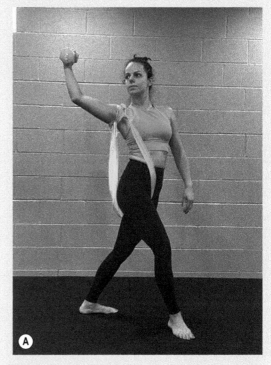

(A)

FIGURE 8.BREAKOUT.5A Photo courtesy of Tetyana Chervinska.

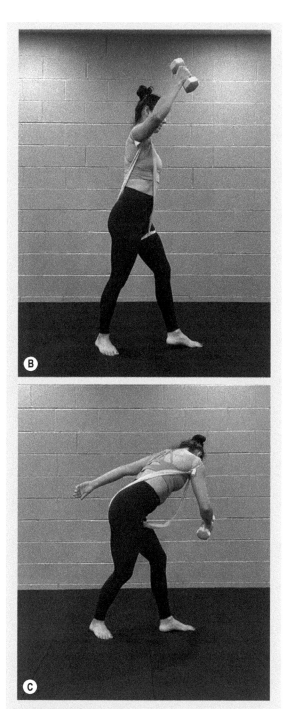

FIGURE 8.BREAKOUT.5B,C Photos courtesy of Tetyana Chervinska.

loading, collagen degradation outweighs collagen synthesis and the athlete's system may be weaker and less able to respond positively to an intense next day workout. However, after 48–72 hours, there is a net synthesis of collagen, which can enhance the athlete's connective tissue strength to better handle heavy exercise loading (Magnusson et al. 2010). Because of the time it takes to have a net synthesis of collagen, it is recommended that fascial training be programmed into a strength and conditioning program only 2–3 times per week to allow for sufficient collagen renewal. Due to this adaptation timeline, coaches may also want to have their athletes engage in fascial training programs prior to the start of heavy resistance training programs. Once fascial conditioning has been established, coaches can intersperse it throughout other cycles of the training program to maintain fascial conditioning with the goal of developing more adaptable and resilient athletes.

References

Bond, M. M., Lloyd, R., Braun, R. A. and Eldridge, J. A. (2019) Measurement of strength gains using a fascial system exercise program. *International Journal of Exercise Science 12*, 1, 825–838.

Magnusson, S. P., Langberg, H. and Kjaer, M. (2010) 'The pathogenesis of tendinopathy: Balancing the response to loading'. *Nature Rev Rheumat.* 6, 262–268.

Myers, T. W. (2020) *Anatomy Trains: Myofascial Meridians for Manual Therapists and Movement Professionals* (4th ed.). London: Elsevier.

Vleeming, A., Snijders, C. J., Stoeckart, R. and Mens, J. M. A. (1995) 'A new light on low back pain.' In *Proceedings from the 2nd Interdisciplinary World Congress on Low Back Pain*, San Diego, CA, USA.

Wilke, J. (2021) 'Myofascial continuity: towards a new understanding of human anatomy.' In R. Schleip and J. Wilke (eds), *Fascia in Sports and Movement.* Edinburgh: Handspring Publishing, pp.221–231.

Zügel, M., Maganaris, C. N., Wilke, J., Jurkat-Rott, K. *et al.* (2018) 'Fascial tissue research in sports medicine: from molecules to tissue adaptation, injury, and diagnostics.' *British Journal of Sports Medicine 52*, 1497. https://doi: 10.1136/bjsports-2018-099308

As noted in our evolution chapter, brachiation is more of a modern choice in the body than a necessity, although many of our favorite sports involve the arms heavily as does our reach to grab an item high on a kitchen shelf. Understanding the cross movement between appendicular limbs (arms to legs) can also make us more efficient in our pedestrian movement (particularly literally walking) to kayaking, golf, and more.

References

Lee, D., Lee, L.-J. and Vleeming, A. (2011) *The Pelvic Girdle: An Integration of Clinical Expertise and Research.* Edinburgh: Churchill Livingstone.

Myers, T. W. (2020) *Anatomy Trains: Myofascial Meridians for Manual Therapists and Movement Professionals* (4th ed.). London: Elsevier.

Stecco, C., Fede, C., Macchi, V., Porzionato, A. *et al.* (2018) 'The fasciacytes: a new cell devoted to fascial gliding regulation: the fasciacytes.' *Clinical Anatomy 31*, 5, 667–76. https://doi.org/10.1002/ca.23072

Further reading

Menon, R., Oswald, S., Raghavan, P., Regatte, R. and Stecco, A. (2020) 'T1ρ-mapping for musculoskeletal pain diagnosis: case series of variation of water bound glycosaminoglycans quantification before and after Fascial Manipulation® in subjects with elbow pain.' *International Journal of Environmental Research and Public Health 17*, 3, 708. https://doi.org/10.3390/ijerph17030708

Stecco, C., Giordani, F., Fan, C., Biz, C. *et al.* (2019) 'Role of fasciae around the median nerve in pathogenesis of carpal tunnel syndrome: microscopic and ultrasound study.' *Journal of Anatomy 236*, 4, 660–667. https://doi.org/10.1111/joa.13124

2

Fascia and the dynamic body
Spatial use and coordination

All living organisms share the ability to negotiate movement in space, and their movement patterns—from a short yoga sequence/vinyasa to a trail run to the larger actions in our work and life—all involve a level of coordination. In essence, we are working with ecology, that branch of science that involves relationship of living organisms, both to each other, as well as to the greater environment. "Spatial coordination" is a term that is used in architecture to describe the process of design and construction. Life, as we have all experienced is far from organized, but coordination creates ease in movement quality. When fascia gets stuck, it can restrict muscle movement as well and use more energy to do any action, and also it is less efficient. In our second part of this book, we are exploring several different movement disciplines as well how the myofascial system shapes differently as we age. Bringing together different elements of either the body or the larger system in relationship to environmental space in a functioning and efficient way is part of the dance of coordination.

Yoga   147

Pilates   158

Training, weight work, and sports specifics   164

Aging process—myofascial efficiency throughout life stages   179

Environmental matters—internal and external space and how we perceive and use it 191

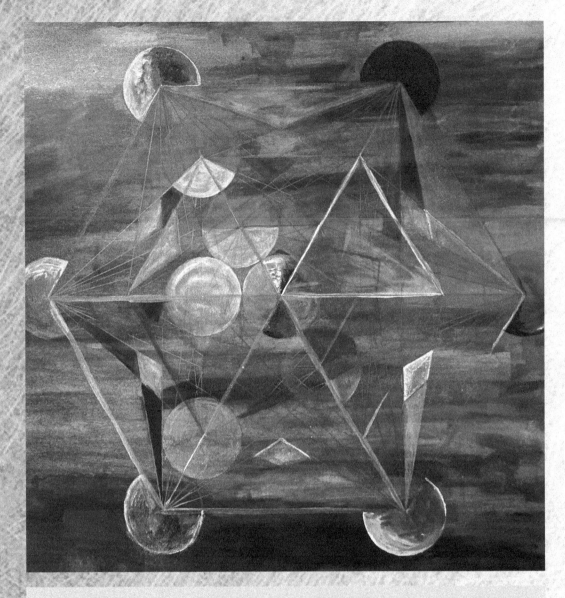

FIGURE PART 2.1 Inner/Outer Space Harmony Series—Field of a Bun Dance. Acrylic on wood by permission of artist Laura V. Ward.

Inner/Outer Space Harmony Series–Field of a Bun Dance is a play on what is seen, what is unseen, what is implied, what we notice, and what our brain decides to interpret for us. In other words, our reality tunnel. For me, painting geometric space and the movement of human fascia both lead to the spectrum of free-dom and form, which I find fascinating. Whether studying anatomy with Gil Hedley, doing Laban's scales that move within the scaffolding of the Platonic solids, or interpreting those Platonic solids through art, something within me is completely caught up, spellbound. I can lose myself with no thought to time. In Effort Theory (from Laban Movement Analysis) there is a drive called Spell Drive. It is a 3 combination of the three Efforts: Space, Weight, and Flow. There is no Time Effort in it–this means we don't see changes of Time. We don't see things speeding up or slowing down. We are lost in our spell. Fascinated–spellbound–bind–bundle–fascia. It all comes around again. Tessellations moving in and out of focus.

Laura V. Ward, artist

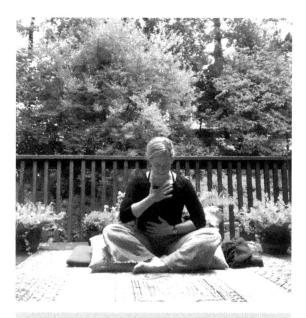

FIGURE 9.1 Yoga has transformed many times from its roots in India to the modern forms focused on asana and more recently to the felt sense of the body.

Photo courtesy of the author.

One of my very first yoga teachers, Karin Stephan, used to tell us the story of how she watched her father, a tailor, hem pants. What appeared to be a shorter leg often was a result of rotation somewhere else in the body. Her father had compassion for his customers no matter what the reason they had need of his skills. This began her journey into observation of the body and care for the person. Years later, when I worked with her after a very difficult car accident, she reminded me not to identify myself as an injury. I would encounter this concept of seeing the whole person over a diagnosis in my later work in myofascial anatomy.

Yoga: a brief history of a complicated practice

Yoga, like fascia, is a system focused on connection and integration. Yoga as a practice extends beyond any one group or belief, but has its original roots in India, where it spread through the Eastern world and eventually gaining a large foothold in the Western world through the 1893 World's Fair in Chicago, and later with interest from pop culture. Placed in the general estimate of 5000–6000 years old (Feuerstein 2008), the practice has evolved or changed branches, particularly in modern times.

The practice has always been about connecting, as noted in the Sanskrit roots of the word yoga, or *yuj*, which means to yoke together in the same way two animals were traditionally yoked together in farm work to be able to work as a unit. Yoga, like fascia, is about the independent components joined together in connection.

The modern branch of yoga has a direct link to Sri Krishnamacharya, who taught many important students including B. K. S. Iyengar (Iyengar yoga which heavily utilizes props to enhance alignment learning), Pattajbhi Jois (Ashtanga yoga which influences other styles of modern vinyasa), Indra Devi (who influenced many in early Hollywood and became a key female teacher), and Krishnamacharya's own son, T. K. V. Desikachar (who influenced modern yoga therapeutics and breathwork). Krishnamacharya is believed to have been influenced by Western styles of movement such as European forms of gymnastics (Singleton 2010). It was Krishnamacharya, and perhaps Desikachar after that, who taught that yoga was about working with the unique person. This is a more holistic view of yoga for the individual person, rather than making a person fit into a certain set of poses or idealistic alignment.

Additional concepts from yoga practice

Patanjali, in the classical yoga text, *The Yoga Sutras*, describes posture as the dynamic between sthira (steadiness) and sukha (openness). This is a description of our anatomy, which, whether on a micro or macro level, needs both stability and openness to function well in movement. Think about this in terms of fascia. If surgery, for example, creates a scar, that action may initially help to immobilize an area from the immediate trauma and create stability. However, if this scar tissue and adhesion of layers remain, the adhesion may restrict movement in the body and cause further injuries.

Additionally, there is the concept that yoga helps humans to focus, and through that focus, things can appear, and in doing so, see things in their true shape (Yoga Sutra 1.2–4). While the yogis may not have been conceptualizing form and function or the fascial system, there is a definite reverberation of the idea that pulling on any part of the system will affect the rest of the whole. Any distortion in the system (mental or physical) results in a distortion of the whole.

Permission to find autonomy in a system

Within the new styles of yoga practice, teachers are looking to help students find more autonomy in the way they respond to directions in their practice and to create a sense of understanding in how movement, asana, feels to them (Figure 9.1). For a while, people wanted to feel a stretch; if we are understanding the fascial science, we can see that sometimes we should be feeling movement instead of hard sensations.

One of my early exposures to "seeing" yoga and visual form artistically was in Vanda Scaravelli's (1991) beautiful book *Awakening the Spine*, which is a holistic way of looking at the body through a lens of nature, holism, and yoga. She learned from both B. K. S. Iyengar and T. K. V. Desikachar and ultimately developed her own yoga, with a leaning toward exploration and away from gurus.

Stretch and the yogi and yogini

There is a common misconception that yoga is about flexibility, but an ideal yoga practice also emphasizes strengthening and work through different movements, both for the muscles and fascia. Originally designed to help prepare the body for seated meditation, the modern yoga practice is often countering a life with smart phones, computers, and more. While there are clear benefits in improving range of motion, particularly in terms of working with connected myofascia, there is also a danger of destabilizing a patient who may need more stability. In other words, starting a yoga practice without addressing underlying postural issues may lead to re-enforcing a pattern. Length, as previously discussed should be strategized before strengthening in poses.

Some teachers may ask a student to "stretch" without a clear understanding of the meaning of the term. For the yogi and yogini, we can look at static stretching, which involves extending muscle groups targeted to their maximum range and holding for 30 seconds or more in active stretch (force is applied by the individual) or passive stretch where the added force is applied by a partner or prop to increase the intensity. However, if a very flexible, fascially "loose" individual hears the word "stretch," they may go well beyond their end range to feel sensation.

Fascia that is stretched quickly will likely tear and be injured, but slow "stretch" can lead to plastic deformation of the tissue, the desired type of tissue deformation we see over a long period of practice in yoga. Fascia is made more mobile through many styles of yoga, from the more active Ashtanga done in a consistent practice to the slow holds of yin yoga.

In terms of fascia, it does appear that "stretch," in different definitions of the term, does make a difference for the body and movement performance. There have been a number of scientific studies that point toward the potential for understanding the importance of stretch in fascia, particularly in terms of lowering the body's inflammation response. Most studies have been tested on rat fascia, with the assumption that a similar response will happen for humans as well. In one study it was noted:

Acute inflammation is accompanied from its outset by the release of specialized pro-resolving mediators (SPMs), including resolvins, that orchestrate the resolution of location inflammation of the back induced by carrageenan, stretching for 10 min twice daily reduced inflammation and improved pain, 2 weeks after carrageenan injection. In this study, we hypothesized that stretching of connective tissue activates local pro-resolving mechanism with the tissue in the acute phase of inflammation.

(Berrueta *et al.* 2016, p.1621)

Muscle spindles are connected to the fascia, and inflammation and pain will be interrelated. If there is dull pain that is relieved by pressure, there may be nociceptive input that is myofascial in character. Any complex syndromes appear to be multisystem in nature affecting the nervous system, muscoloskeletal, vascular, and immune responses, affecting the body on many levels from cells to tissue. In a study by Berrueta *et al.* (2016), rats with subcutaneous inflammation of the back reduced inflammation through 10 minutes of twice daily stretching. Their hypothesis was that stretching connective tissue stimulates mechanisms that reduce inflammatory responses and reduced the migration of neutrophils.

Ultimately, the balance of mobility and strength is also working with and understanding the individual practitioner. No one should be shamed for having a wide range of motion, or barely the ability to touch one's toes (Figure 9.2). Practitioners in asana practice need to work intelligently and with agency in their own bodies.

Fascia connections to poses

An understanding of myofascia can help deepen an understanding of enhancing asana practice. Many of the poses that have developed in yoga may have come about through experimentation. Lion's pose (in which the tongue is stuck out and the eyes roll upwards) helps to connect to the deep myofascial connections from tongue to pelvic floor. While the pose is traditionally done seated, practitioners can feel a connection to the pelvic floor on the exhale.

Tadasana (mountain pose) can be enhanced by placing a lightweight block between the legs. Stand in mountain and then roll the femurs so the volume of the adductors makes contact with the block, which works the full range of the fascial pelvic floor.

Practitioners in warrior 2 (Virabhadrasana 2) often collapse the back foot. We can work the relationship of the foot arch by lifting the inside edge (tibialis anterior) and elongating the outer edge of the leg (lengthening through the peroneals/fibularis).

Additionally, taking multi-vectored approaches to traditionally planar movement can enhance the practice. Ultimately ease and coordination come with myofascial efficiency, which should not be mistaken for range of motion. Each practitioner should look for ease in their own body (Figure 9.2).

Resonant breathing, chanting, and more

Bernardi *et al.* (2001) studied the effects of rhythmic yoga mantras (in addition to rosary recitations) that appeared to match innate cardiovascular rhythms. As noted, "both prayer and mantra caused striking, powerful, and synchronous increases in existing cardiovascular rhythms when recited six times a minute" (p.1446). This is what is called a state of coherence, where things work together and can have a positive physical and psychological effect. In contrast, incoherence, where heart rate is out of sync with breathing, can bring about stress.

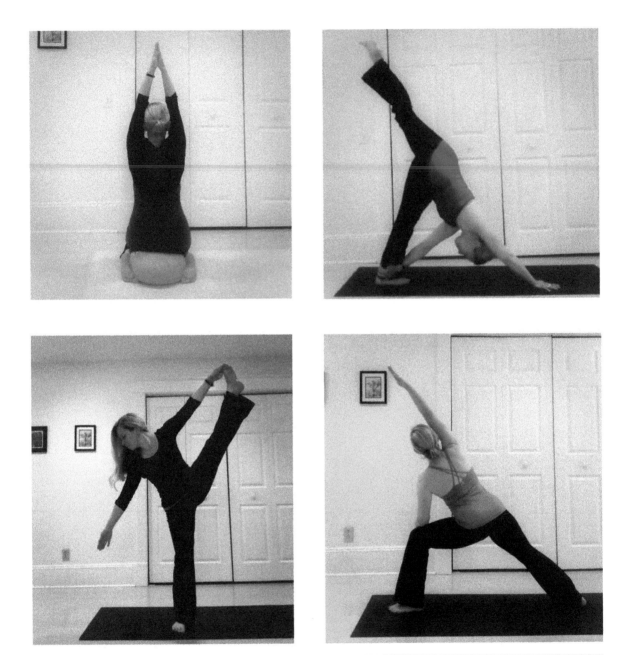

FIGURE 9.2 Variations on classical yoga asanas. Range of motion (ROM) is less important than coordination and ease of movement in the myofascial system. However, both those with lots of ROM and those with limited ROM can face different issues fascially. With greater natural ROM often comes a tendency to overextend in order to feel end range sensation. Tighter bodies may not reach their toes but be prone to fewer fascia injuries. Both types of bodies are to be accepted.

Photos courtesy of the author.

Suboccipital sun salutations

The suboccipitals are a group of four paired muscles (Figure 9.3) that help to extend the head as well as lateral flexion. To see the power of the suboccipitals on the movement of the head and orientation in the body, grab a partner for an observation of suboccipital sun salutations.

One partner will be blindfolded and will perform sun salutations, or another simple sequence of yoga poses. The other will be the observer. The first partner (with eyelids closed) moves the muscles of the eyes either strongly to the right or left without telling the partner which they are doing.

Then they will perform their sequence blindfolded while partner two guesses which direction they were "looking." Often this will pull the head and orientation on the map toward the side of focus.

A high proportion of stretch receptors in these tissues make them very receptive to directional changes. The suboccipitals are powerful orientation muscles of the head and neck positioning and can be damaged in whiplash. They are also quite sensitive to triggering positioning whether or not the eyes are open or closed. Think also about their starlike shape as a group, which allows for many possibilities in range and movement.

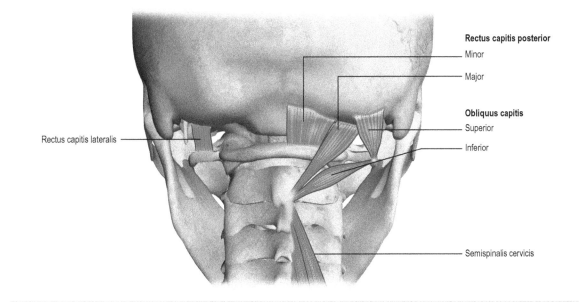

Rectus capitis posterior
— Minor
— Major

Obliquus capitis
— Superior
— Inferior

Rectus capitis lateralis

Semispinalis cervicis

FIGURE 9.3 Posterior view of muscles c1, c2, c3. Innervated by the suboccipital nerve, the star of muscles at the base of the occiput are known as the suboccipital muscles. These have a role in maintaining postural alignment and orienting the body in space. These have a lot of the muscle spindles (or stretch receptors) that help sense changes and rate of lengthening muscles along with the Golgi tendon organ which senses muscle tension changes. The suboccipitals may have 50 times more muscle spindles than the gluteal muscles making them highly sensitive. The four suboccipital muscles are: rectus capitis posterior major, rectus capitis posterior minor, obliquus capitis inferior, and obliquus capitis superior. Three of these—both of the obliquus capitis muscles and rectus capitis posterior form what is known as the suboccipital triangle. In addition to the frame of these three muscles, the "floor" of this triangle is the posterior atlanto-occipital membrane. The "roof" is formed by the semispinalis capitis muscle, and deep to that, a layer of fibrous adipose tissue. These fascial pieces contribute to connections in the fascia.

Chapter nine

Going deeper—the myodural bridge

The link between the connection of the dura mater (hard mother) and the rectus capitis muscles has been explored by Scali *et al.* (2013) as well as von Lanz (1929) and can be considered part of another deep myofascial connection. As noted in Scali *et al.* (2013):

The existence of a true connection between the RCPma and the cervical dura mater provides new insight in understanding the complex anatomy of the atlantoaxial interspace. The presence of a neural component within this connection suggests that it may serve another function aside from simply anchoring this muscle to the dura mater. Such a connection may be involved in monitoring dural tension and may also play a role in certain cervicogenic pathologies. This study also supports previous reports that no true membrane joins the posterior arch of the atlas to the laminae of the axis and contradicts the conventional belief that the ligamentum flavum joins these two structures. (p.558)

Walking meditation

In the traditional practice of the eight limbs of yoga practice from the ancient text of *The Yoga Sutras*, the idea of concentration is a precursor to meditation. Walking meditations are found in numerous cultures and can be a way to practice being both present and increasing the body's proprioception. Our etymological root of proprioception is from the Latin, meaning to take hold of oneself. Sensing the body in the present is often a way to be aware of the here and now. Yoga teaches that emotional distress is often caused by focusing on the past, or projection into the future. By changing a pattern of a walk, even if just slightly, we can focus a level of mindfulness and add a challenge of balance.

In a large empty space or outdoor area, begin with your normal walking pattern and start to change directions, first walking forwards but then backwards and sideways as well as on diagonals. Begin to adapt this pattern, starting with your right foot. Step (right), step (left), step (right), and pause, lifting onto the ball mounts of your feet. Start again, beginning now with the left foot—step (left), step (right), step (left), and pause, lifting onto the ball mounts of both feet. This quiet pattern cultivates

mindfulness and a myofascial smooth quality and softness with the deceleration of movement.

Moving in multidirectionality and challenging coordination

Connection and coordination have been a hallmark of yoga asana (Figure 9.4). When looking at the continuity from one part of the body to the next, the distal range of motion matters less than the overall easiness and clarity of form. Every part of the body, including down to the toes, participates fully and actively.

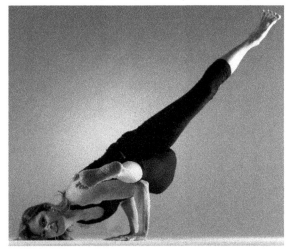

FIGURE 9.4 Mastering length and ease in the body before building strength. In all forms of yoga, particularly in long-holding static forms of yoga, the healthy stress applied to fascia changes the system and the shape of the body.

Photo courtesy of Karen Rider.

Most yoga asanas begin to combine coordination of multiple lines of myfascial connection in the idea of balancing the biotensegral form. Purposely layering traditional asana with variations can be one way to achieve this (Figures 9.5 and 9.6). Unlike manual therapy practices that focus each session on a different area, most movement sessions utilize multiple focuses in the same session or class. However, an emphasis on finding length and space in the body as a starting point is useful in yoga as well as many other movement practices.

Moving in multidirectionality and challenging coordination

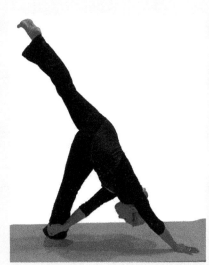

FIGURE 9.5 Combining asana work can challenge multiple myofascial connections in coordination. Taking a down dog into a three point contact and then two can add levels to practicing strength, balance, and coordination of the multiple relationships.

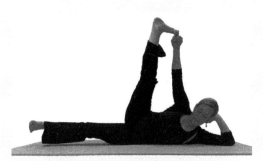

FIGURE 9.6 Variation on Anatasana (Sleeping Vishnu Pose). In this variation of the side lying pose, we again are combining concepts of lateral to deep lines of myofascial connection. Beginning side lying in Anatasana, lift the top leg (knee is welcomed to remain bent and the toe hold is optional). Once that balance is established, the bottom leg can lift. Watch for compensation patterns in rocking forwards or back.

Hand mudras: ancient practices for modern times

Carrie Gaynor

The use of mudras dates back to ancient times when hand gestures were used intuitively to promote healing, concentration, and meditation. Each mudra has its own physical shape and its own intrinsic energy. For example, each of the fingers is associated with one of the five energy centers along the spine, correlating to the universal elements of space, air, fire, water, and earth. When we perform a mudra, we evoke the physical and energetic channels of the body and mind. In fact, this hand–body–mind connection is emphasized in many healing systems, including Ayurveda, qi gong, reflexology, and acupuncture.

As we follow the fascia from the hands through the arms and the shoulders, trunk, and spine, we will see how hand mudras can profoundly influence the healthy interrelationships of these regions.

These relationships are challenged by the extraordinary amount of time we spend with our hands cupped around electronic devices, or at a keyboard with our head and shoulders rounded forward. This posture effectively trains our myofascial tissues to perceive dysfunctional posture and movement patterns as normal.

Hand mudras, practiced consciously and regularly, can effectively counteract these technologically-induced postural and structural dysfunctions. Here is a 5–10-minute daily hand mudra practice to counterbalance the cumulative negative effects of your technological activities.

Mudras can be practiced in a seated position or combined with motions or flows.

The Three Mudra Flows

Mudra flow 1
Mudra flow 1 emphasizes movement in the sagittal plane, involving flexion and extension.

Mudra flow 1—instructions

Sit with your hands in *Salutation Mudra*. Hinging at the hips, lean forward and release your hands from Salutation Mudra, forming *Inner-Om Mudra* as you transition forward to Cat Pose. Just before your hands land on the ground in Cat Pose, release *Inner-Om Mudra* and transition to *Earth Mudra*. As you land, cushion the impact with a cat-like suppleness (Figure 9.breakout.1).

Take a moment to notice the grounded qualities of *Earth Mudra*: your hands stretch open, while your shoulders and trunk stabilize your position.

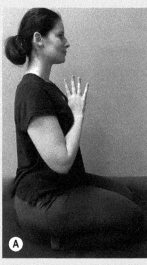

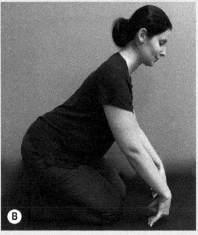

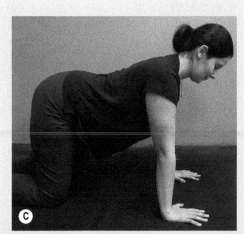

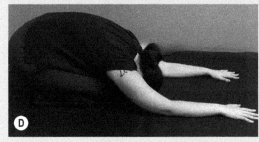

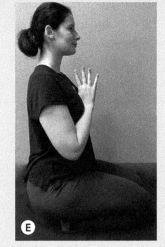

FIGURE 9.BREAKOUT.1 a) Sitting (Salutation Mudra); b and c) Transition to Cat (Inner Om Mudra); d) Settle back into Child (Earth Mudra); e) Roll to Sitting. Mudra flow adapted from ©2020 TriYoga International—Level Basics. Used by permission. (Images from author.)

Then settle back into Child Pose, feeling Earth Mudra in this position. Complete the flow by rolling the spine until you are in an upright sitting position, returning the hands back into *Salutation Mudra*. Repeat this sequence several times.

Mudra flow 2

Mudra flow 2 emphasizes movement in the frontal plane, involving lateral flexion—that is, side-bending. All directions are given as if you were turning to the right.

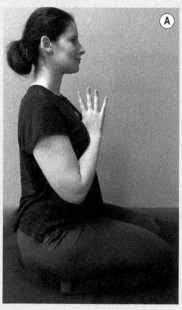

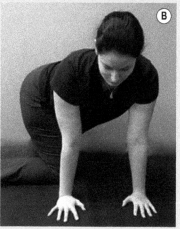

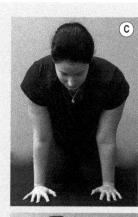

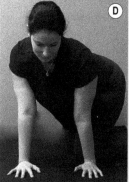

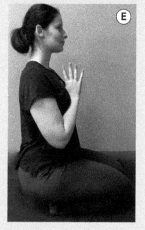

FIGURE 9.BREAKOUT.2 a) Sitting (Salutation Mudra); b) Quarter turn to Side Cat; c) Step legs to Cat (Earth Mudra); d) Step legs to Side Cat; e) Return to Sitting. Mudra flow adapted from ©2020 TriYoga International— Level 2. Used by permission. (Images from author.)

Mudra flow 2 instructions

Sit with your hands in *Salutation Mudra* (Figure 9. breakout.2a). Rotate your upper body a quarter-turn to the right, leading with your hands. Land in Side Cat with your palms flat in *Earth Mudra* (Figure 9. breakout.2b): your right hand will touch first, then your left hand. Leaving your palms in place, rotate your lower legs to the left. Now you are in Cat Pose again (Figure 9.breakout.2c). Finally, move your lower legs to the left: now you are back in Side Cat, on the opposite side (Figure 9.breakout.2d).

Leaving your lower legs in place, rotate your pelvis so you are sitting on your calves again. As you rotate, lift your hands off the floor: the right hand comes up first, followed by the left hand. Return the hands to *Salutation Mudra*. You are now facing the opposite direction (Figure 9.breakout.2e). To complete the movement and return to your original position, perform the entire sequence in the opposite direction: turn to your left, and lead with your left hand. Repeat this sequence several times.

Mudra flow 3

Mudra flow 3 emphasizes movement in the transverse plane—that is, right and left rotation. All directions are given as if you were turning to the right.

Mudra flow 3 is the same as *Mudra flow 2*, with one key difference. As in *Mudra flow 2*, sit with your hands in *Salutation Mudra*. Rotate your upper body a quarter-turn to the right, leading with your hands. Land in Side Cat with your palms flat in Earth *Mudra* (Figure 9.breakout.2b). But this time, both your hands touch the ground *at the same time*. Leaving your palms in place, rotate your lower legs a quarter-turn to the left. Now you are in Cat Pose again (Figure 9.breakout.2c above). Finally, move your lower legs yet another quarter-turn to the left: now you are in Side Cat, on the opposite side (Figure 9.breakout.2d).

Leaving your lower legs in place, rotate your pelvis so you are sitting on your calves again.

As you rotate, lift *both* your hands off the floor simultaneously. Return the hands to *Salutation Mudra*. You are now facing the opposite direction. To complete the movement and return to your original position, perform the entire sequence in the opposite direction: turn to your left, and lead with your left hand. Repeat this sequence several times.

Mudra flows 1, 2, and *3* elegantly demonstrate specific ways we can bring myofascial anatomy into our everyday lives, promoting both physical and mental health. Healthy hands are essential to our wellbeing. We've seen how mudras seamlessly integrate the hands into the shoulder, trunk, and spine. And we've observed that as we develop these connections, we initiate powerful changes in our myofascial system, unleashing our freedom of movement in all three dimensions.

These mudra flows provide spiritual benefits, too, evoking in our bodies and minds the qualities of unconditional self-love, meditative awareness, and groundedness. As we practice these mudra flows, we connect to our higher selves, and we free our upper bodies to move the way they were meant to move—beginning and ending with the hands.

Final relaxation tension, release and yawn and reach

Pandiculation is a wave-like movement of the soft tissues that is observed in many animals, particularly in a gigantic yawn, and "might preserve the integrative role of the myofascial system by (a) developing and maintaining appropriate physiological fascial interconnections and (b) modulating the pre-stress of the myofascial system by regularly activating the tonic musculature" (Bertolucci 2011).

At the end of a yoga class, in the final relaxation pose known as *savasana*, the yoga teacher has an opportunity to fascially work with the relaxed body.

- In final relaxation position, feel the heaviness through the center of the body, middle of the forehead, middle of the throat, middle of the chest, middle of the belly, middle of the tailbone, heavy and relaxed and released.

- Beginning with the toes, squeeze the toes quite tightly, inhale the breath, exhale, and relax and release.

- Squeeze the toes, and the legs now quite tightly, deepen the breath, and relax and release. Squeeze the toes, the legs, up the front of the chest and down the muscles of the back. Squeeze tightly, relax, and release. Continuing, squeeze the toes, feet, legs, front and back of the torso, and through the arms into the fists of the hands. Inhale and exhale, release, and let go. Once more, squeeze toes, feet, legs, front and back of the body, through the arms and fists of the hands and into the muscles of the face, squeezing tightly, deepen the breath and then relax and release, let go.

- Let the body settle into the floor and actively relax. The observation of the breath can be used if anxious. For the next several minutes, you have absolutely nothing else to do. When you begin to return to the space around you, start to slowly wiggle fingers and toes and circle wrists and ankles. Allow a big yawn and allow the body to respond to the movement. When ready, roll to the side and return to a comfortable seated position.

Modern yoga is starting to shed some of its attachments to the larger asanas (poses) and begin (or return to) more subtle work, including breath and body sensation. A new generation of practitioners are particularly interested in exploring this myofascially as a means of understanding how to work with the body in a more integrated way.

Yoga has traditionally been rooted in how things connect together to create something more complete than individual parts.

References

Bernardi, L., Sleight, P., Bandinelli, G., Cencetti, S. *et al.* (2001) 'Effect of rosary prayer and yoga mantras on autonomic cardiovascular rhythms: comparative study.' *BMJ 323*, 7327, 1446–1449. https://doi.org/10.1136/bmj.323.7327.1446

Berrueta, L., Muskaj, I., Olenich, S., Butler, T. *et al.* (2016) 'Stretching impacts inflammation resolution in connective tissue: stretching impacts inflammation resolution.' *Journal of Cellular Physiology 231*, 7, 1621–1627. https://doi.org/10.1002/jcp.25263

Bertolucci, L. F. (2011) 'Pandiculation: Nature's way of maintaining the functional integrity of the myofascial system?' *Journal of Bodywork and Movement Therapies 15*, 3, 268–280. https://doi.org/10.1016/j.jbmt.2010.12.006

Feuerstein, G. (2008) *The Yoga Tradition: Its History, Literature, Philosophy, and Practice.* Chino Valley, AZ: Hohm Press.

Scali, F., Pontell, M. E., Enix, D. E. and Marshall, E. (2013) 'Histological analysis of the rectus capitis posterior major's myodural bridge.' *The Spine Journal 13*, 5, 558–563. https://doi.org/10.1016/j.spinee.2013.01.015

Scaravelli, V. (1991) *Awakening the Spine: The Stress-Free New Yoga That Restores Health, Vitality and Energy.* San Francisco, CA: Harper Collins.

Singleton, M. (2010) *Yoga Body: The Origins of Modern Posture Practice.* Oxford: Oxford University Press.

von Lanz, T. (1929) 'Über die Rückenmarkshäute: I. Die Konstruktive Form der harten Haut des menschlichen Rückenmarkes und ihrer Bänder.' *Wilhelm Roux' Archiv für Entwicklungsmechanik der Organismen 118*, 1, 252–307. https://doi.org/10.1007/BF02108876

Further reading

Fede, C., Albertin, G., Petrelli, L., Sfriso, M. M. *et al.* (2016) 'Hormone receptor expression in human fascial tissue.' *European Journal of Histochemistry.* https://doi.org/10.4081/ejh.2016.2710

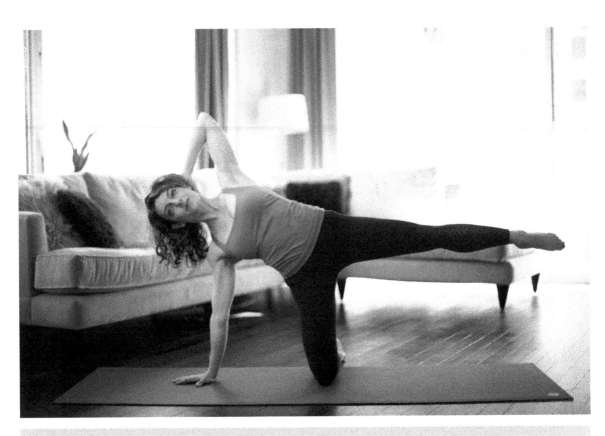

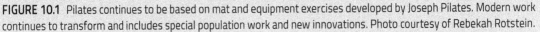

FIGURE 10.1 Pilates continues to be based on mat and equipment exercises developed by Joseph Pilates. Modern work continues to transform and includes special population work and new innovations. Photo courtesy of Rebekah Rotstein.

When I was teaching a lot of myofascial anatomy workshops, my most enthusiastic students were often from Pilates. Fascia-focused work matches well with the original theories and practice and the field continues to innovate in the spirit of its original founder (Figure 10.1). The world of Pilates today is largely dominated by gym mat classes and in dedicated studios that offer more of the apparatus and equipment. Developed by Joseph Hubertus Pilates (1880–1967), his system (which he called Contrology) was first a means of rehabilitation during World War I and then taught to the ballerinas and modern dancers that he trained along with his wife, Clara, in New York City.

He was an inventor and thinker and created the equipment including innovations like the Wunda Chair, which was designed to be functional in form as both home gym equipment and a seat. Transforming to fold into a piece of furniture was especially well-suited to city apartments and a brilliant piece of design. It is interesting to think about where Pilates himself would have taken the field these days, but it is likely he would have continued to innovate and design additional equipment.

Pilates wrote several books (Figure 10.2), and in *Return to Life Through Contrology* (2012), first published in 1945, he introduced six primary principles (Breathing, Centering, Concentration,

Control, Flow, and Precision) considered the foundation to his approach to exercise. His concept of contrology would later be renamed Pilates, much in the same way Rolfing was named after Ida Rolf.

Pilates, in his work as corrective exercise, trained many famous teachers such as Romana Kryzanowska, Eve Gentry, and Ron Fletcher. Second generation teachers include many of the modern leaders who have begun to focus on elements of fascial training in the Pilates method and the next level of their students who are becoming

more creative in their approaches to the work. As noted by movement educator Mary Bond (2018), "Yoga and Pilates are 'fascia' friendly,' but because they don't have a bouncing element, they don't condition fascial elasticity" (p.291). However, the addition of newer add-on equipment, such as the jump board for the Reformer, can change the nature of many of the classic exercises. Additionally, as noted by Larkam (in Schleip 2015), although 29 of the mat exercises are not ideal for developing elastic recoil in weight bearing (due to being open kinetic chain for the lower extremity), "Joseph Pilates performed many of the mat exercises with rather vigorous elastic bounces in the end ranges of available motion (Pilates, 1932–1945) so even his open kinetic chain exercises can be used to develop elastic recoil" (p.455).

We can explore fascial connections through more subtle means. Pilates is known as a whole-body exercise; the classic exercises move the whole body, flowing along myofascial lines and connections, supporting and strengthening slings, and engaging fascial structures particularly around the famous Pilates powerhouse. Pilates is often attributed with connecting mind and body; following the original principles can bring a focus and a calm when moving which could be described as interoceptive in character. Let's invite a few of our Pilates experts to share their views and work in the myofascial body.

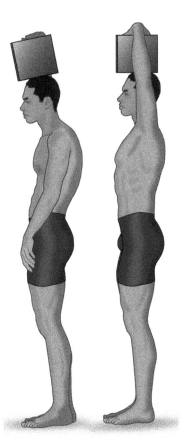

FIGURE 10.2 After the cover of *Your Health*, by Joseph Pilates. The integration of the Pilates image could be conceptualized through the double helix of spiral connections (from Myers's rhomboid/serratus connections for example) winding together to create a sense of lift.

The Pilates Method, linear or tensegril?
Tracey Mellor

One of the criticisms of Joseph Pilates's Method is that it is too linear.

The Pilates industry has worked hard to address this criticism and in the 21st century Pilates Studio we can now call upon an additional 80 years of research into anatomy, new pieces of equipment, new techniques of seeing into the body and a re-appraisal of fascial tissues and their significance in movement and sensory perception. We also have new models to explain how the body moves.

As a studio Pilates teacher, working with the traditional Pilates machines, I would argue that the industry has adapted, and moved on. We have a new vocabulary, that of fascia and tensegrity, to explain why the Pilates Method is still effective.

I want to focus on the connection between body and machine. Not in the old language of describing the body as a machine, but by recognizing the synergy between body and machine, how the combination can allow ease of movement and proprioceptive feedback.

Let me give you an example of this synergy in action. Many clients measure their progress in being able to achieve exercises they originally found difficult or "impossible." One of those "go to" or "test" exercises is the roll back or sit up. Using the push through bar on the Pilates Trapeze table I can show the client that this movement is not just about core strength, it also has a lot to do with spine flexibility, coordination of movement, shoulder blade and head positioning, etc. With the help of the push through bar the impossible movement becomes possible, even easy.

How can we explain how this? Using our new vocabulary, we can explain this magical movement on the machine in a new way.

What we are looking for in a Pilates exercise is dynamic stability or controlled movement. When explaining movement using the language of the tensegrity model, "biotensegrity (tensegrity applied to the body) allows the body to change shape with minimum effort and remain completely stable throughout" (Scarr 2018).

In this example, the ease of movement using the push though bar is not solely due to the strength of individual components (specific muscle strengths and joint range of motion, etc.). It can be explained because the body can now be viewed as and becomes part of a tensegrity/biotensegrity structure.

This tensegral structure can be configured to distribute the forces throughout its entirety. Every part of the body from the macro to the micro works together with the machine, the tensegrity structure can be taken beyond the body to include the machine, thus allowing for a successful distribution of forces.

Breaking this down further we have to consider the four-bar closed system theory which is part of the tensegrity model. In the Pilates studio we are used to working with closed, pseudo closed and open systems. A closed system is the most stable where all limbs are connected to a piece of equipment or the floor, an open system is where limbs are free to move unconnected and is more challenging. A four-bar closed system (there can be more bars), lacks the stability and strength of a three-bar closed system or triangle, because it allows for controlled movement. The bars can be compressive structures or tissues under tension. The bars are linked by joints. When powered by a motor, or in the human body a muscle, one of the bars is held stable. This configuration allows the other bars to move through a range of motions including arcs, circles, and potentially spirals; each of the moving bars influences the behavior of all the others in the system.

Pilates machines already move in arcs, the push through bar on the Trapeze table and chair pedal are examples. Add in the four-bar closed system theory and what we had considered linear movements can now be considered curves, circles, and spirals. The four-bar closed system can both expand and reduce the forces, tempo, and energy transfer in a heterarchical manner. In this example, where the client is taken from supine to sitting with ease, we can expand it to incorporate the immediate environment around the client's body—the machine. At least one joint and one bar (the junction of the upright and the bed on the Trapeze table) is fixed. The other bars and joints, found within the connected body and the machine, can then proceed to move through a series of curves, circles, and spirals to allow the client to move from supine to seated smoothly and effortlessly. This is because the forces are spread not only throughout the client's body but throughout the machine as well. The fixed joint and bar of the machine frees the other bars and joints in the body for movement because they no longer have to find their own stability, the machine becomes part of an extended tensegrity/biotensegrity system. The shoulder blade can rotate and glide rather than "jammed down," the hip flexors do not have to "grip" to stabilize the pelvis, and the spine can be mobile and flexible. The client has dynamic stability and can safely learn the movement and build strength, and will eventually move away from the external scaffold of the machine.

As soon as you start to see the synergy between body and machine, and recognize four-bar closed systems, they are everywhere in the Pilates studio. The body has volume and moves in 3D freedom. From the fibers of collagen of the fascial architecture to the expanded biotensegral system incorporating the Pilates machines, there is movement in curves, circles, and spirals.

Inspiration for this is based upon the following lecture in 2012 attended by the author in Belgium:

"Steve Levin 4 bar biomechanics of a closed chain TAKE 2."

Reference

Scarr, G. (2018) *Biotensegrity: The Structural Basis of Life.* Edinburgh: Handspring Publishing.

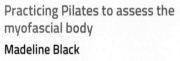

Practicing Pilates to assess the myofascial body

Madeline Black

The Pilates Method mat exercises are designed with a focus on the torso coordination with movements such as torso articulation, the distal-proximal/proximal-distal activations and breathing.

J. H. Pilates's classic mat exercises are performed in supine, prone, side-lying, kneeling, and standing (Pilates and Miller 1934).

Pilates's mat movements are initiated proximally from torso or distally from feet, top of head or hands, and at times simultaneous motion like rolling. The articulation and movement sequencing of each exercise is precise and stimulates a specific neuromyofascial response, as in a flexor response or extensor response (Black 2021). Practicing Pilates is the art of discovering how moving within the Method feels, not only the proprioception but the interoception deep within the trunk. Activating the weave of the myofascial core, the intrinsic as well as extrinsic, requires concentration and consciousness of the less familiar intrinsic sensations of breathing and continuous torso activation response to the limbs. This stimulation is a continuous activation of the myofascial core system in all dimensions-sagittal, coronal, and transverse planes.

For most people, the ability to feel the functional tensional relationships of the torso is limited and entirely unconscious. Guiding a person to move while experiencing this generally unconscious place requires imagery, palpation, and specific positioning of the body to stimulate the response.

Imagery

A physical practice is enhanced when combined with imagery (Kraeutner *et al.* 2016). Elicit imagery through verbal description, using gestures and visuals of bone models in motion. For an example, to stimulate the torso from the lower extremity you may choose to describe how the head of the femur glides posteriorly into the acetabulum prior to lifting the foot. Using a skeletal model of the lower extremity, demonstrate how the femur moves posterior and inferior, facilitating the activation of the flexors.

For myofascial continuous motion, visual imagery is most effective. Imagine a puppet string and puppeteer. The puppet string image is overlapped with anatomical imagery. The top of the string, held by the puppeteer, is at the top where the continuous structures from the LE meet the diaphragm. The puppeteer gently pulls on the string, the tension moves down the string, drawing the head of the femur posteriorly into the acetabulum and continues to the medial aspect of the femur articulating the acetabular-femoral joint into flexion as the foot floats off the mat.

A note: Many Pilates practices teach that the shin needs to be lifted into the habitual tabletop position with 90° knee and hip flexion. When the lower limb is hanging, it facilitates the proximal activation desired, enabling the client to sense the change of tissue tension and centrate the femoral head. The sequential movement travels from proximal the torso, and inferiorly toward the foot. The table top position stimulates a distal to proximal motion potentially inhibiting the femur's posterior/inferior motion at the actetabular–femoral joint. After experiencing the interoception of the tensional activity, advance the training effect by extending the knee.

Palpation for self-discovery (Figure 10. movement.1)

Part 1

- Lie supine with both knees flexed, feet on the mat.
- Use the imagery to move the knee toward the chest in hip flexion with dangling lower leg.
- Place same side hand on top of the femur, the opposite hand near the groin of the same side, to feel the tension change.
- Be sure the hand on the knee is relaxed and feeling heavy.
- Use the weight of the hand into the knee facilitating a force vector toward the posterior acetabular–femoral joint, feeling the deepening of the femoral head into the acetabulum.
- Maintain the force vector posteriorly and move the femoral head in a small circle as if you are rolling a pestle in a mortar.
- Move in both directions.
- Repeat this on the other side.

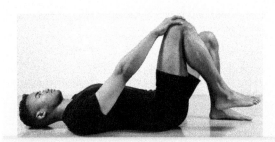

FIGURE 10.MOVEMENT.1 Isometric to feel engagement.

Photo by Cathy Stancil Photography.

Part 2

- Flex one hip with dangling lower leg.
- Place right hand on top of right knee superiorly and medially with arm extended.
- Left hand touches the soft tissue superior of the inguinal ligament on right side.
- Press the knee into the hand, moving toward hip flexion.
- Block the hip flexion with the right hand creating an isometric contraction.
- Notice the femur sinking posteriorly into the acetabulum.
- Left hand is listening for the tissue tension.
  - Was there a change of tension?
  - Was the tension a feeling of pulling up and inward or pressing out into the hand?
  - The sensation of tissue tension is pulling up and in rather than pressing outward.
    - If it is outward, the effort was too great.
    - Or the femur is not seated well into the socket.
    - Experiment with changing the angle of the femur, adduct or abduct more, try less hip flexion.

Incorporating breath

Pilates teachers cue the breath in a variety of ways. Allow the client to breathe naturally without cueing and take note of their pattern of breathing. The pre-exercises above require total concentration from the client on the sequencing and embodiment of the Method. After they are confident with the pre-exercises and feel organized in their body, add a specific cue for the breath. Experiment with the breath pattern to see how it affects the tissue tensions in the torso. You are helping the client to discover their inner connectedness of the breath with the activation of the trunk. Once the client experiences the motor learning of torso to acetabular–femoral joint continuity, the progression may expand more distally toward the feet and head.

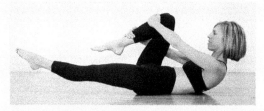

FIGURE 10. MOVEMENT. 2 J. H. Pilates mat: single leg stretch.

Photo by Cathy Stancil Photography.

Move into the single leg stretch position (Figure 10. movement.2). The hand on the bent leg uses the force vector into the femur as in the pre-exercises above to feel the femoral head posterior glide. Rather than reaching the straight leg outward, draw the straight leg into the acetabulum as if you are shortening the leg a small amount. Change sides, pause, and repeat the intention of the femur deepening in the acetabulum and opposite straight leg drawing in. Practice slowly at first to feel the deep sensation of the flexor response from leg to head.

References

Black, M. (2021) *Centered: Organizing the Body through Kinesiology, Movement Theory and Pilates Technique.* Edinburgh: Handspring Publishing.

Kraeutner, S. N., MacKenzie, L. A., Westwood, D. A. and Boe, S. G. (2016) 'Characterizing skill acquisition through motor imagery with no prior physical practice.' *Journal of Experimental Psychology: Human Perception and Performance 42,* 2, 257–265. doi: 10.1037/xhp0000148

Pilates, J. H. and Miller, W. J. [1934] (2021) *Return to Life Through Contrology.* Bristol: Mockingbird Press.

References

Bond, M. (2018) *Your Body Mandala: A Guide to Posture, Perception and Presence.* Maitland, FL: MCP Books.

Pilates, J. H. (2012) *Return to Life.* 2nd ed. Miami, FL: Pilates Method Alliance, Inc.

Schleip, R., Baker, A. and Avison, J. (eds) (2015) *Fascia in Sport and Movement.* Edinburgh: Handspring Publishing.

Further reading

Black, M., Calais-Germain, B. and Vleeming, A. (2015) *Centered: Organizing the Body Through Kinesiology, Movement Theory and Pilates Techniques.* Edinburgh: Handspring Publishing.

Dum, R. P., Levinthal, D. J. and Strick, P. L. (2016) 'Motor, cognitive, and affective areas of the cerebral cortex influence the adrenal medulla.' *Proceedings of the National Academy of Sciences 113,* 35, 9922–9927. https://doi.org/10.1073/pnas.1605044113

Larkam, E. J. (2017) *Fascia in Motion: Fascia-Focused Movement for Pilates.* Edinburgh: Handspring Publishing.

Myers, T. W. (2020) *Anatomy Trains: Myofascial Meridians for Manual Therapists and Movement Professionals* (4th ed.). London: Elsevier.

Training, weight work, and sports specifics

The human body does not wear out with use. On the contrary, it wears down when it is not used.

Christopher Alexander *et al.* (1977)

Training fascia

What is fitness and what is the goal of fitness anyway? Attempting to define "fitness" can bring up many opinions, including efficiency of movement, healthy weight, ability to perform walking or running actions, etc. If we are unable to perform daily tasks, all the exercise in the gym is not serving a purpose. If we are training for a performance athletic task, we want to be able to accomplish that goal with less effort and more efficiency. Timing is everything. We hear that a lot in life and the same is true in fascia. We can also add that context is everything. What may make sense for one type of athlete or body, may not for the next. Immediate movement for the fascia before swimming, for example, may increase the range of motion through tissue hydration.

The way we think and train has changed dramatically, from the aerobics craze of the 1980s to newer ideas of "functional fitness" as well as the growth of yoga, Pilates, and other minded and mindful movements. Our traditional way of looking at the body was to focus on the muscle-based system. Gyms are still filled with machines that highlight the individual muscles, but mindful movement is having its moment. An image can capture a moment or a pose that might look photogenic but lack movement or functional integrity. My friend David Jacobs, a mobility coach, talks about entering every session with the mindset of a "creative-humble-facilitator." As he puts it, "we can't fix humans. They are not broken. Things break. Humans require healing and I just try and help provide a path for someone to reach that state" (personal correspondence).

Fascial awareness has led to new strategies for training the body with multidirectionality, vectors, and more global ways of looking at the body. In late 2020, Emily Harrington became the first woman to free climb El Capitan via the Golden Gate route in one day. Free soloing is a style of rock climbing where no ropes or harnesses are used, other than a rope below used to break a fall, or sometimes without a safety rope at all, as was done by Alex Honnold on his famous ascent. Harrington is reported throughout the climbing community to have kept herself going with the mantra, "slow is smooth, smooth is fast."

Building a body for movement

Fascia trains slower than muscle, but it is more resilient if it is trained well. So, the shape of our fascial organization is important to consider. Forces in the body organize our fascia, and then our fascia organizes what the cells in the body do. We have looked at the general concept of tensegrity, but this concept at the cellular level is important. If collagen is a cell product, the shape of what it becomes is interesting, as it forms a triple helix, like a strong, woven rope. The Golgi tendon organ nerve ending goes into the tendon, and with pull, the helix of the collagen is straightened and unwound a bit. Without the ability to load, the crimp of the fascia loses it shape. Why should we care? If you have a client that hasn't stimulated their fascia in a while, either through inactivity due to injury or mental state, that body is going to have a slower time with new load.

Proprieties of training fascia for the movement professional

Now that we have a basic understanding of fascia, we can start to look at the major concepts in training fascia (Figure 11.1). Healthy fascia has a high ability to slide between layers, and there is an elevated density of proprioception receptors in this area, critical for professional and daily movers alike.

Elasticity

A loss of elasticity in the body means that the tissue can no longer stretch properly. Here, fiber content may be high and there is stiffness in the tissue such as in a plantar fasciitis. In discussing elastic properties, we can use a term called the coefficient of restitution, which is how long you can hold the elasticity, and how fast the elasticity can recoil. Tissue can only hold elasticity for about a second. When you are running, the Achilles tendon stores and returns the energy.

As a kid, I took the time to loop together rubber bands to create a ball made up of the elastic bands gathered from the newspaper and various grocery store items. The coefficient of restitution for any rubber-based ball is very high, but also very short. The surface of both the ball and what it bounces against makes a difference. A superball in its smoothness has a high coefficient of restitution. My kitchen floor may be an ideal place to bounce that ball, but my carpet will quickly absorb the extra energy. Up until recently, there was a poor understanding of the effects of training on tendons and the ability to increase elastic storage. Reeves (2006) found that exercise groups training with resistance had increased elastic storage capacity and implied increased tendon loads.

The example given earlier in the book of an efficient bouncy and elastic quality of movement is that of the kangaroo in its efficient gait (Sawicki *et al.* 2009) as previously discussed. The bounciness of its hop is not adequately explained by muscular action alone. Kram and Dawson (1998) discussed in their studies the catapult mechanism, where the elastic energy is stored in the fascia through pre-loading. In cultivating elastic rebound, we are looking for the ability to control deceleration and acceleration.

Fibroblasts (the cells that create more fascial fibers) respond to load and architecturally remodel the collagenous connective tissue depending on the movement (or the lack of movement) that body encounters. If the body does not get challenged, both a loss of flexibility and strength can occur, and fibrosis can build up.

Plasticity

Plasticity is about the stretch in the tissue that can deform the body system. Consistent stretch will make the fibers slide apart while a sustained stretch will create new bonds and change the tissue. This is why we warn athletes that there is a loss of strength immediately after a sustained stretch session (Magnusson *et al.* 2010). As noted in the abstract of the article from *Nature Reviews Rheumatology*:

Mechanical loading of tendon tissue results in upregulation of collagen expression and increased synthesis of collagen protein, the extent of which is probably regulated by the strain experienced by the resident fibroblasts (tenocytes). This increase in collagen formation peaks around 24 hours after exercise and remains elevated for about three days. The degradation of collagen proteins also rises after exercise but seems to peak earlier than the synthesis. Despite the ability of tendons to adapt to loading, repetitive use often results in injuries, such as tendinopathy, which is characterized by pain during activity, localized tenderness upon palpation, swelling, and impaired performance. (Magnusson et al. 2010)

So what does some of this mean for the movement practitioner? If we put sustained stretch on the fascia, there is a time of weakness after a heavy stretch session or yoga (depending, of course, on the style). After 24 hours there is a deficit in tissue, whereas after a few days the tissue can actually come back stronger. In sports such as football, there is a need for strength during a game. Over the years teaching athletes at the university level, I've been careful to pay attention to the sports activities that they are doing and their schedule of games as well as the style of stretch. "Stretch" includes passive, active, dynamic, ballistic, PNF (proprioceptive neuromuscular facilitation), static, and several more. Diving deeper into this realm of myofascial stretch for performance includes research from authors Frederick and Frederick (2020) and several other of our guests in the following pages.

Multidirectionality

We are looking to load fascia in multidirectional movement and dynamic action in order to increase fascial elasticity (Fukashiro *et al.* 2006). We can think of movement as energy that is directional in nature, like a vector, although of course the body is much more sophisticated than a simple line of force. Luckily, physics can handle these multilayered ideas and vectors can be an interesting and accurate way to describe movement of the fascial tissues. In graphing vectors, the visual represents position, a displacement in position, acceleration, and velocity. These also have relevance in a body of water, as much as in a human body, made largely of water. In water, multiple parts can be in motion in different velocities. A vector field is defined as these different areas of velocity.

Differential movement

When we move, we have layers that slide against each other and move over other layers. The idea of geology is useful here. The slow move and glide of plate tectonics for example, is similar to the shear and glide of muscle and fascia sliding. Ida Rolf has been quoted as having talked about the muscles having the ability to move against each other "like silk stockings" (personal communication, Myers 2018). Differential movement can be thought of as forces from different areas affecting the foundation of another. For example, the tree roots growing under my old house caused changes to the soil that shifted the structure above. Muscles with their fascial compartments may also, in essence, not be working so much with the idea of origin and insertion, but in relationship to everything around them.

Remodeling

Remodeling is done over a slower time. Unlike bone, where the calcium is repairing, in fascia the collagen fibers are knitting together to repair an injury. In the past, bones used to be held in place for a long time, which gave them the opportunity to rebuild, but if you wait too long, the fascia gets weak. Fascia needs reorganization through movement.

In 2002, Järvinen *et al.* found that immobilizing the body after injury creates a felt-like collagen arrangement and lack of "crimp" (the classic wave shape a crimping iron makes with hair); the organizational shape that we look for in healthy tissue. Muscle takes around five to eight weeks to remodel, but fascia takes much longer—anywhere from six weeks to two years. For an athlete that is training quickly, the injuries that develop are fascial tears, as the muscle may have expanded, but the fascial net has not yet had the time to remodel.

If we are training just individual muscles, such as we would do at a traditional gym with machine work, the fascia between the muscles is not trained effectively, nor is the coordination. To train the long myofascial chains or any named connections, there is an important piece to consider. Focusing on the longitudinal lines in force transmission will impact especially postural patterns over long periods of time. Over short periods of time, latitudinal or parallel force transmission is more common in the body.

If you are working out at the gym and isolating and "strengthening" your quadriceps on a machine by pushing your ankle against a bar as you extend the legs while lifting the bar, you are training your body as a machine, not as a body that can be dynamic. In this particular example, one could cause sacroiliac issues if the quads are overtrained without the idea of stabilization as we need in daily life.

Training should also include moving, lubricating, and looking at the intermuscular septums as being part of a new area of training concept that concentrates on the longitudinal force transmission. Peter Huijing's work (2007) furthered the concept that in addition to the longitudinal force distribution of the myofascial meridians, fascia can also be distributed to parallel structures and antagonists. When Huijing loaded rat tendons, the majority of the force (around 70%) was found to go to the proximal attachment, but an additional 30% goes to nearby structures.

In brief, when we use the body effectively, we need less effort to move the body efficiently. As noted by Elphinston (2019) in describing battle ropes:

Many people brace their bodies against the load of ropes, eliminating the potential offered by their legs, and thereby increasing the demand on their shoulders. Some even bob up and down with their knees, assuming that this energy will somehow make it past their rigid midsection. Ultimately, though, the ropes should mirror the ripple of energy moving up through the body, and this can only be achieved by sinking the body into the feet, transforming the legs from tense to elastic, and allowing their energy to transmit up and out through the hands. (Elphinston 2019, p.35)

When we are looking at fitness and sports, we need to also take a moment decide how we train

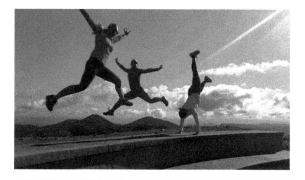

FIGURE 11.1 Training fascia is a relatively new concept. It responds to stimuli and mechanical stretch loading. By creating a myofascially adaptable body, we are able to engage in more areas of human daily and athletic performance with greater ease.

Photo courtesy of Lori Officer.

movement and performance. Noted trainer and fascia enthusiast Dr. Wilbour Kelsick has noted, "You cannot train body parts in isolation and expect to have efficient global functioning and training for runners must be elastically functional and global in its approach, inclusive of the entire body mechanism and not just the lower extremities" (Kelsick in Schleip, Baker, and Avison 2015).

Anyone training quickly at the expense of considering the whole body, will often take the strain in fascial areas (like the Achilles tendon or hamstring insertion), even when the movement correction might involve somewhere quite distant from the area of pain.

Walk this way

Before we get into other sports, the most basic movement that we build upon for other sports and movement is the basic action of walking. As noted by Zorn:

not only is walking, besides running, probably our most natural way of moving, the one that most closely corresponds to our body structure, but it can also be a dynamic form of meditation, that is to say, walking can easily combine movement and contemplation. Now, while it is true that almost anyone can lumber around or shuffle their feet, I believe that walking "correctly" is actually a great challenge. My hypothesis is that to walk "correctly," you need to walk "elastically". (Schleip et al. pp.161–162)

Nutrition and fascia for the body

I knew my university student track athletes were highly interested in how to recover from their own trail runs, and many rehydrated with water and various sports drinks. Not a big fan of the sugar content and artificial colors, I became interested in the latest research in fascial sports and wellness. Bone broth intrigued me for its high collagen content. Could rehydrating after a run or hike with bone broth be a healthy option for sports hydration? This is still a question under debate, but:

Boiling the skin, bones, and other connective tissues of cows, pigs, fish, and other animals results in the release of collagen from within the tissues in the forms of gelatin (denatured but mostly intact collagen protein). To make hydrolyzed collagen, the gelatin is further broken down using acid or enzymes such as pepsin, papain, bromelain, or protease. Therefore, the amino acid content of gelatin and hydrolyzed collagen is the same. The main difference is that one forms a gel, and the other does not. (Steffen and Baar in Lesondak and Akey 2020)

Collagen synthesis also depends on vitamin C, which is generally fairly prevalent in modern culture, which is important as it helps to hold fibers together. Trabold *et al.* (2003) demonstrated that lactate creates collagen synthesis, leading to the interesting question of whether lactate accumulation is, in part, creating fascial fibrosis.

Walking as an "indicator species"

Indicator species can be organisms of any kind that give an indication of the overall health in any environment. In her book *A Field Guide to Getting Lost*, author Rebecca Solnit (2017) discussed walking as an "indicator" species that determines the overall healthy checkup of the system. Walking can be a type of indicator of something larger in the system. If the act of walking is diminished or lost, it may be an indication of what is possible for the body in larger levels.

Fascial tensioning for the weight-bearing athlete

If we consider some of our actions in sports from launching a javelin to swinging a hockey stick backwards in anticipation of hitting a puck, we are myofascially tensioning the body like a spring, ready to change its state from potential energy to kinetic energy. As noted by Lesondak (2017):

Energy storage in tissues around the shoulder allows the human to throw at speeds over 100 miles an hour, compared to 20 miles per hour in primates. Pre-contraction of the muscle stretches connective tissues, which then explosively release to accomplish a movement for which muscle power alone would be insufficient. The storage is diffused across a network of as yet undefined tissues, but the "wind up" for the baseball pitch indicates the whole body is involved. (p.141)

Through proper training of the tensile work of the fascial system we can actually create more power. Stabilization of the joints is important before we get to mobility in the rest of the body. Having a mix of strength, but letting it go when we need to, is key. Fascial tensioning may be more the felt sensation than muscle tension.

Can you grab the cereal box on the top shelf?

As we start to look into different forms of movement, we will also keep this idea in mind for myofascial movement and its application: Does the movement we do have a purpose in the functionality of the myofascial body? The push in the modern fitness (starting in the 1960s) and movement industry has focused on machines designed for the "body as machine" concept. The very first patent for a treadmill was issued in the US in 1913 and gained momentum through the following decades. Repetitions of exercises such as preacher curls might make one strong in a very limited way but lacks the multidirectional training and unpredictable load that is important to a body that lives in the world and contends with picking up children or running down a city street to catch a bus. "Functional fitness" is prepping the body in movement to have better resiliency for common daily life situations.

Fascia is an organizer of shape, and movement organizes through patterns and rhythm but needs a wide range of challenges. If the structure is unable to sustain a movement, injury will occur. This is an important piece in understanding our healing and training. Fascial injuries (including cartilage, tendon ligament, and joint capsules) take longer to heal because of the lack of vascularity in the fascia.

Most of our clients don't get injured in a big athletic event. Instead, they injure themselves reaching for the box of cereal on the high shelf or turning in the car to retrieve an item from the back seat.

Functional fascia training for indoors and outdoors

If most of our waking hours are spent indoors, how can we incorporate fascia training into a relatively static environment? During the pandemic, for many, this indoor time increased during periods of lock down.

Some thoughts:

1. Change the way you move in dynamic shifts. Think like a choreographer. Do you usually stay at eye level as you move through your house? Could you shift to crawl, or stand on tiptoe? Can you move quietly? Can you occupy space when you enter a room? Vary your movement drivers, but also vary your movement levels.

2. Use your counters and furniture to explore climbing. Stimulate the skin for proprioception.

3. Vary the way you approach a typical task or space. If you always sit in the same seat, change your place. Better yet, change the furniture or vary tasks without furniture.

4. Think of linking two activities together for more dynamic changes and to challenge coordination.

Using myofascial concepts in building a varied approach to movement

Mike Fitch, Creator of Animal Flow

When people ask me what Animal Flow (AF) is, I'll usually tell them, "If you were to see someone practicing Animal Flow, it would look like a mix of yoga, breakdancing, modern dance and gymnastics." But the experience of AF is completely different to each practitioner. To some, it's their daily workout, while to others it can vary from a movement

meditation, mobility training, cardiovascular conditioning, skill practice, or something they use to fill in the gaps of their other go-to exercise strategies.

Over the years, the program has evolved and while the movements have become even more finely tuned, the inception of AF was deeply based on my understanding of anatomy and the needs of the human body (Figure 11.2). The entire program is set to achieve the following goals and concepts:

1. Articular variability: move every joint in as many directions as possible, especially those angles that the person would not explore on a daily basis.

2. Ground based movement: the majority of AF movements are quadrupedal. Closed chain, quadrupedal movements are excellent for creating a proprioceptively rich environment, where the participant must move their body around an object (i.e. the floor) versus move an object around their body.

3. Load the body globally: the AF movements were designed with the goal of loading the muscular subsystems and fascial lines in both shortened and lengthened positions. This creates a variety of loading patterns that focus on tissue synergies versus single muscles.

4. Body/brain challenge: there is an entire language built around AF that allows the instructor to "call out" a command, which encourages a speedy reaction time of the participant. Even without the call outs, it was proven that a four-week AF program improved markers of cognition in the study "Quadrupedal movement training improves markers of cognition and joint repositioning" (Matthews *et al.* 2016).

5. Fun: it's widely known that if a person enjoys the exercise task, then the adherence to the program is higher.

Reference

Matthews, M. J., Yusuf, M., Doyle, C. and Thompson, C. (2016) 'Quadrupedal movement training improves markers of cognition and joint repositioning.' *Human Movement Science, 47,* 70–80. https://doi.org/10.1016/j.humov.2016.02.002

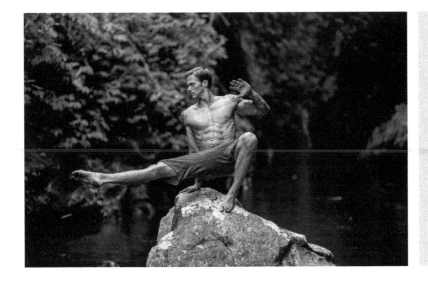

FIGURE 11.2 Animal Flow is a practice built from goals and concepts of articular variability, ground based movement, loading the body globally and challenging the brain and body through fun.

Photo courtesy of Mike Fitch, Animal Flow.

Biomotor abilities and fascia adaptation

The focus on biomotor abilities has gone in and out of style over the years among athletic trainers. These abilities are critically important if the goal of the training is to improve a practice for overall performance, not just for the drill itself. Depending on the source, there are anywhere between three to eight biomotor abilities defined as critical to practice from strength (optimal, absolute, limit, and relative), power (starting, reactive, eccentric, and optimal), endurance, speed, coordination, flexibility, agility, and balance. As interest in fascia has continued to grow, more sports scientists are looking at the relationship of fascial restrictions and kinetic chain issues. In one study by van Pletzen and Venter (2012), the researchers used the Bunkie Test (Brumitt 2015) to determine performance in selected physical areas (agility, speed, explosive power, and muscle endurance). This designed test involves simple stabilization with a chair or bench in the following named lines: posterior power line, anterior power line, posterior stabilizing line, lateral stabilizing line, and medial stabilizing line.

The strength of cumulative sub-maximal load

Travis Johnson PhD, FAFS, CSCS, CFSC, Kinetikos

I landed on Kodiak Island, Alaska, in the spring of 1993 and nearly had my hand broken. At least that's what it felt like. I stepped in for a cordial handshake with the captain of the fishing boat I would be working on for the next four months and found myself caught in a vice grip the likes of which I had not experienced before. About two hours later I met his neighbor and made the same mistake. It was even worse: bones grinding as I struggled to generate the barest amount of opposing force to uphold my end of the greeting.

Interestingly, neither of these men was particularly large nor imposing in size and stature. In fact, I was taller and probably outweighed them both. The term that comes to mind is "wiry."

They were not anomalies either. Over the course of that summer, I met lots of people that were far stronger than one would imagine, and the common denominator seemed to be many years of continuous work in the fishing industry.

Similar observations have been noted in farming communities. Renowned Canadian exercise physiologist Michol Dalcourt frequently mentions that the farm kids on hockey teams were overwhelmingly stronger than their city-dwelling counterparts, regardless of the weightlifting the city kids did at the gym.

To explain this, people often focus on the complex movements and load variability the fisherman or farmer is exposed to that creates better integrations and linkages through the body overall (compared to classic strength lifts).

However, it was RKC instructor Troy Anderson that really got me thinking about sub-maximal loading and volume over time. Having grown up on a farm, Troy explained that work on the farm is not about doing a couple max weightlifting efforts and then resting the remainder of the day. Nor is it done 2–3 times per week with rest days in between. Rather, farm work is hours of sub-maximal loading all day, every day involving a variety of tasks.

Consistent repetition of these workdays over many years leads to the kind of strength associated with farmers, as well as the fisherman I met in Kodiak and many other manual labor professionals.

To keep the discussion simple in a limited space, I should clarify that I am considering maximal loading to be repetitively working at one's maximal effort and/or taking muscles to total failure. Thus, sub-maximal loading would NOT involve repetitively working at maximal effort or taking muscles to total failure. For a visual reference: imagine chopping and stacking a bunch of firewood or digging a 4-foot-deep trench for 20 feet in length.

Considering that the fascial network organizes force created by muscles, it behooves us to have fascial integrity that can aptly support the forces muscles generate (in addition to the forces we face from gravity, ground reaction, and mass and momentum). One could even speculate that in the absence of sufficient support structures, the nervous system would down-regulate the force-generating capacity of our muscles.

While it is widely recognized that a resistance training program will create adaptation first in the nervous system, followed by the muscular system, and finally in the fascial/connective network. It is often overlooked that months and years are required to achieve even moderate thickening and strength adaptations in connective tissue. Long-term, frequent, and consistent exposure is necessary.

Achieving frequent and consistent exposure to load can be difficult in the face of popular belief that load based training should always be followed by a 36–48 hours rest period. In fact, when considering collagen degradation and synthesis following bouts of exercise, the research seems to suggest that training should only be done 2–3 times a week.

However, what people usually do in exercise bouts is strive to work near maximal effort and repeatedly take muscles or regions to failure ... in which case, of course, longer recovery periods are mandated.

To achieve the frequency and consistency found in physical labor populations (and dare I say, reap some of the same structural strength and resiliency benefits), sub-maximal loads can be used every day, with maximal or failure loading occurring periodically at planned instances throughout the week, month, and year.

From the perspective of practical application, making time to train every day is feasible, though day-long work/training sessions are an impossibility for most people. But a similar training effect might be possible by simply creating more time under constant load during a typical 45–75 minutes training session.

Try this with an Ultimate Sandbag (DVRTFitness.com):

- Pick up the Ultimate Sandbag and do 10 reps of each: Clean, Overhead Press, Good Morning, Bent Over Row, MAX Lunge. Then walk around carrying the bag for 2–3 minutes. Return to where you started and begin again with the Cleans, etc.
- Keep doing this for about 30 minutes and try to not set the Ultimate Sandbag down.
- Hint: you are going to want a light bag ... this is supposed to be sub-maximal loading over time.
- Feel free to add some variability by stepping laterally during the Cleans, rotating as you Press, offsetting the bag during Row, putting the bag on a single shoulder as you walk, or anything else you can think of to mix things up.

Maximal effort work can still be done. However, rather than avoiding all load on the following day in your attempts to recover, perhaps do something like the above example or simply walk for 60 minutes wearing a 25 lb backpack.

Load is essential to our development and our ongoing physical health (as we have learned from astronauts). Thus, I truly feel the more frequently we can put ourselves under some amount of load the more favorably our body will develop and maintain the structural integrity we all need and desire. The strongest people I have ever met in my life did exactly that as a matter of course. And with grip strength now correlated to longevity, it looks like those fisherman and farmers will be around a long time.

If I consider training in a more fascially focused running style, I am going to vary my speed and intensity, and, for much of the past few years, I've focused on changing my footwear with every other run. Our storage capacity for elastic energy can be cultivated, particularly through the plantar aponeurosis and Achilles tendon.

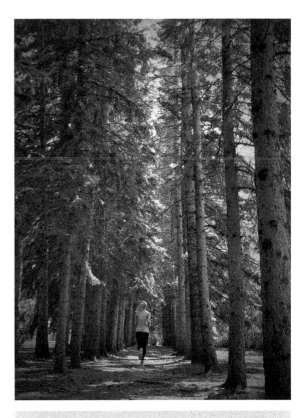

FIGURE 11.3 Running smoothly is an act of myofascial efficiency in coordination.

Photo courtesy of Gail O'Reilly, Zenergy.

Zenergy Running
Gail O'Reilly

Running requires balanced fluid motion. I advocate that you should run with kindness, patience, and always lead with an open heart. Run with the intention to feel unified and connected, because every part of the body must perform together to create harmonious and healthy movement (Figure 11.3).

Developing an integrated, whole, and mindful approach will enable a natural, responsive, and efficient encompassment of the body's fascia webbing and myofascial meridians. To help runners perform to their true potential as well as produce more elasticity, improve energy expenditure, reduce injury, and create feedback of positive sensations, I propose adopting a methodology of small refinements and adjustments based upon the whole body and interconnectivity of myofascial meridians.

A small adjustment in the position of the upper body, for example, "elevates" from the arches of the feet upwards, bringing the spine into neutral alignment, lengthening the myofascial connections, stabilizing, and decompressing. This simple change in posture while running is the basis upon which the other adjustments and refinements in technique build upon.

Adjustments to the chin and eyes intensifies the inner focus; adding a smooth arm glide creates essential rhythm in association with the leg stride and a shift of weight into the balls of the feet generates a springing effect.

A change in breathing technique helps restore healthy functioning in all myofascial meridians.

Finally, the icing on the cake is a technique I call dissolve, that powerfully connects the mind and the body on a deeper level.

All these small improvements add up to bigger gains and make running more enjoyable and efficient for the runner.

Stretch to Win
Chris Frederick
Dynamic Stretching for Movement

Dynamic stretching is one choice among several that can help a person warm up and prepare pre-activity or cool down and help recovery post-activity. On a spectrum of preparing for any full body movement, fitness training, or sports, a common dynamic protocol would be to start with range of motion (ROM) exercises, then progress to dynamic stretching before participating in more specific drills for a physical fitness session, competitive athletic, or dance event. Adding and ending with ballistic movements for an even more complete warm-up (e.g. in fitness—partial squat progressed to full squat progressed to burpees) would be appropriate if preparing for performing power movements in any physical training, sports, or dance (Frederick and Frederick 2017).

A full body (or isolated torso and/or limb) movement performed through a partial or full ROM without encountering tissue or joint resistance would qualify as a ROM drill, practice, or exercise.

If one feels and then moves through any resistance that is felt beyond the normal ROM for a specific movement, then that experience qualifies as dynamic stretching in contrast to static stretching. It is often easier to feel this resistance in one's body when movement is done at slower tempos.

It is noteworthy that based on consistent, recent research that has emerged regarding warm-up and stretching protocols (Behm *et al.* 2016; Kallerud and Gleeson 2013; Opplert and Babault 2018), dynamic stretching has been newly prioritized as an essential element in fitness training by leading evidenced based educational institutions for fitness professionals (Sutton 2021).

This author has educated and trained professional dance companies and individual dancers in the importance of replacing a dominance of traditional passive static stretching before practice and training in favor of dynamic stretching. Anecdotally, this change was immediately successful in all cases by greatly reducing injuries, early fatigue, and chronic strain in addition to improving proprioceptive awareness.

Dynamic stretches are commonly done while standing. Here I present more options, done on the floor. I have devised a dynamic stretch program called the Core 4 to be used pre- or post-activity. The following stretches make up a dynamic progression from ground movements that can be added preparatory to more vigorous standing movements. It is best to do them after a light warm-up such as an easy jog/run, stationary bicycle, or other relatively effortless activity for 5–10 minutes—just enough to generate very light perspiration.

The stretches engage entire myofascial kinetic chains and nomenclature in therapy, fitness, and sports may vary. Terms such as slings, links, lines, and nets are currently in common use. For this program, stretches are named after the targeted general anatomical regions.

General guidelines for dynamic mobility preparation:

- Compare how you feel and move before and after these stretches. Over time, you will know which ones are the most beneficial and how to vary based on need.
- Make your movements flow.
- Exhale into the stretch, and inhale coming out of the stretch.
- Don't count reps; rather, finish the movement when no longer making gains in flexibility.
- If the movement doesn't loosen you up enough to perform, then do SMR (self-myofascial release) on the problem spot and try the stretches again.
- Never let your spine sag, but never hold your core so tight that you can't move well during the stretches.
- These are dynamic stretch movements; you should not feel a big stretch. Use less intensity and faster tempos and do as many reps as are needed to feel more mobile but still strong and ready to perform.
- For cool downs, perform the same movements but about 3x slower by taking slower and longer breaths resulting in prolonged stretches. Make the stretch

movements last longer so that you are still moving and not holding the stretch (unless you are doing a static stretch for different reasons and purposes). Explore different angles in each movement to customize your needs at that moment.

Core 4 on the Floor™

The Core 4 program has been successfully used as both an assessment and a flexibility exercise program on thousands of clients and students. It focuses on dynamic flexibility preparation of the core myofasciae of your lower body and progresses to your upper body. The initial focus is dynamic core mobility, and the progression integrates motor control and dynamic core stability. This routine applies to most activities and sports that require optimal core control (Frederick and Frederick 2017).

The Core 4 is made up of the power-generating regions for most movement in fitness and sports. In terms of bones and joints, this would be your lower lumbar–pelvic–hip area. In terms of myofasciae, this would be all your core muscles and fascia (lumbodorsal or thoracolumbar fascia, transversus abdominis, obliques, deep and superficial back extensors, iliopsoas, glutes, and deep hip rotators). These muscles and associated fasciae, especially those surrounding the hips, provide the foundation for many athletic movements that athletes depend on for performance. Therefore, it is extremely important to achieve balance in mobility in the Core 4 to generate the energy-efficient, powerful functioning that is required in most sports, dance, and in high-level fitness training.

Dynamic stretching to improve mobility in the lower body first makes sense because it is the base or foundation for most sport and athletic movements. Four key lower-body muscles and their kinetic chains are identified that can be focused on to improve mobility:

- Glute, hip, and back warm-up (includes myofasciae below in the proximal hamstring and above in the lower to upper back and neck).
- Rotation warm-up for hip, back, and neck (includes quadratus lumborum bilaterally and myofasciae

around the entire waist and hips below and into the torso rotators and neck above).

- Hip flexor warm-up (includes iliopsoas and the myofasciae below in the thigh and groin and above along the entire front of the abdominals and neck).
- Lat to low back warm-up (includes latissimus dorsi and myofasciae from the low back and pelvis on up to the shoulder and chest).

Note that the latissimus dorsi is included in this group because it attaches to both the lower back and the pelvis, as well as to the shoulder. It functions as a kinetic bridge that connects the lower body to the upper body.

The Core 4 program opens areas that may be causing restriction around your hips and low back, which will also help regions higher up (e.g. the spine and shoulders) and lower down (e.g. the knees, ankles, and feet) because of the long, extensive connections through your connective tissue network or fascial net. Complete the entire Core 4 on one side of your body before stretching the other side.

1. Glute, hip, and back warm-up

Instructions

1. Sit on the floor and place one leg in front and one behind and bring the front foot inward until the foot touches the back knee, or as close as possible (Figure 11.breakout.1a). Position your weight so you are sitting more on the glute of the front leg. Adjust for comfort. Place your hands in a push-up position in front of you with the arms straight.

2. As you inhale, lengthen the whole spine up through the top of your head; then, exhale and move down and forward over the knee, keeping the spine long (Figure 11.breakout.1b).

3. Roll up through the spine back to the erect starting position. Repeat 3x or as needed.

4. From the last repetition above, take the torso forward to the left and right of the knee at different angles to target the different glute fibers

(Figure 11.breakout.1c and Figure 11.breakout.1d). Repeat both directions 2x or as needed.

Tips

- Breathe and wave into and out of the stretch until you feel your tissues release.
- Drop your body closer to the floor and move from side to side.
- Complete the rest of the following stretches before doing the other side.

FIGURE 11.BREAKOUT.1A

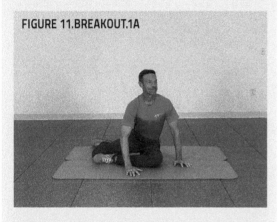

FIGURE 11.BREAKOUT.1B

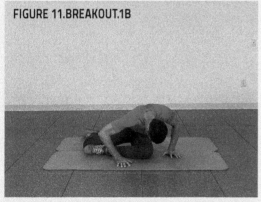

2. Rotation warm-up for hip, back, and neck

Instructions

1. From the glute stretch position, turn, and walk the hands toward the rear until you feel a slight stretch in the back, hips, and/or legs (Figure 11. breakout.2a).

FIGURE 11.BREAKOUT.1C

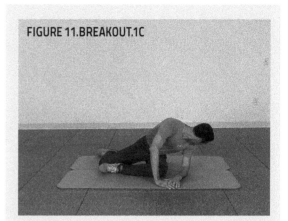

FIGURE 11.BREAKOUT.1D

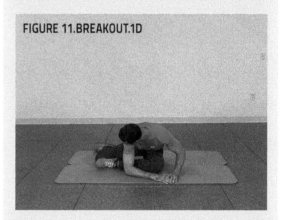

2. Keep the hands still and lean toward the hand that is on the same side as the front leg, and inhale (Figure 11.breakout.2b).
3. Exhale as you lean back again.
4. Repeat 3x or as needed.

Tips

- Walk the hands out a little farther with each repetition to progress the stretch.
- Complete the rest of the following stretches before doing the other side.

3. Hip flexor warm-up

Instructions

1. From last position in the previous stretch, place the back forearm on the ground and find

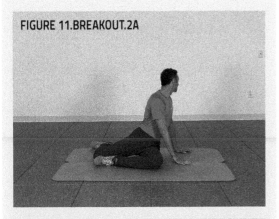

FIGURE 11.BREAKOUT.2A

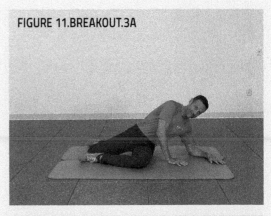

FIGURE 11.BREAKOUT.3A

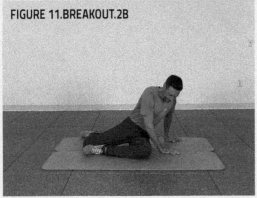

FIGURE 11.BREAKOUT.2B

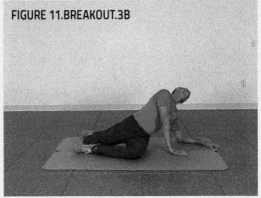

FIGURE 11.BREAKOUT.3B

a stable position for the shoulder, where you can balance on that arm with your full weight. Slide the forearm to the rear as your back starts to arch and stop when you feel a mild stretch. Inhale and lean forward on both hands (Figure 11.breakout.3a).

2. Exhale while you arch the back and look up to ceiling (Figure 11.breakout.3b) feeling the stretch in your hip flexors (and sometimes the back).

3. Repeat 3x or as needed.

- Lean back farther to progress the stretch.

- Find the stretch by arching the back rather than twisting it.

- Complete the last stretch below before doing the other side.

4. Lat to low back warm-up

Instructions

1. From the last position in the previous hip flexor stretch, inhale, and reach your arm overhead (Figure11.breakout.4a).

2. Extend the arm out from the hip as you reach. This looks like you are swimming in the air (Figure11.breakout.4b).

3. Exhale as you rotate the chest toward the floor while you reach the arm out (Figure11.breakout.4c).

4. Circle your arm down and back up overhead.

5. Repeat 3x or as needed.

Tips

- Keep reaching the arm throughout the stretch for maximal effect.

- Try to get the chest more parallel to floor with each rep.

Repeat entire series from beginning on other side.

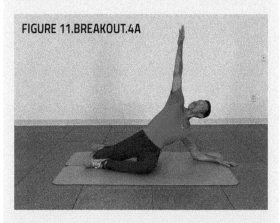

FIGURE 11.BREAKOUT.4A

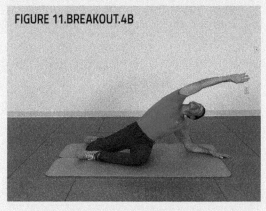

FIGURE 11.BREAKOUT.4B

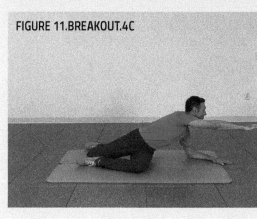

FIGURE 11.BREAKOUT.4C

A complete warm-up before activities such as fitness training and sports progress from a 5–10 minute activity like a light jog or stationary bike or full body ROM before progressing to dynamic stretches. Dynamic stretches can be done on the ground and progress to standing with increased tempos and frequencies (repetitions) until one feels sufficiently warmed-up to engage in the intended activity. The person should feel alert, mobile, and ready for high intensity activity. They should not feel tired, relaxed, or too mobile to perform.

Dynamic stretches can also be used to cool down after activity to support a complete and efficient recovery. Tempos are slow so that breathing and duration of stretches are longer to help oxygenate and rehydrate tissues, flush metabolic waste, and restore flexibility. The person is encouraged to keep moving in the stretches to explore various angles in order to individualize the stretch for their specific needs. This protocol will both increase and maintain flexibility and mobility for an active lifestyle.

References

Behm, D. G., Blazevich, A. J., Kay, A. D. and McHugh, M. (2016) 'Acute effects of muscle stretching on physical performance, range of motion, and injury incidence in healthy active individuals: a systematic review.' *Applied Physiology, Nutrition, and Metabolism 41*, 1, 1–11. https://doi.org/10.1139/apnm-2015-0235

Frederick, A. and Frederick, C. (2017) *Stretch to Win*. 2nd ed. Champaign, IL: Human Kinetics.

Kallerud, H. and Gleeson, N. (2013) 'Effects of stretching on performances involving stretch-shortening cycles.' *Sports Medicine 43*, 8, 733–750. https://doi.org/10.1007/s40279-013-0053-x

Opplert, J. and Babault, N. (2018) 'Acute effects of dynamic stretching on muscle flexibility and performance: An analysis of the current literature.' *Sports Medicine 48*, 2, 299–325. https://doi.org/10.1007/s40279-017-0797-9

Sutton, B. (2021) *An explanation of the new updates to the OPT™ model*. Accessed on 03/16/2022 at https://blog.nasm.org/new-opt-model-updates

References

Brumitt, J. (2015) 'The Bunkie Test: descriptive data for a novel test of core muscular endurance.' *Rehabilitation Research and Practice 2015*, 1–9. https://doi.org/10.1155/2015/780127

Elphinston, J. (2019) *The Power and the Grace: A Professional's Guide to Ease and Efficiency in Functional Movement.* Edinburgh: Handspring Publishing.

Frederick, A. and Frederick, C. (2020) *Fascial Stretch Therapy™.* Edinburgh: Handspring Publishing.

Fukashiro, S., Hay, D. C. and Nagano, A. (2006) 'Biomechanical behavior of muscle-tendon complex during dynamic human movements.' *Journal of Applied Biomechanics 22*, 2, 131–147. https://doi.org/10.1123/jab.22.2.131

Huijing, P. A. (2007) 'Epimuscular myofascial force transmission between antagonistic and synergistic muscles can explain movement limitation in spastic paresis.' *Journal of Electromyography and Kinesiology 17*, 6, 708–724. https://doi.org/10.1016/j.jelekin.2007.02.003

Järvinen, T. A. H., Józsa, L., Kannus, P., Järvinen, T. L. N. and Järvinen, M. (2002) 'Organization and distribution of intramuscular connective tissue in normal and immobilized skeletal muscles. An immunohistochemical, polarization and scanning electron microscopic study.' *Journal of Muscle Research and Cell Motility 23*, 3, 245–254. https://doi.org/10.1023/A:1020904518336

Kram, R. and Dawson, T. J. (1998) 'Energetics and biomechanics of locomotion by red kangaroos (Macropus rufus).' *Comparative Biochemistry and Physiology Part B: Biochemistry and Molecular Biology 120*, 1, 41–49. https://doi.org/10.1016/S0305-0491(98)00022-4

Lesondak, D. (2017) *Fascia: What it is and why it matters.* Edinburgh: Handspring Publishing.

Lesondak, D. and Akey, A. M. (eds) (2020) *Fascia, function, and medical applications.* Boca Raton, FL: CRC Press.

Magnusson, S. P., Langberg, H. and Kjaer, M. (2010) 'The pathogenesis of tendinopathy: balancing the response to loading.' *Nature Reviews Rheumatology 6*, 5, 262–268. https://doi.org/10.1038/nrrheum.2010.43

Reeves, N. D. (2006) 'Adaptation of the tendon to mechanical usage.' *Journal of Musculoskeletal & Neuronal Interactions 6*, 2, 174–180.

Sawicki, G. S., Lewis, C. L. and Ferris, D. P. (2009) 'It pays to have a spring in your step.' *Exercise and Sport Sciences Reviews 37*, 3, 130–138. https://doi.org/10.1097/JES.0b013e31819c2df6

Schleip, R., Baker, A. and Avison, J. (eds) (2015) *Fascia in Sport and Movement.* Edinburgh: Handspring Publishing.

Solnit, R. (2017) *A Field Guide to Getting Lost.* Edinburgh: Canongate Books.

van Pletzen, D. and Venter, R. E. (2012) 'The relationship between the Bunkie-test and physical performance in Rugby Union players.' *International Journal of Sports Science & Coaching 7*, 3, 543–553. https://doi.org/10.1260/1747-9541.7.3.543

Further reading

Alexander, C., Ishikawa, S. and Silverstein, M. (1977) *A Pattern Language: Towns, Buildings, Construction.* Oxford: Oxford University Press.

Anderson, B. (1981) Flexibility testing. *NSCA Journal 3*, 2, 20–23.

Baechle, T. R. (1994) 'Neuromuscular adaptations to conditioning.' In *Essentials of Strength Training and Conditioning.* Champaign, IL: Human Kinetics.

Barker, V. (1993) *Posture Makes Perfect.* Tokyo: Japan Publications.

Lesondak, D. (2017) *Fascia: What it is and why it matters.* Edinburgh: Handspring Publishing.

Trabold, O., Wagner, S., Wicke, C., Scheuenstuhl, H. *et al.* (2003) 'Lactate and oxygen constitute a fundamental regulatory mechanism in wound healing.' *Wound Repair and Regeneration 11*, 6, 504–509. https://doi.org/10.1046/j.1524-475X.2003.11621.x

We are connected fascially from early in our embryological development throughout our entire life. Understanding how fascia affects us at different ages and stages can help us train better at every age and be more resilient for the various stages of life. Life itself shapes our form and understanding myofascia throughout the stages of life can help navigate each of those stages better. If the fascial web begins approximately two weeks into embryological development (and is still intact when we die), how we treat that web can create a sense of health or challenge the body profoundly. What if, as therapists, coaches, parents, and society members, we can look at the myofascial work of the body as the framework for movement programs, and design elements for building and play. We are using the concept of encouraging multidirectional and multivectored movement to create balance between the large and fine myofascial connections in the body; using this concept encourages mobility development to keep the body resilient at any age. We want to thoughtfully use our knowledge to support our changing human form.

Additionally, we need to keep in mind that just as a movement pattern that serves one person may not serve another, patterns that we utilize at one age of development may not be who or what we are in years to come. As noted by the dancer and longtime movement explorer Andrea Olsen:

Perception is a construct, and attitudes change. It can be useful to take a look at familiar views and values, and discern how those ideas were formed. Patterns that you established at age twelve, eighteen, or even last week may no longer be appropriate for who you are now. Conditioned habits in coordination can result in overcontraction of muscles (think tight hips). Mental sees about the dancing body manifest in action. We choose what to plant and what to nourish. This requires uncoupling biography and biology—personal story and genetically endowed structure. Receiving sensory signals, updating interpretation, and allowing communicative expression changes us. The ways we construct meaning are impacted: our view of the world and what we think is real. (Olsen 2014, p.8)

In other words, our shape changes, as does our perception of the world. This in turn, reworks us.

Early childhood development

Babies have no movement agenda (aside from basic needs such as food) and motivation is through need and unstructured play. Early childhood interaction for the majority of humans on earth still begins with breastfeeding, which has a large impact on oral pharyngeal work. Up until kindergarten (around age five for most children in the US), most children easily perform squats and sit easily on the ground as well as navigate the monkey bars. Children move naturally through the space around them and don't edit themselves in their movement behaviors in very early ages. In other words, they fall and squirm and move and recover easier than adults.

Spirals, so critical as a movement motif and shape in the universe, is also critical to the beginning development of a child. As a start, we can conceptualize the human body lying on the ground supine as having seven main weighted places in the body (two arms, two legs, the pelvis, the head, and the chest). Between these weighted places we have rotational capacity (think of giving yourself a hug and rotating between the pelvis and the chest). In this position on the back, the weighted areas can remain all on the floor, or curled up, picking up arms and legs off the floor. The first major change of posture a baby will make is rotating the head to follow a desired object and that can turn the rest of the baby into rotation with the head with the ability to lift and lengthen. The eyes (or for some the ears) drive the shift and change.

Another spiral brings the baby from the belly to the seated position with two large masses off the floor (chest and head off the floor). Turning in another spiral brings the baby to a crawling position with the weights of the trunk in the air (head, chest, and pelvis). Kneeling comes next with a knee and one foot, and the final rotation into standing takes the final stage of walking with the weight on essentially one and a half feet.

Climb a tree or out to the playground

Several years ago, when I injured my right arm and had a brief issue of lateral epicondylitis, I became fascinated with the profound lack of grip strength and as I was healing, began to re-engage in utilizing the local playground equipment at the end of my trail run for additional rehabilitation, a part of my daily play these days. Any adult who has spent time away from swinging will definitely understand that grip is critical to mastering the monkey bars or other gym equipment. We do not technically have a need any longer for overhead reach, but certainly there are aspects of our anatomy that still respond well myofascially to utilizing the arms in multiple ways.

Children still do this to climb trees (although less available to many kids). Louv (2008) explored the relationship of environment to play and noted:

Within the space of a few decades, the way children understand and experience nature has changed radically. The polarity of the relationship has reversed. Today, kids are aware of the global threats to the environment—but their physical contact, their intimacy with nature, is fading. That's exactly the opposite of how it was when I was a child. (p.1)

Play, in an unstable environment, trains the body both muscularly and fascially. Parkour, developed in France by urban young adults interacting with the built environment, still offers a means to engage the body and balance through maximizing efficiency of movement and relaxing that tensegral body during the inevitable falls that come in play. As we know, a tense body bracing for a fall (as often happens in the elderly worried about injury) will often leave a wrist or stiffened area vulnerable

to breaking. The Parkour practitioner, or kid who is able to fall and roll through, distributing pressure throughout the body, will often come away without any injury.

There are times when straightening a myofascial chain makes sense to help efficiency and force transmission. To note:

Watch a gibbon's elegant swinging from branch to branch; they hardly bend their elbows in horizontal deviation movements. The same is true for children in the playground (Figure 12.1). They are able to catch bar to bar, but as a result

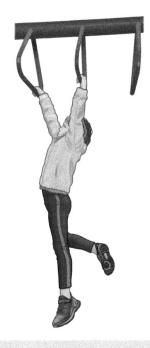

FIGURE 12.1 Girl on playground equipment. When our arms are by our sides, both pectoralis major and the latissimus dorsi muscles have a twist before their connections to the arm bone. Bringing the arms overhead unwinds the twists and allows the arms to work fully into brachiation. Adding the myofascial connections, the arm continues its pull through the torso, especially when the arm is straight. Children developing coordination and strength actually are able to work this action through a line of force transmission with each arm grab they perform.

of their lack of upper arm strength, they are unable to bend their elbows. Nevertheless, in order to train fascia you definitely need strong muscles. This gives us a hint for the importance of muscular strength training as a pre-requisite in order to exercise fascia connective tissues properly. (Heiduk in Schleip and Wilke 2021, pp.407–408)

Early school age

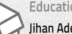

Row, row, row your boat...
myofascial efficiency through play

Children benefit from play and the basic concepts of movement play can target the myofascial system. In working with early childhood development, kids work through song, movement, and play. Impulse control skills and rhythm and coordination are all being developed. Let's take a movement exercise and then break it down for its benefits.

Organize in a circle of children (pre-school age through early elementary) around a large stretch band (many are sold commercially under materials such as elastic covered by fleece or terry cloth, but any stretchy fabric can be made into a large loop). Everyone can get into their boats by putting feet over the band while holding on (using the yoga boat pose), feet either grounded (the boat is at the dock!) or off the ground (balancing like a boat in the water). We will start singing, "Row, row, row your boat gently down the stream. Merrily, merrily, merrily, merrily, life is but a dream." First time through is practice, but now we've encountered a sticky molasses river, so we will have to work hard and move through slowly... "Roooowww, roooowww, roooowww your boat," and so on, until we get through the sticky river. We've now opened up to a lake, but we spot an alligator, so we are going to row as quickly as possible (paddling and song get very fast!). Finally, we are through the dangers and onto clear waters (paddling once more).

If we look at this myofascially, we are working coordination above all, as well as physical and emotional regulation.

Emerging adulthood

There is a need for the field of research in the areas between young adulthood and fully realized independence. Legally, adulthood (particularly in the US) begins with significant rights at age 18 with additional legal separation of health information, voting, etc. However, most college kids are less equipped these days at navigating a world without the constant interference of smart phones. There is an equal bias on parents that children should be able to succeed well on their own. There is a new area of psychology of the age between adolescence and adulthood that therapist Jeffrey Jensen Arnett terms "emerging adulthood" (Arnett 2014). After a large study in 1995, interviewing 300 young adults, he was surprised at the response of how, for many, that question of personal identity was a common theme.

Education of fascia for kids
Jihan Adem

Fascia anatomy education, even for adults, is a relatively new concept, especially for the average Joe. So, to think about fascia anatomy education for children? Well, that's pretty much an entirely new concept.

As our understanding of fascia grows and new research presents continuing ideas of the potential properties and strengths of this fascinating connective tissue, I can't help but imagine what a world we could create if there were ideas and ways of demonstrating the interconnectedness of our being to our children, how they may understand their bodies more wholly, and themselves in a way that took us many years to appreciate.

The concepts of fascia currently being presented go a long way to explaining the functional relationships of the human body, effectively. Thoughts about fascia, being considered as a body-wide system, are relatively new in the day-to-day world of the average person walking along the street. And for those of us who have been working within the field of movement and manual therapies for the past few decades, we will be amongst a specific group who are actively seeking information on understanding more about how our bodies are connected and how we function as an integrated form in movement and life. For some, this will include how both body and mind are interrelated, and how the study of fascia holds key understandings for this conceptional idea and how fascia is being researched as a sensory and emotional organ. This is a far cry from history when Cartesian dualism played a fundamental role in wrestling the practice of medicine away from church oversight. The formal separation of the "mind" from the "body" allowed for religion to concern itself with the non-corporeal "mind," while dominion over the "body" was ceded to medical science and the academic study of physiology and anatomy that followed.

From the moment we come into existence, our environment influences us for the good and as a challenge. As a friend said to me:

> Watch a young child run and play and we notice how they are free of the restrictions of movement of that of an older child... Fascia in the young could be free of the emotion and life events of the old. It could be the blueprint of the ideal—before we carry out our lives in a non-ideal way—most of the time uneducated in the ways of our intrinsic system of systems. (Zaranko 2020)

What benefits could there be in introducing functional anatomical learning, at a young age, in a wider circle; with the addition of, fascia anatomy to support healthier growth and empowerment of each young individual?

When we think about the future of fascia anatomy education, it becomes really clear to me that the way in which we educate our youngest children is crucial so they have the chance to treasure and embody the knowledge that we have only just come to understand. From there, take their views, experience, and passion to further develop understandings and knowledge for their generation and beyond.

Reference

Zaranko, A. BDA 2020 Personal communication.

What's in a name?

These days the biological identifiers of "male" and "female" are perhaps more accurately falling on a spectrum, and that even biologically, our hormone levels or certain organ attributes may greatly vary from person to person. Non-binary, trans, intersex, and more all have a place in the fascia world and at the table.

Pregnancy, menopause, and more...

For many identifying as women, the fascial changes in the body vary due to estrogen levels changing throughout the lifetime, so understanding both our evolutionary heritage as well as the changes through your own or a client's lifetime, it is important to understand the effects of the body system, particularly on stability and appropriate mobility around the pelvis. For women in different life cycles of menstruation, pregnancy, and post-menopausal life, the levels of estrogen appear to have a direct effect on the mobility of the fascial tissues. What does this mean for exercise, especially for movement? With the wider hip, the body is over engaging and overutilizing muscles like the quadratus lumborum. We need to consider integrating the body at a neuromuscular level. This can lead to IT band syndrome, pelvic floor disfunctions, and more. For women, in particular, there is a great need to focus on stability in the body system, and not mobility of dysfunctional patterns.

Most women have instability in their gait stabilization and this translates to other common exercises like fire hydrant (leg laterally rotated out to the side). This may show up as wobbling in quadruped position due to instability in the fascial pelvic floor and the lower lumbar spine. Organize the inner stability along this line, and other movement and lines can balance from this as well.

A pregnant woman has more elasticity in the fascia. In a study headed by Caterina Fede, the relationship between fascia and hormone levels was correlated during the different stages of menses (Fede *et al.* 2019). Basically, hormones can increase flexibility during ovulation, and during the menses themselves there is a stiffening effect. What does this mean for movement? Maybe there is a need to be careful on joint loading during ovulation, and at minimum, more awareness for alignment. Additionally, Fede and her team noted the ability of fascial cells to modify components of the extracellular matrix. One example is Relaxin-1, known to pregnant and breastfeeding mothers as it allows more flexibility in the body. It reduces the matrix synthesis and, as such, has an anti-fibrotic effect.

Type 3 collagen fibers and fibrillin are produced in pregnancy and make one more elastic than in other periods of the circle. This allows for the shape of the abdominal cavity to accommodate the growing fetus. However, along with this comes a reduction in balance and an increase in instability, such as in the sacroiliac (SI) joint. So, the increased range of elasticity comes with a cost to balance. We know sex hormones affect connective tissue like the pubic synthesis. After pregnancy, for example, there is a level of the hormones that takes time to come back to "normal." When Tamoxifen is used in breast cancer treatment, it can affect the fascia, making it more rigid and also affecting pain. The expression of collagen remodeling is also different in women than in men, and has a role in the extracellular matrix (ECM) remodeling. While the research in contraceptive use and its effects on fascia have been limited, there is strong evidence that oral contraceptive use depresses collagen synthesis (Hansen *et al.* 2009).

In post-menopause, the receptors for sensitivity to estrogen are decreased. Eiling *et al.* (2007) found there is higher laxity in the knee, for example, in the ovulatory stage due to this loss of stability. This has important implications for movement, where female athletes may need to consider fascia training and movement at different stages of their circle. Their suggestion was also for future studies to investigate the effects of the contraceptive pill on the lower limb musculotendinous stiffness (MTS). Given the high rate of anterior cruciate ligament (ACL) injuries among young female athletes, this would be an important area to investigate.

The abdominal wall brings up some issues, particularly with women and aging. As noted by Zorn (in Schleip 2015) the rectus abdominis has work to do: "In fact, this large muscle should *pull up* the pubic bone with agility and, thereby, adjust the balance of the pelvis and fine-tune its position with respect to the quickly changing forces during movement" (p.165). Likewise, the SI joint is often considered a vulnerable area, although it is prone to similar issues as any other fascial joint and needs a balance between freedom of movement and stabilization.

Caesarean sections (CS)

One in four women have a caesarean section, whether elective or emergency. While c-sections can be necessary, they are also associated with a higher risk for challenges in the mother's health (The Lancet 2018) including ramifications from c-section scarring, which is a fascial issue. Any surgery destroys the continuity of the tissue quality of fascia. Scar tissue implies the scar tissue forces will be redistributed along the path of least resistance. We know that women tend to have umbilical hernias, while men have inguinal each due to the region where the fascia is at its weakest. While the research is currently lacking, there may prove to be a connection between c-section scarring and the prevalence of umbilical hernias nearby for women in their later years.

Fascia in the aging body

Healthy aging should be an accessible concept especially if one keeps in mind how to keep fascially nourished and allow the slide and glide of myofascia to continue to work well. Two pieces above all may be the most important part of aging both on the micro and global level: first, as we age, it is important to continue to stay resilient to what life continues to offer and, second, connection is important both in terms of the form of the body and form of the larger culture.

Supporting healthy aging changes us on a very basic level. Nobel Prize winner (2009) Elizabeth H. Blackburn observed that inflammation, cell damage, and more literally shorten the telomeres that cap the DNA strands. The number one way that we can engage in healthy living is working in connected communities. It is important to find the connection in your community. After that, movement is also a prescription for good health.

Aging is, in essence, the process of the body drying out. A healthy ECM is full of water, but an aging ECM is less hydrophilic. If interstitial fluid helps in tissue remodeling, fascia under healthy action is responsive, but without could cause issues such as lymphoedema or tumor growth. However, it may be the wrong thought process to try to "counteract" aging. The bigger challenge is perhaps to overcome the assumption that aging means inevitable pain and disease. One of my yoga teachers, Tao Porchon Lynch, lived until the age of 101 and, in part, her resiliency may have been helped by her endless curiosity. She started studying yoga at eight years old, and took up ballroom dancing in her eighties.

The beauty industry likewise focuses on fascia, although the names are the building blocks of fascia such as collagen, hyaluronic acid, etc. Aging for many is the time of deeper wrinkles and joint achiness. As we get older, the connective tissue, in general, becomes stiffer, especially in the ECM which adds the decrease in elastic recoil. This loss of elasticity in the body also includes the lens of the eye that often stiffens by middle age. When we are younger, the lens behind the iris flexes in a process called "accommodation," literally being able to adapt to changes in near and far distances. When the lens becomes more rigid, this condition is known as presbyopia.

What is clear, is the current model for aging is based on chronic pain and problems, rather than healthy aging. As noted by Huber *et al.* (2011):

Ageing with chronic illnesses has become the norm, and chronic diseases account for most of the expenditures of the healthcare system, putting pressure on its sustainability. In this context the WHOs [World Health Organization] definition becomes counterproductive as it declares people with chronic diseases and disabilities definitively ill. It minimises the role of the human capacity to cope autonomously with life's ever changing physical, emotional, and social challenges and to function with fulfilment and a feeling of wellbeing with a chronic disease or disability. (p.343)

Trindade *et al.* (2012) showed in their work that the deep temporal fascia is less resilient and stiffer in the elderly than in younger people. While there are advantages to age creating more stability, there is a distant decrease in the range of flexibility in older people.

In many ways, this follows Dr. Ira Byock's thought process that, "it is not easy to die well in modern times." He explains that:

Death is the most inevitable fact of life. But the experience of dying has changed over the course of history, especially within the past fifty years. In many ways dying has become a lot harder. We are the benefactors and victims of scientific success. Serious, chronic illness is an invention of the late twentieth century, the fruit of our species' intellectual prowess, the culmination (at least so far) of millennia of scientific progress. (Byock 2013, p.2)

Twyla Tharp is known as a force in modern dance for her volume of work and her longevity in an often time-limited career. Seventy-eight years old at the time of publication of her 2019 book *Keep It Moving*, her point is not to keep movement going, but to move even better. As she writes, "age is not the enemy. Stagnation is the enemy. Complacency is the enemy. Statis is the enemy... all animate creatures are destroyed when frozen. They do not move. This is not a worthy goal" (p.6). Sounds a lot like a plan for working fascia.

A large part of healthy aging is a satisfaction with life and the ability, on a realistically level, to move through it. If the long stride is both a sign of youth as well as the necessary means for the tissues to gain the transfer of kinetic energy, we have to think of what we are doing to our elderly population by limiting the environment both in terms of pathways to walk on, and movement that can accommodate the range of ankle movement needed for functionality, particularly in terms of walking.

New research in aging, particularly in relationship to the extracellular matrix (Pavan *et al.* 2020) notes there is an increase in passive stiffness as we get older. The study executed by Pavan and colleagues compared the passive stress that generated elongation of fibers in young and old groups of subjects. They concluded that "in human skeletal muscles, the age-related reduced compliance is due to an increase in stiffness of the ECM, mainly caused by collagen accumulation" (Pavan *et al.* 2020, p.1). Additionally, as learned in our fascial anatomy, hyaluronan is responsible for the slide and glide in tissue and is noticeably diminished in the aging body. Back pain is often another common complaint in adult populations and part of the reason can be the fascial set-up of the thoracolumbar fascia that is full of a high proportion of nociceptors (free nerve endings) as well as sympathetic nerves. This may, in part, explain a heightened feeling of pain as a response to stress.

How can we can age better myofascially is a question a lot of us are asking as we want the best possible quality of life for as long as we can. What is intelligent aging? The average age of Nobel Prize winners had been 60 and is continuing to trend higher, but intelligent aging is also about being able to participate in the things we enjoy and want to do.

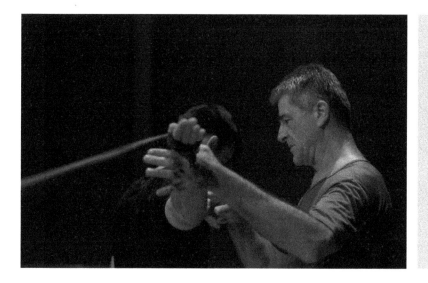

FIGURE 12.2 Active aging involves working with the myofascial system and dynamic training to decrease stiffness and improve strength and range of motion.

Photo courtesy of Johannes Freiberg.

Aging well through a dynamic fascial system

Johannes Carl Freiberg Neto

Aging is a natural process, but the term "old age" is a historical and socially constructed category, produced by industrial modernity (Correia *et al.* 2011).

The term "Active Aging," conceptualized in a multi-dimensional way by the WHO (2005), justifies that the elderly should be involved in activities that require physical and mental effort, in order to improve the quality of life (QOL) as they age (Centro Internacional de Longevidade Brasil 2015) (Figure 12.2).

Understanding yourself in your aging process and developing sufficient knowledge about cardiorespiratory, nervous, muscular, and fascial system training, can assist in the evaluation and analysis of the aging process itself and how to properly adjust physical practice. In addition to teaching movement-related content, learning about the functional advantages of training the fascial system in particular, together with your health and physical capabilities, can elevate the enjoyment of self-managing your own physical, cognitive, motor, and emotional reality. Put another way, think about what it means to grow old, allowing yourself to review your concepts and to build a more positive view of old age.

Studies show that the time to climb stairs, get up from a chair, and walk a defined distance increases significantly in the elderly. Tests show that the volume, strength, and power of the quadriceps muscle decrease significantly. These changes are associated with muscle tone, stiffness, and elasticity (Agyapong-Badu *et al.* 2016), which can vary progressively by about 1.5% per year in this population (Kocur *et al.* 2019).

With aging, there is compelling evidence that many of the age-related negative changes related to muscle function and metabolism are caused by lifestyle changes secondary to aging, especially physical inactivity (Distefano and Goodpaster 2018).

The fibrous muscular fascial system is organized in three layers, presenting internally as an endomysium, related to muscle fibers; the perimysium, resistant sheaths that transmit strength to the tendons and support the neurovascular system; and the epimysium, which involves the muscle giving form and resistance to muscle contraction (Purslow 2010). Its gelatinous component, a fundamental substance, is responsible for hydration and cellular nutrition, as well as the ability to slide extra- and intramuscularly, providing ample capacity for directing strength (Stecco *et al.* 2013).

There is a direct relationship between strength and collagen fibers, which with different stimuli, and if subjected to mechanical overloads, alter their composition and, consequently, the movement performance (Zullo *et al.* 2020), thus restricting muscle extensibility and decreasing the range of motion (Wilke *et al.* 2019).

With advancing age, there is an increase in the amount of crosslinking, decreasing elasticity, and stiffening of the ECM, consequently causing muscle stiffness, impairing muscle function (Etienne *et al.* 2020).

Among many alternatives, Fascial Fitness (or Fascial Wellness) exercises can provide a tensional, neuronal, and vascular coordinative activity, improving the quality of the movement, as well as its mobility (Guzzoni *et al.* 2018).

The challenge is how to assist the elderly to recover functionality, rehabilitate and regenerate fascial tissue. The use of physical practices focused on the fascial system allows an intervention that increases the possibility of success, speed, and self-efficacy of the exercise, as well as changing and maintaining changes in behavior of these elderly people (Schleip *et al.* 2021).

Active dynamic stretches of the fascial system are potentially a way to train the fascia during aging. Decreasing stiffness through a program of aerobic exercises, improving strength by including eccentric–concentric muscle contractions and maintaining a good range of motion.

Basic active dynamic stretch training is used to influence the fascial skeletal muscle system by increasing its ability to transmit extra and intramuscular strength. Basic exercises oriented toward fascia are designed to involve many variations with low loads (up to 1 kg maximum), rhythmic/cyclical in nature, with low repetitions (maximum of 15 repetitions) and few sets (from 1 to 4), with pauses for tissue rehydration, including movements full of quasi-isometric states and where elastic bounce movements are interposed.

Four basic principles for dynamic fascial training are designed to improve the motor skills of the elderly:

1. all activity is global/local
2. must be performed from the peripheral to the center, followed by center-peripheral balances
3. a state of basal fascial tone (tensegral) must be established to improve focus
4. the movements follow the eccentric–concentric principles, with encouragement to maintain good positioning and balance that has been established in the initial phase of the movement to be performed.

The movements happen in the three classic planes, starting with the sagittal plane, then frontal and followed by diagonal and spiral movements. It starts with homologous, ipsilateral activity and ends with contralateral activities that involve three-dimensional actions.

References

Agyapong-Badu, S., Warner, M., Samuel, D. and Stokes, M. (2016) 'Measurement of ageing effects on muscle tone and mechanical properties of rectus femoris and biceps brachii in healthy males and females using a novel hand-held myometric device.' *Archives of Gerontology and Geriatrics 62*, 59–67. https://doi.org/10.1016/j.archger.2015.09.011

Correia, M., Miranda, M. and Velardi, M. (2011) 'The practice of physical education for elderly anchored in Freire's pedagogy: reflections on a problem-dialogic experience.' *Movimento: Revista Da Escola de Educação Física 17*, 281–297.

Distefano, G. and Goodpaster, B. H. (2018) 'Effects of exercise and aging on skeletal muscle.' *Cold Spring Harbor Perspectives in Medicine 8*, 3, a029785. https://doi.org/10.1101/cshperspect.a029785

Etienne, J., Liu, C., Skinner, C. M., Conboy, M. J. and Conboy, I. M. (2020) 'Skeletal muscle as an experimental model of choice to study tissue aging and rejuvenation.' *Skeletal Muscle 10*, 1, 4. https://doi.org/10.1186/s13395-020-0222-1

Guzzoni, V., Ribeiro, M. B. T., Lopes, G. N., de Cássia Marqueti, R., de Andrade, R. V., Selistre-de-Araujo, H. S. and Durigan, J. L. Q. (2018) 'Effect of resistance training on extracellular matrix adaptations in skeletal muscle of older rats.' *Frontiers in Physiology 9*, 374. https://doi.org/10.3389/fphys.2018.00374

Kocur, P., Tomczak, M., Wiernicka, M., Goliwąs, M., Lewandowski, J. and Łochyński, D. (2019) 'Relationship between age, BMI, head posture and superficial neck muscle stiffness and elasticity in adult women.' *Scientific Reports 9*, 1, 8515. https://doi.org/10.1038/s41598-019-44837-5

Purslow, P. P. (2010) 'Muscle fascia and force transmission.' *Journal of Bodywork and Movement Therapies 14*, 4, 411–417. https://doi.org/10.1016/j.jbmt.2010.01.005

Schleip, R. with Bayer, J. (2021) *Fascial Fitness: Practical Exercises to Stay Flexible, Active and Pain Free in Just 20 Minutes a Week.* Berkeley, CA: North Atlantic Books.

Wilke, J., Kalo, K., Niederer, D., Vogt, L. and Banzer, W. (2019) 'Gathering hints for myofascial force transmission under in vivo conditions: are remote exercise effects age dependent?' *Journal of Sport Rehabilitation 28*, 7, 758–763. https://doi.org/10.1123/jsr.2018-0184

Zullo, A., Fleckenstein, J., Schleip, R., Hoppe, K., Wearing, S. and Klingler, W. (2020) 'Structural and functional changes in the coupling of fascial tissue, skeletal muscle, and nerves during aging.' *Frontiers in Physiology 11*, 592. https://doi.org/10.3389/fphys.2020.00592

Chapter twelve

Integrative approach to exercise as we age
Sue Lembeck-Edens

Photography by Stacie Bird

Our bodies are designed to move. Children freely use their bodies to learn about themselves and the world around them. As we age, this freedom and curiosity often diminishes, and our movement repertoire narrows; "exercise" becomes limited to sports or the gym. The physical effects of repetitive actions and a more sedentary lifestyle can lead to patterns of imbalance, injury, and chronic pain. Healthy movement, on the other hand, encompasses much more. Comprehensive movement is not only about building strong bones and muscles, but also about improving brain function and memory, gaining kinesthetic awareness and self-expression.

Creating body ease, maintaining balance, and adapting to mental and physical changes are a central focus for the older student, which means specifically addressing the health and function of the myofascial system. As we age, our fascia often dries, stiffens, and becomes inflexible and proprioceptive communication slows. A different approach to exercise selection is necessary to maintain and increase strength, flexibility, balance, and endurance. Mindful and integrative exercises such as yoga and t'ai chi provide older students options.

These somatic traditions of yoga, t'ai chi, and qi gong are restorative because students practice slow, flowing, movements paired with conscious breath, strengthening the parasympathetic nervous system. Participants reduce the reactive fight/flight/freeze response of the sympathetic nervous system and welcome a more receptive, focused, and calm experience. These mindful qualities can bring the student into a flow state that enhances proprioception and hydration to myofascial tissue in a safe way.

Props, such as a chair, are used for safety, and to accommodate physical limitations such as a hip or knee replacement. Exercises are introduced sequentially, first establishing simple patterns to create a solid foundation on which complexity is later built.

Picture series descriptions (from Meditation Through the Seasons class by S. Lembeck-Edens)

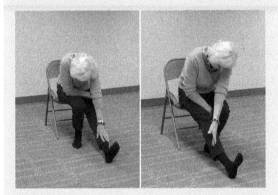

FIGURE 12.BREAKOUT.1 Seated forward fold and the added vector variation.

1. **Seated forward fold** (Figure 12.breakout.1)
   Beginning position: Sit toward the front edge of the chair with one leg straightened and heel well-connected to floor.

   a. Inhale: Raise the same arm as outstretched leg overhead.

   b. Exhale: Reach the extended arm up, out, and then downward toward the toes on the extended leg.

   c. Inhale/exhale: Remain in the forward fold for several breaths, allowing the back of the body to open and lengthen with each exhale.

   d. On an inhale: Return upright again reaching the arm out and up overhead.

   e. Release and repeat on the other side.

   Variation: stretch load with additional vector

   Beginning position: Sit toward the front edge of the chair with one leg straightened and heel well connected to floor.

a. Inhale: Raise the opposite arm as outstretched leg overhead.

b. Exhale: Reach the extended arm up, out, and then downward toward the pinky toe or outer shin on the extended leg.

c. Inhale/exhale: Remain in the forward fold with slight rotation for several breaths, allowing the back of the body to open and lengthen with each exhale.

d. On an inhale: Return upright again, reaching the arm out and up overhead.

e. Release and repeat on the other side.

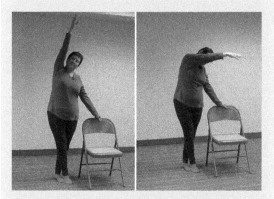

FIGURE 12.BREAKOUT.2 Standing thread the needle and variation.

2. **Standing thread the needle** (Figure 12.breakout.2)
   Beginning position: Stand to the side of the chair with the outer leg crossed over the leg closest to the chair. Plant/ground both feet on the floor and place hand to the back of the chair for stability.

a. Inhale: Raise the outer arm overhead while that same hip leans away from the chair in a full body side bend.

b. Exhale: Maintaining the lengthened spine and hips, gently curve the upper body forward, creating space between the shoulder blades.

c. Inhale: Open the chest, shoulder, and arm to starting position or into a slight upper back extension.

d. Exhale: Return to starting position.

e. Release and repeat on the other side.

Variation: thread the needle balance

Beginning position: Stand to the side of the chair with the inner leg bent and foot placed securely on the chair seat. Plant/ground the foot still on the floor and place hand to the back of the chair for stability.

a. Inhale: Raise the outer arm overhead allow the eyes to follow the arm if balance allows.

b. Exhale: Gently curve/round the upper body forward and "thread" the hand between/through the bent knee and chair. Allow the eyes to follow the hand if balance allows.

c. Inhale: Return to open the chest, shoulder, and arm to starting position or into a slight upper back extension.

d. Exhale: Return to starting position.

e. Release and repeat on the other side.

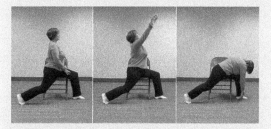

FIGURE 12.BREAKOUT.3 Seated Warrior sequence.

3. **Seated Warrior** (Figure 12.breakout.3)
   Beginning position: Sit toward the front of the chair, turn the body and legs to one side. Extend the "front" leg as far behind you as possible, stretching through the ball of the foot. Ground through the feet, add a squeeze in the buttocks and engage the core to sit tall. Place both hands on either side of the bent knee.

a. Inhale: Raise both straight arms up overhead. Allow the eyes to follow the hands.

b. Exhale: Continue reaching skyward, lengthening the spine, engaging the entire front fascia, keeping shoulders relaxed.

c. Inhale: Engage the upper back and chest to add a greater spinal extension or backward bend, opening the heart and front of the throat.

d. Exhale: Lengthen the arms and spine outward and then down toward the floor.

e. Inhale/exhale: Remain in the forward fold, lengthening through the back body.

f. Inhale: Press into the feet, engage the core and return to the body and arms overhead into the backward bend.

g. Exhale: Slowly release the backward bend and lower the arms to the starting position.

h. Release the legs and repeat on the other side.

References

Arnett, J. J. (2014) *Emerging Adulthood: The Winding Road from the late Teens through the Twenties.* Oxford: Oxford University Press.

Byock, I. (2013) *The Best Care Possible: A Physician's Quest to Transform Care through the End of Life.* New York, NY: Avery Publishing.

Eiling, E., Bryant, A. L., Petersen, W., Murphy, A. and Hohmann, E. (2007) 'Effects of menstrual-cycle hormone fluctuations on musculotendinous stiffness and knee joint laxity.' *Knee Surgery, Sports Traumatology, Arthroscopy 15*, 2, 126–132. https://doi.org/10.1007/s00167-006-0143-5

Fede, C., Pirri, C., Fan, C., Albertin, G. *et al.* (2019) 'Sensitivity of the fasciae to sex hormone levels: modulation of collagen-I, collagen-III and fibrillin production.' *PLOS ONE 14*, 9, e0223195. https://doi.org/10.1371/journal.pone.0223195

Hansen, M., Miller, B. F., Holm, L., Doessing, S. *et al.* (2009) 'Effect of administration of oral contraceptives in vivo on collagen synthesis in tendon and muscle connective tissue in young women.' *Journal of Applied Physiology 106*, 4, 1435–1443. https://doi.org/10.1152/japplphysiol.90933.2008

Huber, M., Knottnerus, J. A., Green, L., Horst, H. v. d. *et al.* (2011) 'How should we define health?' *BMJ 343*, 2, d4163–d4163. https://doi.org/10.1136/bmj.d4163

Louv, R. (2008) *Last Child in The Woods: Saving our Children from Nature-deficit Disorder.* Chapel Hill, NC: Algonquin Books.

Olsen, A. (2014) *The Place of Dance: A Somatic Guide to Dancing and Dance Making.* Middletown, CT: Wesleyan University Press.

Pavan, P., Monti, E., Bondí, M., Fan, C. *et al.* (2020) 'Alterations of extracellular matrix mechanical properties contribute to age-related functional impairment of human skeletal muscles.' *International Journal of Molecular Sciences 21*, 11, 3992. https://doi.org/10.3390/ijms21113992

Schleip, R. (2015) *Fascia in Sport and Movement.* Edinburgh: Handspring Publishing.

Schleip, R. and Wilke, J. (2021). *Fascia in Sport and Movement.* 2nd ed. Edinburgh: Handspring Publishing.

Tharp, T. (2019) *Keep It Moving: Lessons for the Rest of your Life.* New York, NY: Simon and Schuster.

The Lancet (2018) 'Stemming the global caesarean section epidemic.' *The Lancet 392*, 10155, 1279. https://doi.org/10.1016/S0140-6736(18)32394-8

Trindade, V. L. A., Martins, P. A. L. S., Santos, S., Parente, M. P. L. *et al.* (2012) 'Experimental study of the influence of senescence in the biomechanical properties of the temporal tendon and deep temporal fascia based on uniaxial tension tests.' *Journal of Biomechanics 45*, 1, 199–201. https://doi.org/10.1016/j.jbiomech.2011.09.018

Further reading

Hargrove, T. (2019) *Playing with Movement: How to Explore the Many Dimensions of Physical Health and Performance.* Seattle, WA: Better Movement.

Jessen, K. R. (2004) 'Glial cells.' *The International Journal of Biochemistry & Cell Biology 36*, 10, 1861–1867. https://doi.org/10.1016/j.biocel.2004.02.023

We react, consciously or unconsciously to places we live and work, in ways we scarcely notice or that are only now becoming known to us... In short, the places where we spend our time affect the people we are and can become.

Tony Hiss, *The Experience of Place* (1991)

Part of the reason I enjoy travel so much is that I get to put myself into new spaces, both in terms of natural environment and architecture. These spaces may be somewhat challenging in their unfamiliarity, or stimulating and thrilling in a different way of experiencing color, texture, and space. Have you ever noticed how after a trip, you return home suddenly aware of the height of your cabinets, or the placement of your light switches? Simple changes in environment may make us reach our arm at a different height or grip a door handle differently. We may wonder what makes a space feel comfortable and peaceful or chaotic.

Having grown up initially in the very flat Midwest of the United States, I noticed my ears popping constantly when my family moved to the up and down hills of New England. I felt like I had landed on Mars the first time I hiked in New Mexico and I gasped at the intensity of the colors of blue sea and sky in Costa Rica and washes of red in Sedona, Arizona. I have made myself shrink in dangerous urban areas and expanded in quiet pathways.

Anatomy itself is not a static two-dimensional construct; it lives in the three-dimensional body, which exists in the larger world. In brief, environment shapes us in numerous ways and what we create in terms of designed environmental space shapes us. This can be from the ways houses are designed or occupied to the paths we walk on. This can challenge the entire fascial system in positive or negative terms.

The etymology of "environment" can be traced back to the Middle French preposition *environ* "around." "Environment," in its most basic meaning, is "that which surrounds." … In a less physical,

more extended sense, it may signify the circumstances and conditions that make up everyday life ("He grew up in a loving *environment*.") The word may also be applied in highly specialized ways, denoting, for example, "the position of a linguistic element." (Merriam-Webster n.d.)

From these definitions we can begin to form an understanding that "environment" has a shape (i.e. the spatial relationship surrounding us) to the more esoteric relationship psychologically or spatially between concepts and ideas. On a micro level we have seen how interstitial space helps shape the relationship between fibers and ground substance. The ECM (Extra Cellular Matrix) is, after all, about the scaffolding shape of fascia without its cells. On a larger scale, how we interact with our environment affects our bodies deeply.

Environmental understanding has begun to be studied more intensely, from the effects of taking a walk in nature (forest bathing) to the stress of how our office space or computer video streams

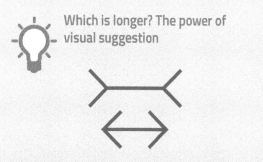

Which is longer? The power of visual suggestion

FIGURE 13.1 Perception is tested through what is known as the Muller-Lyer illusion in which two lines appear to be different lengths due to the addition of the arrows. Once we recognize the illusion, we can understand it the next time we encounter it. Understanding how we perceive both our connections internally and externally helps us apply our learning quicker the next time it is met.

can affect our body alignment and wellbeing. In terms of our fascial anatomy, the positioning of our bodies is highly tied to the concept of proprioception and our sensation of the emotional being tied to the concept of interoception.

As noted by Johnson (2008):

acknowledging that every aspect of human being is grounded in specific forms of bodily engagement with an environment requires a far-reaching rethinking of who and what we are... Change your brain, your body, or your environment in non-trivial ways, and you will change how you experience your world, what things are meaningful to you, and even who you are. (p.2)

The map is not the territory

You may have heard, "the map is not the territory." This phrase came from Alfred Korzybski (1879–1950), a philosopher and thinker who created the field of semantics. Central to his ideas is the thought that we are limited by what our body system can perceive. In other words, we don't truly see the entire picture of the world around us, or what is truly reality. Take a look at Figure 13.2, of the clouds and landscape. If I look up a map of this particular region, I can find land elevation and measurements and yet that model is not the reality I experience as I walk along this trail, or even in taking this picture, or the description of it as "Clouds in New York's Hudson Valley."

Fascia as a sensory organ: proprioception, interoception, and more

We can consider fascia a communicating network of information for the body and its relationship with the world internally and externally. The fascial mechanoreceptors are all about detecting stimuli that come from internal and external environments and are a family of nerves (Ruffini, Pacini, Golgi tendon organ/Golgi receptors, interstitial as well as muscle spindles). They all have different roles in order to respond to types of movement and load. *Ruffini* receptors respond well to shearing of tissue, which is done in manual work through relaxing the tissue. In movement, this is achieved less easily but is possible through

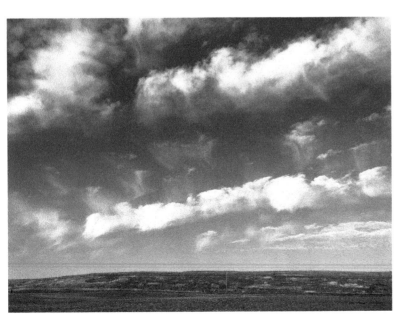

FIGURE 13.2 Clouds in New York's Hudson Valley.

Photo courtesy of the author.

slow, sustained stretch and sometimes with myofascial tools. The dura mater also is home to these receptors. These receptors are sensitive to and help control finger movement and position and are involved in grasping actions. They appear to increase the parasympathetic response and downregulate the sympathetic nervous system. *Pacini* receptors are stimulated by pressure and vibrational changes as well as temperature. They may also play a part in perceiving texture of smooth versus rough surfaces and helping to adjust the body's response. Curiously, sound, particularly in the low-frequency ranges, affects these receptors. A Balkan brass band with the accompaniment of a deep drum might be affecting folk dancers who are simultaneously rapidly changing pressure in the stomping and stepping style of these dances.

Also known as the GTO, neurotendinous organ, or neurotendinous spindle, *the Golgi tendon organ* is involved in sensing changes in muscle tension and is found at the musculotendinous junctions. They are located in the deep fascia but also in areas like the retinacula of the ankle where they are thickenings of the deep fascia formed from two to three layers of parallel collagen fiber bundles. Here is the important part: "the retinacula are not static structures for joint stabilisation, like the ligaments, but a specialisation of the fascia for local spatial proprioception of the movements of foot and ankle" (Stecco *et al.* 2010). *The interstitial receptors*, also known as free nerve endings, give temperature, stress, and tension feedback throughout the body, even to the level of the periosteum, the fascial covering of bone. They are considered the most abundant of the mechanoreceptors and are particularly important in the gliding areas between the superficial and deep fascia. If we consider both their abundance and relationship to the autonomic nervous system, their importance comes into play in both increasing proprioceptive awareness with training as well as modulating an overactive autonomic nervous system. Finally, muscle spindles are wrapped in fascia and located in the belly of muscles and respond to contraction and lengthening.

Proprioception

All of these mechanoreceptors (sometimes also called sensory nerves) help to give us our feedback for understanding where we are in space and how we should respond to that information. Proprioception appears to come from feelings in the tensioning and shearing of the superficial fascial layers. Pattern and form, as we have seen, overlap in the world of science, structure of anatomy, and design in architectural space. Both are very intertwined into perception, proprioception, interoception, and also exteroception. As a reminder, proprioception has been called the sixth sense (the other five being hearing vision, taste, smell, and touch) and describes how we know where we are in space. The Latin word, *proprius*, means self. According to Freeman and Wyke (1966), the three keys to proprioceptive input and also for posture are the soles of the feet, the sacroiliac joint, and the cervical spine.

In movement, we can think of proprioceptive awareness for practical and performance level sense. Joint proprioception comes from the connective tissue giving a proprioceptive awareness. Joints need to have sensing ability in the micromovement. Whether standing on a paddleboard or standing on one's hands, small proprioceptive readjustment helps to maintain balance. If you are about to sprain your ankle, having proprioception will allow you to sense your joint position and this is important in getting dynamic movement. With age, we sometimes lose the ability of recreating spatial relationships and the proprioceptive ability to organize the body can diminish.

Information on processing movement goes through several steps and responses from the posterior insula to the anterior insula. The brain first unconsciously processes what is going on in the body through a primary interoceptive representation. Then motor functions are triggered in the hypothalamus and amygdala. All of this coordinates with the muscles; nervous system and particularly the fascia, which is wealthy in terms of its mechanoreceptors and responds to and needs stimulation.

The web of fascia in the body can be thought of as a medium through which force is distributed. The shear vibrations and tension in the most superficial fascial sheets appear to be the source of a lot of our proprioceptive feedback. By training the body three-dimensionally, we are helping the health of the whole net as well as helping the communication for proprioceptibility. So, what is the takeaway? We need a movement to help the body learn how to understand its relationship in the environment around us. Movement that emphasizes multidirectionality in particular will help train and enhance proprioceptive abilities in the body.

The small nerve proprioceptors are prevalent in the soles of the feet and the palms of the hands and in fascia throughout the body, which helps with that orientation in space. If the fascia as an overall net is blended throughout the body, it will be affected by muscle tension as well. In tensioning the body, we may be creating more microstability in the fascia as well as in the joint positioning. Wobble boards, BOSUs and other fitness equipment are specifically training the proprioception of the body. Kinesthesia is body awareness in navigating the moving body. Specifically, the proprioceptors create awareness of the positioning of body.

Interoception

While we look to proprioception as being how we orient in space, interoception is felt sensation in our viscera or the sense of the internal environment of the body. Emotions can arise from the perception of felt changes in the body and is particularly important in felt sense of anxiety and more. Our sense of homeostasis is important and may be our felt sense of temperature or a racing heartbeat. If we connect a felt sensation with past

trauma or discomfort, an emotional response may be equated to a feeling.

What do we mean when we say we have a "gut" reaction? We learn through the eyes, through the ears but rely on gut instincts to respond to many emotional situations. In terms of our fascia, the Golgi tendon and stretch receptors in the gut are part of the awareness of self that gives us warning of a dangerous situation, as well as awareness.

Interoception is more about the "felt" body, or the emotional side of fascia, as well as the subjective feelings of our body. As previously noted, it is clear that motion and emotion are linked in fields from dance/movement therapy to sports psychology. Interoception is what is thought to be at the core of our need for socially appropriate touch and light massage techniques. Interoception is the awareness of the body's own felt internal signals. Interstitial receptors help to construct the feelings of hunger, pain, cold and hot, and more.

In terms of the general population, motion and emotion are also closely connected. The environment has clear connections to this as well.

We can view interoception as a way to correlate connections between fascia, specifically receptors and sensation. In the past several years, the research in interoception has been rapidly growing, particularly in terms of contemplative movement practices (Farb *et al.* 2015), body psychotherapy, emotional processing, and more.

Our new understanding of these relationships between fascia (an organ of wholeness and connection) and our felt sensation of placement in the world and with each other comes at an interesting time of an increase in separation from the body and a great longing to come back to a positive sense of body self.

Neuroception

Neuroception is what helps orient to danger and cures of what may be unsafe. The term was coined by Stephen Porges (2009) as part of his polyvagal theory which gives a possible new perspective, although still scientifically unsubstantiated. As a general premise, the theory focuses on the neural regulation of the two vagal systems. For example, by noticing the danger sounds in nature, we orient to what might harm us, whereas observing a beautiful sunset for too long may lull us into a relaxation response that may actually put us into danger. However, in our modern lives we often misread and misinterpret danger and are unable to let the stress go. When the human body is startled, the brain's amygdala alerts the sympathetic system, but it may misread memories, or even give a response based on a reaction to a horror film, for example. If we cannot accurately read a situation and respond appropriately, the body can feel chronically stressed.

If you have ever had a migraine, you may have experienced nociceptive pain, which is linked with the trigeminal nerve. The nerve gets its name from its three (tri) branches, the ophthalmic division (going to the eye), the maxillary division (to the cheek), and the mandibular division. This is often called the great sensory nerve of the face because of all of the sensation. The trigeminal nerve also controls the dura mater, which is the connective tissue known as the "hard mother" surrounding the brain. The nociceptors (which are pain receptors) in the dura mater can be sensitized by pain. The stimulus may be coming from the dura mater, but the sensory neurons can be an area of converging neurons, so essentially it is a similar phenomenon of referred pain.

Exteroception

Exteroception is the perception of sensation outside of the body, and is commonly related to the five senses that we commonly learn about (sight, sound, smell, taste, and touch) and how the outside stimuli come back into the inner body.

Fine-tuning the proprioceptive body can mean the difference between playing an instrument with finesse, judging how much force is needed to throw a ball, or pick up a glass of juice. Most of us perform thousands of proprioceptive movements throughout the day without a second thought. The sense of kinesthetic, or movement body, is tied in with our nervous system and also into our sense of space and our perception of time.

What you can see, hear, and feel at any given moment, the movements you made to get there, and your memory of those movements and knowledge of local geography all contribute to your sense of your position in the world. Your brain's different sensory and motor systems all work in concert to produce this sense. Not only does your memory and knowledge help you know where you are, but where you are triggers memories and knowledge. So when you have forgotten what's on your grocery list, going back to the kitchen will help you remember what you were planning to cook. (Groh 2014, p.4)

Repatterning movement may be part of training the proprioceptive body in space. Yoga teachers in the vinyasa style will have students move in a sequenced pattern. Perhaps the return to a familiar asana within a new sequence helps the body increase proprioception. Familiar sports drills might also benefit from a return to a known movement exercise before challenging a new combination.

Modes of perception
Dr. Neil Theise

It is through one's senses that one creates the world. And since everyone's sensorium is probably a little different, our worlds differ; in part, this is the mechanism whereby human diversity flowers creatively. Some sensorial differences are what we are born with. Typical deviations from norms, such as color-blindness, make clear that such variability exists. But early in life, we begin taking note that someone might hear things we can't or that we can see details that pass others by, revealing a natural variation.

And then there are occasional astonishing leaps beyond the norm. For example, my friend and collaborator Maureen Seaberg, writer and tetrachromat, "the girl with kaleidoscope eyes" (Seaberg 2014), has four cone classes in her retina for perceiving color rather than the normal three. The result is that while most humans can distinguish 1 million colors, she can distinguish up to 100 million! So, the range of different inborn sensory capacities between humans is vaster than many of us may realize.

Things get even more wondrous when you consider synesthetes, people with synesthesias: interconnections between different senses, such as experiencing colors when hearing music, or tasting flavors when regarding different shapes. Maureen is also a synesthete with multiple synesthesias, which even before she became aware of her tetrachromacy, led her to write the book *Tasting the Universe* (Seaberg 2011) and to publish her "Sensorium" blog on PsychologyToday. com. So, in fact, the worlds people experience are often as different, in subtle or extreme ways, from each other as those between humans and animals.

But the senses we are born with are not necessarily the ones we are stuck with. Of course, one can lose sensory abilities; one can become blind or deaf through acquired illness or injury or through changes of aging. But one's senses can also sharpen, become more sensitive, in response to our behaviors. If you think about it, you can probably recognize some way in which this is true for you. Through practicing the piano, your ability to discern fine differences in music or be aware of fine sensations of touch and movement in your fingers grows. Playing baseball, the ability to see the details of the pitched ball approaching you increases, the ball seeming to slow down, its motion becoming vivid to your eye. Becoming a practiced cook, one's senses of smell and taste sharpen, becoming more subtle.

It is my guess that those senses that are most refined as inborn characteristics probably condition, to some extent, what activities interest you. But then, once you begin to practice such an activity, further refinements can happen.

I think of a remarkable moment with a massage therapist I once saw on a regular basis. He had amazing intuitions about where the issues in my body were and how to use the most subtle engagements—fingers to flesh—to coax me into suppleness and flexibility and freedom from pain. One day I was on the table, and he was working on me. I was in the usual blissed out, dream like state when he chuckled a little. He sometimes did that when he found a peculiar knot in my back, but this time there was no knot. I asked him what was so funny? He said, "The lights just came back on." The power had gone out for about 10 minutes! Face down, eyes closed I hadn't noticed. And he just kept on working as though nothing had happened, but when they came on again, he chuckled. I said to him afterwards: "It's like your fingers are eyes." He nodded, agreeing, indeed they were. He didn't need sight to know how to touch and manipulate and heal me. His fingers could do it all on their own. Were they extra-sensitive from the beginning and that helped him discover the pleasure of being a body worker? Quite possibly. But were those senses refined by his long practice? I'm sure. And those skills helped make him a healer—or at least find the best way to exhibit his capacity for healing.

Proof of this comes from first person reports. I personally know that when I started as a pathology trainee, there were cell types I could not see under the microscope at low power. I had to go from 2x magnification to 100x magnification to identify them confidently. Six months into my training, I was tutoring a medical student and realized I could now see them at 2x. My practice had changed my sensory abilities.

Dr. William "Bill" Bushell, another friend, colleague, and collaborator of Maureen and mine, is an MIT biophysical anthropologist who documents astounding sensory abilities in adept practitioners of diverse cultural traditions such as Tibetan Buddhism. Adept meditation practitioners, for example, claim they can train themselves to see the tiniest sensory inputs (e.g. single sparks of light in a dark room from 30 feet away). While this seems unlikely for ordinary human abilities, it turns out, as Bill has noted, that it is possible indeed, for laboratory-based investigations prove that the human retina can detect a single photon of light. As he recently wrote with Maureen:

> A profound movement is underway in physics and related disciplines, one which has been accelerating. The public has not heard much about it, nor has the wider physics community. It is a groundswell of research focused on the discovery of the human potential for directly perceiving key aspects of what can genuinely be referred to as the "fabric of the universe." What is astonishing about this news is that science is moving toward a day when human direct, sensory perception of the quantum may answer lingering questions about physics. (Bushell and Seaberg 2018)

And:

> human beings have the proven potential to see light on the level of the single photon, essentially the most irreducible unit of light that exists; hear at the level of vibrations with amplitudes on the atomic scale, and discriminate auditory time intervals within the range of millionths of a second; *experience acute tactile discrimination on the nanoscale—i.e. billionths of a meter...* [Emphasis added] (Bushell and Seaberg 2019)

In fact, he has gathered vast documentary evidence regarding how non-technological human practices, such as meditation, can achieve profound changes in sensory perception, even including spontaneous development of synesthetic capabilities.

Maureen speaks of having synesthesia-dar—that she has a gift for recognizing a synesthete even before she's told it. Much of her blog consists of interviews with people she has read about or met who she "guesses" are synesthetes and they admit yes. She has written one such piece about me (Seaberg 2012). Bill introduced me to Maureen originally, and after spending time together she told me she thought I was a synesthete. I demurred. No flashy mixes of colors and sounds and tastes and shapes and numbers and letters for me! Just regular, ordinary, slightly sharper vision of the trained pathologist and long-term Zen Buddhist meditator, but that was all! But she poked and probed until she asked me about what time "looks like." I said it was a little hard to describe, but then made my best try—it's kind of like wheels in space around me. She exulted in her success: I am a spatial sequence synesthete! For me time has not only location, but movement. I was shocked. I thought everyone experienced time the way I did. Apparently not... Maureen wrote this about me:

> He is known as a creative researcher and wonders if his synesthesia plays a role. "The ease with which I can conjure images and this sense of being in an alternate space in my imagination is part of my creativity." He became interested in physics as a 12-year-old boy and was captured by Einstein's method of conducting "thought experiments." He realized later the ways he works things out in research now are very similar to that construct. [...] the space in which I was traveling [in thought experiments] was the same kind of space as the space in which I experience time: open, unbounded, freely rotated. (Seaberg 2012)

I experience time and all my sensations in an internal spaciousness that while I can't point to it, I know is all around me. The questions and curiosities that arise from my clinical and scientific practices I work out in that "imaginal space." After Maureen and Bill brought me into awareness of this habit, this capacity, I discover that it's not something I share with a lot of people and deeply appreciate that it is a kind of grace that I have it.

Of course, that leads me to ask you, the reader: What are your special sensitivities and gifts, however subtle? How did they lead you into the practices that define your life? And how do you use them to affect the world around you for the better?

References

Seaberg, M. (2014) 'Girl with kaleidoscope eyes.' *Vogue*, December 2014.

Seaberg, M. (2011) *Tasting the Universe*. Pompton Plains, NJ: New Page Books.

Bushell, W. C. and Seaberg, M. (2018) 'Experiments suggest humans can directly observe the quantum.' *Psychology Today* December 5, 2018.

Bushell, W. C. and Seaberg, M. (2019) 'Experiments suggest humans can directly observe the quantum, Part II: It would be useful to add adept perceivers to the studies.' *Psychology Today*, May 31, 2019.

Seaberg, M. (2012) 'Dr. Neil Theise's magnificent time wheels.' *Psychology Today*, February 14, 2012.

The world is all gates, all opportunities, strings of tension waiting to be struck...

Ralph Waldo Emerson

Fascia as rebar

I studied architecture with great interest as part of my art history training, many years ago. Structure, even of a built kind, is not all static. Buildings prone to areas with earthquakes and hurricanes are built with rebar as a means to distribute weight and strain. Let's explore this design principle and create a connection to see how our fascia network is a type of vibrant, adaptable rebar.

Rebar is a contraction of reinforcing bar, usually made of steel or a gathered mesh of steel wires. In other words, it is a type of fascia in the non-anatomical sense of the word. It is used with modern buildings, in particular, as concrete is strong in terms of compression, but not in tensile force. By adding rebar into a structure, it is able to distribute stress and strain more readily, similar to the concept of biotensegrity via the myofascial system.

Fascia, the "wood wide web" and mutualism

In 1997, scientist Suzanne Simard was featured on the cover of *Nature* for her work with the symbiotic relationship between fungal filaments, or hyphae, and tree roots. The scope of the relationship is vast, both in terms of physical size and its critical importance to both species. This is a fantastically complex connective system. This supportive network was labelled the "wood wide web" and the work continues to explore the relationship between tree species as well as their exchange of carbon dioxide. As noted by MacFarlane (2018):

> If there is human meaning to be made of the wood wide web, it is surely that what might save us as we move forwards into the precarious, unsettled centuries ahead is collaboration: mutualism, symbiosis, the inclusive human work of collective decision-making extended to more-than-human communities. *You look at the network, and then it starts to look back at you...* (p.113)

This woven network of interconnection and collaboration has lots of similarities to our fascial network just under the surface of our bodies. Simard (2021) herself made the connection between the mycorrhizal network, or the symbiotic relationship between plant and fungus and the neural network (p.229).

What has intrigued me further is that the "wood wide web" has a relationship with tree roots to fungus that are important to consider that is similar to the fern-like colloids in fascia. As noted in Simard (2021), trees and fungus have the relationship, "out of the fungus flowed a whole underground apparatus—truffles, cords, and strands that in turn grew fans of ultrafine hyphae that infiltrated the soil pores. These pores were where water was held so tightly that it would take a million of the microscopic threads to suck up enough to make a drop. The fans could be soaking up the water from the soil pores, then funneling it to the strands that formed the cord, which then passed it to the attached for root" (p.58–59). In essence, the fungus brings the water and nutrients to the tree and the tree helps give sugars to the fungus via photosynthesis.

There is another piece to this equation in our perception of knowledge being tied into the perception of what we experience and can see. As someone who spends a lot of time outdoors, I'm amazed at how little experience many people have with nature. According to the Mayo Clinic's Well Living Lab, the average American spends 90% or more of their day indoors. The indoor environment may have little relationship to the outdoor environment and indeed, many people, whether in the gym or in an office space, will work or work out without a large awareness of their surroundings. In this new era of lower contact with the physical world, we may well be losing our sensitivity for varied tactile surfaces due to lack of stimulation.

We also are increasingly living in a two-dimensional world. The latest generation of children is having difficulty with spatial relationships. Dr. Dimitri Christakis, the lead author of the American Academy of Pediatrics' latest screen-time study (Council on Communications and Media 2016) has been sounding the alarm for a while that play is needed, and less time with media. The COVID pandemic has resulted in increased screen time, and there is a high increase in stress and anxiety, particularly in children and young adults. The position of typing at a computer screen (as well as driving a car, or texting on a cell phone) tends to shorten the immediate front of the body and pull the sternocleidomastoids forward, collapsing the chest—the same response we have to trauma. It might be not such a far leap to wonder if our technology is enhancing a position that our bodies anatomically associate with stress.

Challenging the body in balance

Let's play with challenging our bodies in space (Figure 13.3 and the sequence of Figure 13.4). From our previous chapters, we know the anatomy of the sides of the body is both designed for stabilization and also involved in side-bending. Let's up the ante by challenging both at the same time but slightly changing the environment. Start with one foot on a yoga block (try with different textures from foam to cork) and stand as if your other foot was on a second, invisible block. Bring your arms up above and then lean over to one side, and then the other. Drop one arm down by your side, and then the other, all while maintaining your balance.

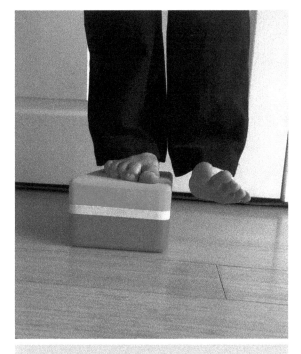

FIGURE 13.3 Balance on a yoga block.

Photo courtesy of the author.

Balancing on a block (Figure 13.3) challenges the myofascial connections in multiple ways and also creates a different surface for foot sensation. In this series, play with leaning side to side while hovering one foot in space. Our relationship with the space and gravity itself will be affected by the objects we chose to interact with for this exercise through soft or hard surfaces. Up the ante again by closing your eyes. Almost immediately, we start to lose our balance without a horizon-line to focus on.

Our suboccipitals (SBL) are tied neurologically to our vision, and when we close our eyes, the balance again is challenged unless we fine-tune our body's sense of finding place. Whether I am working with athletes or weekend warriors, I like to challenge the body by introducing changes in the environment, including textures and spatial use. Nature often provides this for free. Kayakers often notice a change in balance when paddling in twilight or near dark, and learn to adjust to the loss of visual cues.

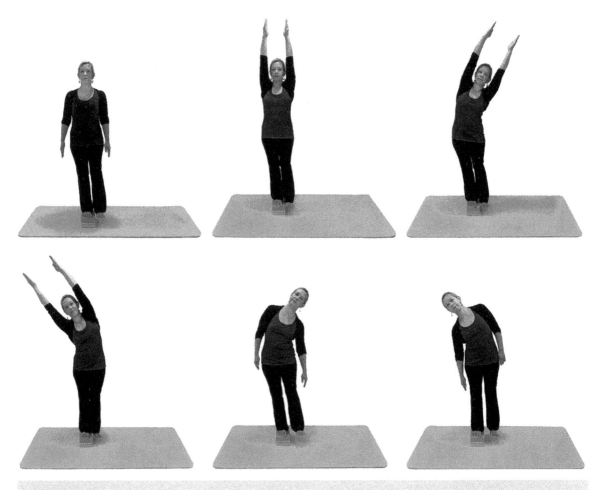

FIGURE 13.4 Balance sequence on a yoga block challenges the body to stabilize in a different relationship to gravity.
Photos courtesy of the author.

Our environmental space and how we play with it matters in maintaining a healthy body and mind. In the 1980s, Harvard psychologist Ellen Langer created what is known as the "counterclockwise" study, later repeated by Pagnini *et al.* (2019). Her basic concept centered around bringing a group of men in their seventies into a time-warped recreated environment that brought them back to an era of when they were in their twenties. Not only were the decorations of the era, but the expectations were that they were vital and capable of doing the same activities they did at that time. Within a week, the group had noted gains in strength, posture, perception, and memory.

Use it or lose it
Robert Schleip

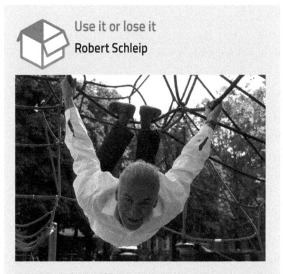

FIGURE 13.BREAKOUT.1 Dr. Robert Schleip has researched fascia both as a scientist and mover and encourages playful movement for our health.

Photo courtesy of Robert Schleip.

One of my personal heroes is the late medical radiological researcher Colin James Alexander from New Zealand. He observed that chimpanzees are usually immunized from joint degenerations like osteoarthrosis or rheumatoid osteoarthritis in old age, contrary to us humans. However, if they are captives in a not species appropriate environment—i.e. in a forbidden cage environment in which they can't use their body in a normal monkey-like manner like swinging, climbing, and chasing each other—then they are prone to exactly the same joint pathologies that are considered normal in human aging. Dr. Alexander's genius question: Could it be that these frequent pathologies in us humans are less due to "wear and tear," but to insufficient loading of our joints over their genetically available range of motion?

He called this the "unused arc hypothesis" and investigated this novel explanation by detailed video recording and analysis of the loading-range of different joints of chimpanzees in their natural jungle environment and comparing that with our human behavior in our current typical sedentary lifestyle. While this extensive study took several years, the final result was very clear and provocative: we humans are prone to joint degeneration at exactly those joints which we tend to load only over a small portion of their full available range of motion in contrast to our monkey siblings who tend to load them over their full range of motion. Best examples are our hip joints or shoulder joints, which we typically load only within a small fraction of their available range of motion. In contrast, those joints, like the elbow joint, that we still tend to use over their full range of motion, we then tend to stay "monkey-like" healthy even in old age.

Modern networks

Similar to the networks of our fascial system, we can expand the metaphor of communication networks to a large-scale level with the rise of the Internet and social networking sites, re-enforcing the concept that we are dealing with three-dimensionality. Think of the languaging of the modern network, which includes switches, routers, bridges, and firewalls. These devices are all interconnected, each processing and passing along information, connected to the other components along numerous, multi-connected paths.

The three-dimensionality of our world and our bodily structures is too often overlooked in rehab and training protocols—our gym, studio floors, homes, and office work environments are all flat and hard, yet the activities people enjoy like hiking, skiing, walking on the beach, and outdoor running is all done on variable terrain (shape, texture, density, temperature).

David Jacobs, trainer

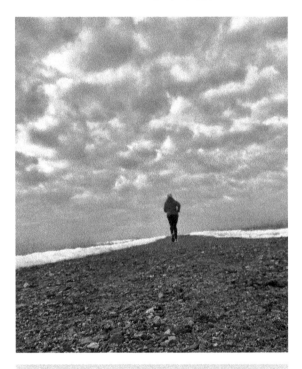

FIGURE 13.5 Trail running. Daily walks and runs can challenge the myofascial form through surface and environmental variations day-to-day (such as running against the wind). An older female runner like me experiences a reduction of resiliency and fat padding in the foot due to lower levels of estrogen. However, stimulation from the environment can help keep mechanoreceptors responsive to positional feedback and help keep balance and proprioceptive control. Coordination is a neuroplastic skill that improves with training at any age and skill level.

Photo by the author.

Additional (foot)notes

I have had my share of trying out different shoes and surfaces, from the rocker surface shoes (somehow meant to invoke the African bare-footed person) to the minimalist fingered sleeve for every toe (in both the sock and shoe version). In the end, I personally realize that while I work mostly barefoot teaching yoga and movement, my time walking or running is mixed between supportive to minimalist footwear, depending on my own judgment. Reality of time also impacts the foot functionality, especially in terms of the fat pad cushioning the calcaneus.

There are numerous benefits to walking on varied and different surfaces (Figure 13.5). Constantly changing terrain requires the ankle joints and their soft tissues to adapt, causing the ankle tendons to glide below the retinaculae, a thickened portion of the fascia profundis which acts as a sleeve to contain and guide the muslces and tendons as they pass around the adapting joints. These fascial thickenings not only help hold the tissues in place but they are also densely innervated to assist with proprioception. Training multidirectionally in these areas makes sense so when the unexpected slip on a driveway happens, the ankle is responsive because it has been trained to be so. Circling wrists and ankles, either as part of a warm-up or coming out of a yoga *savasana* (final relaxation) may also be helping to awaken these proprioceptive areas, and at minimum, likely helping with the glide in this area.

I have been interested in how we as people are shaped by environmental space, and in turn, how we shape our environment around us. Where we live geographically (hilly terrain or urban jungle), office or outdoors impacts our anatomy. I have also found that cultures have preferences toward spatial use that is reflected in both their movement expression and architecture.

One example is the flying buttresses of a Gothic cathedral that echoes the movement aesthetic of a ballerina en pointe (Figure 13.6a,b). To add to this, Kemp (2016) notes:

A construction can both follow certain necessary principles if it is to stand up and also be a particular expression of social forces. A Gothic flying buttress and a twenty-first-century bridge by Cecil Balmond are very much of their period, but they share underlying mathematical rationales in how they handle the resolution of forces of tension and compression that endow the structures with stability. (p.3)

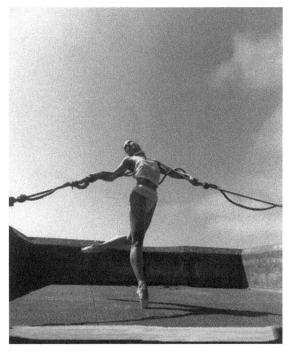

FIGURE 13.6b Dancer. The aesthetic of the ballet dance mimics the architecture of the gothic cathedrals with an emphasis on height and lift.

Photo courtesy of Marilyn Miller.

Larger implications of environmental space on the body

Where we move and where we train has further implications on how we train our body. The modern world lacks natural stressors on the body system. The implications for our myofascial body are important.

Humans have created and shaped environmental space since the beginning of civilization. Humans are reshaping internal anatomy as well as the external environment. Within the field of cognitive science, Andy Clark and David J. Chalmers wrote about the concept of "extended cognition" in their article, "The Extended Mind" (1998) in which they question:

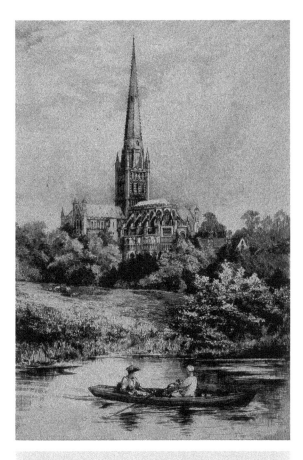

FIGURE 13.6a Norwich Cathedral, Norwich, Norfolk: from the river. Etching by E. Slocombe.

Credit: Wellcome Collection. Public Domain Mark.

Chapter thirteen

Where does the mind stop and the rest of the world begin? The question invites two standard replies. Some accept the boundaries of skin and skull and say that what is outside the body is outside the mind. Others are impressed by arguments suggesting that the meaning of our words "just ain't in the head" and hold that this externalism about meaning carries over into an externalism about mind. We propose to pursue a third position. We advocate a very different sort of externalism an active externalism, based on the active role of the environment in driving cognitive processes. (p. 7)

Get grounded

Find an area of natural surface (be mindful if you live somewhere that has danger of broken glass or other health risks). Remove socks and shoes and take time to feel the sensations to your feet. Feel free to add in hands and other parts! Is the ground hard, yielding? Are there different textures and sensations that you are experiencing? How do you move differently against a natural surface? Set a time for yourself just to be present in this environment. A few minutes, maybe five or ten, and see if you can check in on your body sensations.

Art, architecture, and spatial relationship

The concept of "space" is one that is shared by many fields but with different definitions and connotations between them. In psychology, the concept of personal space is critical in establishing cultural and psychological norms of acceptability. In terms of architecture, the choice of where to place a structure and where to leave open space is critical and likewise reflects (whether well or poorly designed) on the culture it serves. In anatomy, the body system itself is constantly changing shape. Spatial use becomes important for how humans move, live, and express themselves in the world. For example, the Latin phrase *solvitur ambulando* translates

roughly as "it is solved by walking." Believed to have been first uttered by Diogenes of Sinope (Carrette 2013), it was his response to an argument that motion is unreal, upon which he got up and walked away, proving his belief system through nonverbal action. Where we have space to move is both a physical and psychological question.

Architecture can be a manifestation of a cultural identity, as well as forming individual reaction to the space around. As the writer Tony Hiss (1991) notes:

we don't just adapt to places, or modify them in order to ease our burdens. We're the only species that over and over again has deliberately transformed our surroundings in order to stretch our capacity for understanding and provoke new accomplishments. And our growing and enhanced understanding is our most valuable, and our most vulnerable, inheritance. (p. xvi)

By recognizing the importance of how public and health spaces are created, societies can enhance the mental health of the overall group. Anatomical needs shape an environment and, in turn, reshape the human body. The connection between environment and the creation of movement is an important one. In this case, the environment serves as the relative constant, where the dance is created as the fleeting form. Of course, as environment or architecture changes, the dance will reflect the landscape it comes from; if we think of traditional dance, its form has a critical connection to the environment and space. European folk dance, for example, is full of stamping and shuffling movements, developed from agricultural farm work, whereas high-stepping dances reflect the landscape of mountainous regions where the need to climb rocky terrain placed a value on these movements (Lomax 1978). Although folk dance forms are regionally fading, there is an increase of urban styles of dance in the United States, such as krumping, seen in the movie *RIZE* (LaChapelle 2005).

These styles are clearly influenced by the urban environment in which they developed. Movement efforts are strong, quick, and free, while the actual "performance" of krumping is limited to a small, confined space.

In 2016, I presented a poster on some of my work about spatial relationship, environment, and anatomy at a regional meeting for the American Association for Anatomy. Besides presenting on a passionate topic, what I enjoyed the most was that it was held at the Roy and Diana Vagelos Education Center, part of Columbia University's Medical College in the Washington Heights neighborhood. Designed by Diller Scofidio + Renfo, the building has huge windows to open up to views of the neighborhood and the Hudson River. It also has a variety of stairs, sloping ramps and classrooms or "academic neighborhoods" that can be reconfigured as needed. The architects clearly understand that space matters for learning and moving through an environment.

This concept has been echoed by progressive architects who understand that "…human beings fashion an environment for themselves, a space to live in, suggested by their patterns of life and constructed around whatever symbols of reality seem important to them" (Scully 1991, p.1). Architecture can be thought of as part of the larger cultural ego can in turn affect individual psyche. It becomes important not only for the individual to find a place that resonates with personal wellbeing, but there is also a larger responsibility for public places to be designed well to ease psychological stress and frustration. For those in our mental health communities, it becomes even more critical that the community supports and nurtures the construction of places that can support us.

The concept of community takes on a shape and threads of attachment as a network of its own.

Feelings of community are based on the sharing and commonality of space, attitude, and behavior. Community spirit, or sense of community, is a form of place attachment that begins when people share with others a physical space or environment (e.g. a neighborhood or workplace). (Kopec 2012, p.297)

What traditionally might have been the central square, serving as an intersection of communal space and utilized for dancing and music, is now replaced with meaningful places that provide a sense of identity, whether the local coffee shop, or the regrowth of a community farmer's market.

The idea of place depends on how individuals conceptualize the world around them. In the field of environmental psychology, the word *place* encompasses more specific notions: place identity, sense of place, and place attachment. Each of these terms attempts to describe a host of emotions that define the meaning of place, which is, essentially, how we see ourselves in relation to others and a particular environment and explains the emotional bond to that place that may develop over time (Kopec 2012, p.61–62).

When utilized effectively, the integration of the natural environment can be therapeutic. Louv (2008), in his pivotal book *Last Child in the Woods: Saving Our Children From Nature Deficit Disorder*, noted that the space allowed for children to explore freely in the natural world has greatly diminished over the course of even just the last generation. The space for creative interaction with the natural world is important in maintaining not only a healthy relationship with the environment, but with humans as a species within it.

As noted by Ackerman (1991):

When we describe ourselves as "sentient" beings (from Latin sentire, "to feel" from Indo-European sent-, "to head for," "go"; hence to go mentally) we mean that we are conscious. The more literal and encompassing meaning is that we have sense perception. (p.xvii)

A sense of place, of belonging, is a sign of psychological attachment to environment. We also seek pattern in ourselves and in our environment.

This could explain why the sequences like the Fibonacci sequences we encountered at the beginning of this book feel comforting, and have often been reproduced in art and architecture. As noted by a Luca Pacioli, who lived during the same time period as Da Vinci, "without mathematics there is no art," alluding to the concepts of divine proportion (Meisner 2014).

Humans impact their environment through their interaction with it, and how they choose to shape it. We have previously treated movement in the West from a primarily mechanistic point of view, and our buildings likewise are viewed for their functionality rather than psychological impact. However, if the emphasis on movement is treated as more profound, our dance interaction with the world will have a chance to flourish.

Over the years, several architects have begun to explore ways to engage the body that can be seen as challenges to the fascial system, even if they did not envision it that way. One example is the architect Arakawa, born in Japan and settled in New York after an early life studying both art and medicine. Along with his wife, Ms. Gins, he has expanded the concept of living in buildings that challenge the body system. Their house, the Bioscleave House, challenges balance and features undulating bumpy floors to keep the body working in unexpected ways. Similarly, in 2016, Lauren Friedrich, of Harvard Graduate School of Design, worked at creating interior spaces that could anatomically challenge the body instead of providing comfort.

Complexity theory and the importance of the connected body as environment

If we look at complexity theory, it can be a framework to view anatomical space on a micro and macro level. Ants are an example of self-organizing from a bottom-up type of system in the same way traffic on a crowded sidewalk. Cells form in the same way, with different cells group together into different types of neighborhoods. A cell "reads" the environment but processes information in complex systems with some sense of randomness. Too much randomness and the ability to organize becomes lost. Too little randomness in the system and the body responds always in the same way and is unable to adapt if there is a change in the environment. We need to train the body environment for randomness and multivectors to create resilience in the body. We are actually designed with a need to be physically challenged in a healthy way to stay adaptive for change.

Randomness plays a part whether we are discussing complexity theory or a spontaneous dinner conversation that is created by unexpected spatial arrangements. Our guests throughout this book have been part of this joined conversation. While mindfulness is a concept many are familiar with, we are still often disconnected from the body and how to move with a sense of ease and comfort. Ultimately, no matter our sport, discipline, or occupation we are looking toward building a resilient system. Understanding that environment matters may give us a reason to look closer at its role in our connected body.

Take your myofascial form out into the world

Draw a picture of the connections important to you in your body. Maybe it is a myofascial connection rooted in specific anatomy. Maybe it is a more general connection of layers or metaphoric threads. Now draw your connection into the larger environment. What is that space for you? Is it a woody path, a river for kayaking, a swimming pool, or skating rink? Does it involve other people (athletics, colleagues or friends and family)?

Now take the paper and turn it over and draw something about your ideal space in the environment you picked. What would you design as a piece of exercise equipment in an outdoor training center? For a home office? Be creative! Think about how space, place and relationships can shift your movement and your mood.

Finally, we can note that we are living in a time period of great discord, and the excitement for fascia has perhaps expanded rapidly because there is a desire for connection. The new (or rediscovered) realization is that the spaces we often have separated in traditional anatomy are actually areas of interest in creating treatment strategies for health. Many of us want to see what ties us all together, and how patterns and form shape us on the small and larger scales. The anatomist in me recognizes that not everything is fascia and that words can matter. Definitions of anatomy from the Terminologia Anatomica with the agreement of people (in this case the International Federation of Associations of Anatomists) are still being debated and updated. Likewise, our larger round table of physical therapists, chiropractors, osteopaths, fitness trainers, movement practitioners, and many others are adding to ideas of this topic. However, we are all still working on how to have that conversation with each other so that growth in our areas of knowledge can continue to expand. Life is ultimately about movement, whether in the tissues of the body or stimulating ideas that spark and shape.

Everything is interwoven, and the web is holy; none of its parts are unconnected. They are composed harmoniously, and together they compose the world. One world, made up of all things. One divinity, present in them all.

Marcus Aurelius, *Meditations*

As we begin to close our movement feast together, we will listen to one last guest for a bit, philosopher, dissector and poet, Gil Hedley. Poetry

is a framing of space as well as an enjoyment. We nourish ourselves with movement and food to feed the basics of functioning in life. Words can also be both practical communication and a way to reach another level of connection with our internal and external environments.

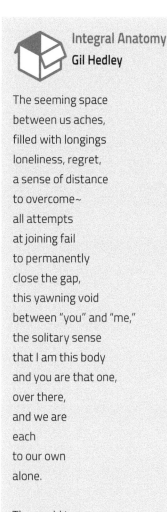

Integral Anatomy
Gil Hedley

The seeming space
between us aches,
filled with longings
loneliness, regret,
a sense of distance
to overcome~
all attempts
at joining fail
to permanently
close the gap,
this yawning void
between "you" and "me,"
the solitary sense
that I am this body
and you are that one,
over there,
and we are
each
to our own
alone.

The world too
seems
a thing apart
and we upon it
every solitary creature

standing separate
unalterably so
as if by some
cruel fate
all in proximity
disconnected,
afraid.

What is born
must die.

Yet the space
we imagine
between us empty,
perhaps is full as
our hearts
overflowing
for a lover
or a child.

The palpable texture
of that "space,"
the irrefutable sense
of one being one
may be more real,
wrap you more perfectly,
than bone-anchored
sinews,
collagenous ropes
and silvery sheets,
the sails and rigging
to navigate within.

Nobody can be
lost at sea

when the ocean
is within you~
What if?
What if
the space we imagine
between us quiet
rings out resonant
to our beating hearts
life plucking strings,
cords echoing
the first sound,
the subtle substance
of that space,
waves weaving us
together,
one fabric
clothing all.

Perhaps the so-called
parts, fitted together
this to that
form a machine
of our mind's
making only
and the truth lies
not in the words
and actions
that divide, dissect
and separate, but
in the seeming space,
the teeming space
between those bits
and pieces,
in the tissues
that continue,

envelope,
connect and relate.

It's in that subtle space
between the two
where we find
the proof that
we are one,
and can only
be so,
mirrored there
as we are
in our flesh
inseparable
and whole.

(Gil Hedley for Berlin Fascia Congress, 2018 and reprinted with kind permission)

References

Ackerman, D. (1991) *A Natural History of the Senses*. New York, NY: Vintage.

Aurelius, Marcus. (2014) *Meditations*. CreateSpace Independent Publishing Platform.

Carrette, J. (2013) *William James's Hidden Religious Imagination: A Universe of Relations*. Abdingdon, UK: Routledge.

Clark, A. and Chalmers, D. (1998) 'The extended mind.' *Analysis 58*, 1, 7–19. https://doi.org/10.1093/analys/58.1.7

Council on Communications and Media (2016) 'Media and young minds.' *Pediatrics 138*, 5, e20162591. https://doi.org/10.1542/peds.2016-2591

Farb, N., Daubenmier, J., Price, C. J., Gard, T. *et al.* (2015) 'Interoception, contemplative practice, and health.' *Frontiers in Psychology 6*. https://doi.org/10.3389/fpsyg.2015.00763

Freeman, M. A. R., and Wyke, B. [1966] (2005). 'Articular contributions to limb muscle reflexes. The effects of partial neurectomy of the knee-joint on postural reflexes.' *British Journal of Surgery 53*, 1, 61–69. https://doi.org/10.1002/bjs.1800530116

Groh, J. M. (2014) *Making Space: How the Brain Knows Where Things Are*. Cambridge, MA: Belknap Press.

Hiss, T. (1991) *The Experience of Place: A New Way of Looking at and Dealing With our Radically Changing Cities and Countryside*. New York, NY: Vintage.

Johnson, M. (2008) *The Meaning of the Body: Aesthetics of Human Understanding*. Chicago, IL: University of Chicago Press.

Kemp, M. (2016) *Structural Intuitions: Seeing Shapes in Art and Science*. Charlottesville, VA: University of Virginia Press.

Kopec, D. (2012) *Environmental Psychology for Design*. London: Fairchild Books.

LaChapelle, D. (dir.) (2005) *Rize*. Lions Gate Films.

Lomax, A. (1978) *Folk Song Style and Culture*. Piscataway, NJ: Transaction Books.

Louv, R. (2008) *Last Child in the Woods: Saving our Children from Nature-deficit Disorder*. Chapel Hill, NC: Algonquin Books.

MacFarlane, R. (2018) *The Lost Words*. Toronto: House of Anansi Press.

Meisner, G. (2014) *Golden Ratio in Art Composition and Design*. The Golden Ratio: Phi, 1.618. Accessed on April 2, 2022 at www.goldennumber.net/art-composition-design

Merriam-Webster (n.d.) *Environment*. Accessed on December 29, 2019 at https://www.merriam-webster.com/dictionary/environment

Pagnini, F., Cavalera, C., Volpato, E., Comazzi, B. *et al.* (2019) 'Ageing as a mindset: a study protocol to rejuvenate older adults with a counterclockwise psychological intervention.' *BMJ Open 9*, 7, e030411. https://doi.org/10.1136/bmjopen-2019-030411

Porges, S. W. (2009) 'The Polyvagal Theory: new insights into adaptive reactions of the autonomic nervous system.' *Cleveland Clinic Journal of Medicine 76*, 4 suppl 2, S86–S90. https://doi.org/10.3949/ccjm.76.s2.17

Scully, V. J. (1991) *Architecture: The Natural and the Manmade*. New York, NY: St. Martin's Press.

Simard, S. (2021) *Finding the Mother Tree: Discovering the Wisdom of the Forest*. New York, NY: Alfred A. Knopf.

Stecco, C., Macchi, V., Porzionato, A., Morra, A. *et al.* (2010) 'The ankle retinacula: morphological evidence of the proprioceptive role of the fascial system.' *Cells Tissues Organs 192*, 3, 200–210. https://doi.org/10.1159/000290225

Further reading

Almond, L. and Whitehead, M. (2012) 'Physical literacy: clarifying the nature of the concept.' *Physical Education Matters 7*, 68–71.

Andrews, K. (2020) *WANDERERS: A History of Women Walking.* London: REAKTION Books.

Bartenieff, I. and Lewis, D. (1980) *Body Movement: Coping with the Environment.* Philadelphia, PA: Gordon and Breach Science Publishers.

Carter, A. and O'Shea, J. (eds) (2010) *The Routledge Dance Studies Reader.* Abingdon, UK: Routledge.

EPILOGUE

Final Thought Box... for now

Humankind has not woven the web of life.

We are but one thread within it.

Whatever we do to the web, we do to ourselves.

All things are bound together.

All things connect.

Chief Seattle, 1854

Science studies the structure of the world from the micro to the macro. It has a curiosity about how it all works. Far from being static, it is continuing to ask questions, make predictions and see how the answers hold up. Our understanding of fascia is an evolving process, and in any good conversation there is a dialogue that is both observational and active. By looking at anything in detail we do put our own lens on to that subject, but we might also discover what that subject can reveal about us.

No doubt, our knowledge of fascia will continue to expand and far from being definitive, this book is meant to spark ideas and conversations that I hope you'll continue in thoughtful ways. We are just beginning to understand the myriad of ways the body is connected on a myofascial level and reaching out wider into the world.

I like the scientific spirit—the holding off, the being sure but not too sure, the willingness to surrender ideas when the evidence is against them: this is ultimately fine—it always keeps the way beyond open—always gives life, thought, affection, the whole man, a chance to try over again after a mistake—after a wrong guess.

Walt Whitman, *Walt Whitman's Camden Conversations*

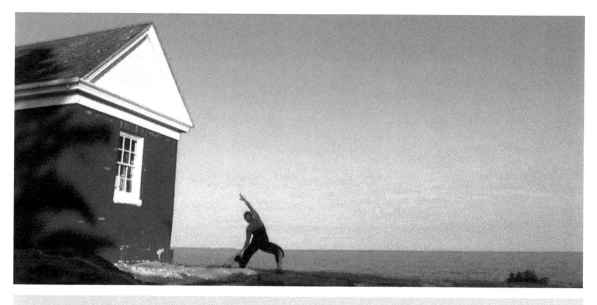

FIGURE EPILOGUE.1 Pemaquid Point, Maine. Self-timer by the author.

APPENDIX 1 Building a tensegrity model

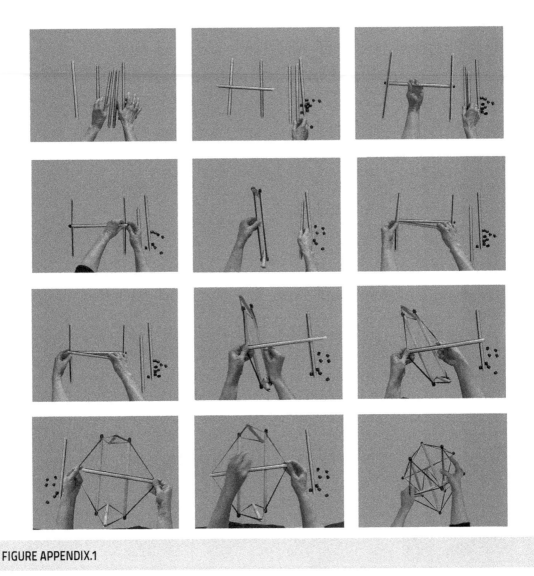

FIGURE APPENDIX.1

In this model, bones are represented by the wooden struts, which are suspended in the tensional rubber bands, acting as myofascial tissues. In the form of a body, strain is distributed in a closed system that creates simultaneous compression and tension and works as a self-organizing shape. The tensegrity model can demonstrate strain in one area will travel to other areas in the structure. A well-balanced model can handle a fall or bounce with resiliency.

INDEX

Note: Page numbers in italics indicate figures.

A

Achilles tendon   165
Act of myofascial efficiency   *172*
Acupuncture points   9
Aging process   179, 186
Anastomosis   35
Anterior cruciate ligament (ACL)
     injuries   183
Anterior oblique sling (AOS)   133
Arm swing   *135*
Articular variability   169
Ashtanga yoga   147

B

Back
  functional line   138
  pain   185
  rotation warm-up for   175
Bartenieff fundamental x movement   *140*
Biomotor abilities and fascia
    adaptation   170
Biotensegrity   36
Board certified dance/movement therapist
    (BC-DMT)   69
Body analysis   78
  assess the body   82–83
  balance   93
  body communication   88
  changing the body   93–94
  fascia holds form   86
  function in motion   91
  Laban movement analysis   88
  meander map   *83*, 83–84
  movement and rest   87–88
  movement toward health   94
  trace-forms and rhythmic patterns   92–93
  whole body mapping   78–81
Body awareness   68
Body/brain challenge   169
Body in motion and emotion   66–67
  appropriate touch   73
  context and shape of the system   75–76
  dance/movement therapy   67–69

  group movement structure   69–70
  ideokinesis   74
  kinesthetic empathy   70
  mirror neurons and mirroring   70
  myofascial middle layer   70–73
  somatics   73–74
  take care of the inner body   76
Body   123–124
  front to back   108–109
  lateral and side body connections   109–113
  metamerism and segmentation   99–102
Bound water   6–7
Breath   120
Breathing body   125

C

Cactus extracellular matrix   *23*
Caesarean sections (CS)   183
Cartesian dualism   182
Catapult mechanism   60–61, 165
  see also Human evolution
Central myofascial body   130–131
Cinderella tissue   5
Collagenase   26–27
Collagen degradation   143
Collagen synthesis   168
Complexity theory   206
Core   119, *119*, 128
  body/mind   123–124
  defined   119
Core 4 program   174
Costovertebral fascia   73

D

Dance/movement therapy premises   67–69
  principle   68
Deep adipose tissue (DAT)   28
Deep fascia   13, *13*
  aponeurotic   13
  epimysial   13
Deep investing fascia   19
Dermatomes   99
Designed test   170
Desikachar, T. K. V.   147
Diaphragms   128
  horizontal dissection   126

Differential movement   166
Dural reflections   50
Dynamicity   89
Dynamic stretching   173

E

Earth Mudra   154
ECM (Extra Cellular Matrix)   191
Écorché   4
Elasticity   165
Emotions   194
Eosinophils   28
Exercises fire hydrant   182, 183
Exteroception   195–198
Extracellular matrix (ECM)   183

F

Falx cerebri   50
Fascia   3
  bound water   6–7
  and categories   7
  comes from   23–24
  compartments, circles, spheres   19–23
  compression   7
  conceptualized as fabric   5–6
  costovertebral   73
  deep   7, *13*, *14*
  deep investing   19
  defined   4–5
  fascicular   7
  fiber   6
  fibroblasts and creating fascial
    architecture   6
  form   10
  function   5
  functional load training and   38–39
  healthy   6
  liminal space   42
  linking   7
  location   27–28
  medical descriptions   4
  metaphor   5
  movement guidelines   58
  myofascial links   7–10
  net plastination project   12
  origin   4

plantar   20
scarpa's   20
sea squirts movement and   47–48
as a sensory organ   192
separating   7
septa   *11*
sibson   73, *74*
superficial   7, *12*
in traditional medical language   20
undulations and waves   41–42
visceral   7, *14*
Fascia anatomy education   181
Fascial awareness   164
Fascial continuities   140
Fascial Net Plastination Project
        (FNPP)   10, 12
Fascial system   140
Fascial tensioning   168
Fascia Revealed: Educating Interconnected
        Anatomy   18, *18*, 19
Fibonacci sequences   206
Fibroblasts   6, 165
"Fitness"   164
Force damping   60
Four-bar closed systems theory   160, 161
Fractals and form   36–37
Front functional line (FFL)   138
Functional fascia training   169
Functional fitness   164, 168
Functional magnetic resonance
        imaging (fMRI)   124

G

Ghost organs   24
"Global stabilization system"   120
Glycoaminoglycans (GAG)   6
Golden Gate route   164
Golgi tendon organ   164, 193
Graphing vectors   166
Ground based movement   169
Ground reaction force (GRF)   60

H

Hand mudras   153
Harrington, Emily   164
Healthy aging   184
Hip

flexor warm-up   175
rotation warm-up for   175
Human evolution
anatomy   57–58
catapult mechanism   60–61
embryology   49–50
fascial foot and facile foot   53–54
fascial forces   59
force damping   60
further thoughts   61–63
genetics and DNA   48
ground reaction force   60
hydraulic amplification   59–60
interaction with the world   50
myofascial force transmission   59
quadruped to biped   50–51
recent evolution   52–53
Hyaluronan   7
Hydraulic amplification   59–60

I

Iliotibial band   6, 112
band syndrome   182
Indicator species   168
Inner-Om Mudra   154
Intermuscular septums   166
Interoception   194
Interstitial receptors   193
Interstitium discovery   30

J

Jing kieng jri bridges   34–35
Joint proprioception   193

K

Kayaking   *137*
Keep It Moving   185
Kinesthetic empathy   70

L

Laban movement analysis (LMA)   88
*Last Child in the Woods: Saving Our Children
    from Nature Deficit Disorder*   205

Latissimus dorsi dissection   *16*
Life form   46–47

M

Major depressive disorder (MDD)   67
Matrix
metalloproteinases (MMP)   26
Meander map   83–84, *83*
Mechanoreceptors   192
Mental imagery (MI)   71
Metamerism and
        segmentation   99–102
Mirror neurons and mirroring   70
Movements
applications   133
Bartenieff Fundamental x   *140*
breathing   161
cross-patterned   133
differential   166
distal-proximal/proximal-distal
        activations   161
elastic quality of   165
ground based   *170*
programs   179
single leg stretch   *163*
tennis elbow   133
torso articulation   161
wave-like   142 156
western styles   147
Mula bandha   123
Multidirectionality   166
Myodural bridge   152
Myofascia   149
Myofascial
alignment   105–106
connections   9, 206
middle line   71
Myxoid liposarcoma   48

N

National Academy of Sports Medicine
        (NASM)   120
National Wildlife Federation   46
Nature   126
Neck, rotation warm-up for   175
Neuroception   194–195

Neutrophils   28
Nutrition and fascia   167–168

P

Pacini receptors   193
Pandiculate   58
Pandiculation movement   156
Patanjali   147
Pectoralis minor   *135*
Pharyngeal pouch   *127*
Pilates
   exercise   160
   machines   160
   mat movements   160
   method   158, *158*, 159, 161
Plantar fascia   20
   and the moving body   102–104
Plasticity   165
"Platonic solids"   88
Playground equipment   180
Posterior oblique sling (POS)   133
Profound movement   197
Proprioception   193

Q

Quality of life (QOL)   186

R

Range of motion (ROM)   150
Remodeling   166
Repatterning movement   195
Resonant breathing
   chanting   149–150
Return to Life Through Contrology   158

Rhythmic yoga mantras   149
River jumping   138, *138*

S

Sacroiliac (SI) joint   88
Salutation Mudra   *154, 155*
Savasana   157
Scarpa's fascia   20
Scar tissue   183
Sea squirts   47–48
Seated forward fold   188, *188*
Seated Warrior   189
Sibson's fascia   73
Six chakras of tantric yoga   *122*
Spirals   114–118
   loops in motion and stability   115
   movement   *117*
   muscles and fascial connections   *116*
   staircase   118
Standing thread the needle   189, *189*
Stick mobility   *134*
Stretch and yogi and yogini   148–149
Suboccipital sun salutations   151
Superficial adipose tissue (SAT)   28

T

Tamoxifen   183
Tasting the Universe   196
Tennis elbow   133
Tensegrity   32–33
The Curves of Life   114
The Pelvic Girdle   133
The Yoga Sutras   147, *152*
Traditional Chinese medicine (TCM)   9
Trail running   *202*
Training fascia   *167*
Trapeze table   160

Trunk dissection   *121*
Type 3 collagen fibers
   and fibrillin   183

U

Undulations and waves   41–42
   see also Fascia
"Unused arc hypothesis"   201

V

Vitality, Performance, Reconditioning
   (ViPR)   38

W

Walking meditation   152
Wave-like movement   142, 156
Weight-bearing athlete   168
Well-balanced model   212
Western styles of movement   147
Whole-body exercise   159
Wunda Chair   158

Y

Yoga   147
   asana   152, *152*
   asanas   *150*
   block   *199*
   pilates   159
   practice   147
   savasana   202
   teachers   147
   variations   *150*